COGNITIVE THERAPY WITH INPATIENTS

Cognitive Therapy with Inpatients

Developing a Cognitive Milieu

Jesse H. Wright
Michael E. Thase
Aaron T. Beck
John W. Ludgate
Editors

THE GUILFORD PRESS
New York London

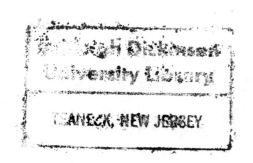

A Division of Guilford Publications, Inc.
72 Spring Street, New York, NY 10012

Printed in the United States of America

This book is printed on acid-free paper.

Last digit is print number: 9 8 7 6 5 4 3 2

Library of Congress Cataloging-in-Publication Data

Cognitive therapy with inpatients: developing a cognitive milieu / edited by Jesse H. Wright . . . [et al.].
p. cm.
Includes bibliographical references and index.
ISBN 0-89862-890-3
1. Cognitive therapy. 2. Milieu therapy.
3. Psychiatric hospital care. I. Wright, Jesse H.
[DNLM: 1. Cognitive Therapy—methods. WM 425 C6766]
RC489.C63C644 1992
616.89 14—dc20
DNLM/DLC
for Library of Congress 92-1529
CIP
r92

Contributors

Curtis L. Barrett, Ph.D., Professor, Department of Psychiatry and Behavioral Sciences, University of Louisville School of Medicine; Director, Psychological Services, Norton Psychiatric Clinic, Louisville, KY

Aaron T. Beck, M.D., University Professor of Psychiatry, Department of Psychiatry, University of Pennsylvania; Director, Center for Cognitive Therapy, Philadelphia, PA

Duane S. Bishop, M.D., Associate Professor, Department of Psychiatry and Human Behavior, Brown University School of Medicine; Director of Rehabilitation Psychiatry, Rhode Island Hospital, Providence, RI

Wayne A. Bowers, Ph.D., Assistant Professor and Director of Psychological Services, Department of Psychiatry, University of Iowa, Cedar Rapids

Kathleen A. Bowler, Ph.D., R.N., C.S., Program Coordinator, Affective Disorders Research, Mood Disorders Module, Western Psychiatric Institute and Clinic; Adjunct Assistant Professor of Nursing, University of Pittsburgh, PA

Susan Byers, Ph.D., Coordinator of Cognitive Therapy Units for CPC Hospitals, CPC Santa Ana Psychiatric Hospital, Santa Ana, CA

Glenda F. Camp, Ph.D., Clinical Psychologist and Director, Cognitive Therapy Program, St. Albans Hospital, Radford, VA

David A. Casey, M.D., Associate Professor, Department of Psychiatry and Behavioral Sciences, University of Louisville School of Medicine; Director, Edward E. Landis Geriatric Psychiatry Center, Norton Psychiatric Clinic, Louisville, KY

Mary Helen Davis, M.D., Assistant Professor, Department of Psychiatry and Behavioral Sciences, University of Louisville School of Medicine; Director, Adult Treatment Program, Norton Psychiatric Clinic, Louisville, KY

Nathan B. Epstein, M.D., Professor Emeritus, Department of Psychiatry and Human Behavior, Brown University School of Medicine, Providence, RI; Psychiatrist-in-Chief, St. Lukes Hospital, New Bedford, MA

Arthur Freeman, Ed.D., Professor, Department of Psychiatry, University of Medicine and Dentistry of New Jersey, Camden, NJ

Mark Gilson, Ph.D., Clinical Psychologist and Director, Atlanta Center for Cognitive Therapy, Atlanta, GA

Robert W. Grant, Ph.D., Assistant Professor, Department of Psychiatry and Behavioral Sciences, University of Louisville School of Medicine; Clinical Psychologist, Norton Psychiatric Clinic, Louisville, KY

Gabor I. Keitner, M.D., Professor, Department of Psychiatry and Human Behavior, Brown University School of Medicine; Associate Medical Director for Inpatient Services and Director of Affective Disorders Program, Butler Hospital, Providence, RI

John W. Ludgate, Ph.D., Consultant Psychologist, Department of Psychiatry, Warneford Hospital, Oxford, England

Robert G. Meyer, Ph.D., Professor, Department of Psychology, University of Louisville, KY

Ivan W. Miller, Ph.D., Associate Professor, Department of Psychiatry and Human Behavior, Brown University School of Medicine; Director of Research and Director of Psychology, Butler Hospital, Providence, RI

Lisa J. Moonis, M.S.N., R.N., C.S., Psychiatric Clinical Nurse Specialist, Allegheny Hospital, Pittsburgh, PA

Christine A. Padesky, Ph.D., Director, Center for Cognitive Therapy, Newport Beach, CA

Christine E. Ryan, Ph.D., Research Associate, Department of Psychiatry and Human Behavior, Brown University School of Medicine; Associate Director of Family Research, Butler Hospital, Providence, RI

G. Randolph Schrodt, Jr., M.D., Associate Professor, Department of Psychiatry and Behavioral Sciences, University of Louisville School of Medicine; Associate Clinical Director, Norton Psychiatric Clinic, Louisville, KY

Jan Scott, M.B., B.S., M.R.C.Psych., Consultant and Senior Lecturer in Psychiatry, University of Newcastle Upon Tyne, England

Tom Sensky, Ph.D., M.B., M.R.C.Psych., Senior Lecturer in Psychiatry, Department of Psychiatry, Charing Cross and Westminster Medical School (University of London), West Middlesex University Hospital, Isleworth, Middlesex, England

Michael E. Thase, M.D., Associate Professor, Department of Psychiatry, University of Pittsburgh School of Medicine; Director, Mood Disorders Module, Western Psychiatric Institute and Clinic, Pittsburgh, PA

Douglas Turkington, M.B., B.S., M.R.C.Psych., Consultant Psychiatrist, St. Nicholas Hospital, Newcastle Upon Tyne, England

Jesse H. Wright, M.D., Ph.D., Professor, Department of Psychiatry and Behavioral Sciences, University of Louisville School of Medicine; Medical Director, Norton Psychiatric Clinic, Louisville, KY

Preface

The introduction of cognitive therapy to inpatient settings comes at a critical juncture in the history of hospital psychiatry. Older treatment models, such as the therapeutic community, have become impractical in an era of vigorous utilization review, strict cost containment, and sharply reduced lengths of stay. Inpatient psychiatric units are under steadily increasing pressure to achieve significant results in the minimum amount of time possible. A new form of inpatient psychiatric treatment—the cognitive milieu—has emerged to meet these challenges.

Over the past decade, cognitive therapy (CT) has been adapted for inpatient use by a number of psychiatric hospitals in the United States and Europe. A sample of these programs is listed in the Appendix. Some of the advantages of CT that have fueled this development include a short-term format, established efficacy, compatibility with biological psychiatry, and evidence for relapse prevention effects. Hospital-based therapists also have found that cognitive therapy is a pragmatic model for treatment that can be understood and used by the wide range of professionals who work in the inpatient setting.

Cognitive therapy is utilized in the psychiatric hospital in two major ways: as a specific treatment method for individuals, families, and groups and as a theoretical construct that guides the entire hospital milieu. The goals of this book are to provide the reader with practical knowledge on (1) how to perform CT with inpatients; and (2) how to develop a cognitively oriented treatment milieu. Wherever possible, detailed instructions and case illustrations are given, so that this volume can be used as a treatment manual for inpatient cognitive therapy programs.

The first section of the book describes general principles of inpatient cognitive therapy. Chapter 1 presents basic cognitive therapy theories and techniques. This material will be especially useful to the reader who does not have extensive experience with using cognitive therapy in clinical practice. Knowledge of fundamental CT procedures is required for understanding the inpatient applications described elsewhere in the volume. The second chapter, "Hospital Psychiatry in Transition," examines the evolution of treatment methods for inpatient psychiatry. After reviewing contributions from earlier models, it describes the unique features and advantages of cognitive therapy units. In Chapter 3, the authors explain and illustrate several different models for using CT in psychiatric hospitals. Step-by-step procedures are outlined for constructing a cognitive milieu.

Detailed instructions for using individual, group, and family cognitive therapy with inpatients are given in the second section of the volume. Significant modifications in standard CT techniques are often required for performing therapy in a hospital environment. In Chapter 4, individual therapy procedures are defined, and strategies are outlined for problems encountered frequently in work with inpatients (e.g., high suicide risk, sexual abuse, depression with psychotic features, social skills deficits). Many cognitive therapy units devote a large part of their resources to the group treatment format. Chapter 5 contains information on how to utilize a variety of inpatient cognitive therapy groups. Particular attention is paid to procedures that can make group therapy a meaningful experience during a brief hospital stay. Chapter 6, "Inpatient Family Therapy," is divided into two segments. In Part I, several different family therapies that are compatible with the CT approach are identified, and general procedures for inpatient family therapy are described. Part II of this chapter illustrates family cognitive therapy in the hospital setting.

The volume then turns to a series of chapters on "The Biomedical Interface." The theoretical and clinical issues involved in combining cognitive and biological treatments are examined in Chapters 7 and 8. The authors describe a cognitive–biological treatment perspective that can effectively join together these two powerful therapeutic approaches. The important role of the psychiatric nurse in implementing a cognitively oriented treatment program is discussed in Chapter 9.

Cognitive therapy has been used for a number of special applications in the psychiatric hospital. The next segment of the book is devoted to describing CT interventions for specific populations or disorders. Methods are articulated for using cognitive therapy for adolescents, substance abusers, geriatric patients, and for those who suffer from eating disorders, chronic depression, personality disorders, and schizophrenia. Recentlv developed cognitive therapy procedures have made a significant impact on hospital care of these types of patients.

The final section of the volume deals with methods of enhancing the effectiveness of inpatient cognitive therapy. Guidelines for educating therapists and patients in cognitive therapy are discussed in Chapter 15. Ongoing training and supervision are an essential component of a well-functioning cognitive milieu. The final chapter of the book describes procedures for the transition and aftercare phases of treatment. One of the most important features of cognitive therapy is its focus on learning new ways of thinking and problem solving. Thorough preparation for discharge and a coordinated outpatient follow-up program can solidify the gains from hospitalization, reduce risk for relapse, and help the patient use cognitive therapy skills in the community.

We hope that this description of inpatient cognitive therapy will assist therapists with meeting the increasing demands of hospital-based treatment and will serve as a stimulus for further development of the cognitive milieu.

Jesse H. Wright, M.D., Ph.D.
Michael E. Thase, M.D.
Aaron T. Beck, M.D.
John W. Ludgate, Ph.D.

Acknowledgments

Colleagues from many inpatient treatment programs and centers for cognitive therapy joined efforts in producing this work. The editors are particularly indebted to their coworkers from the cognitive therapy units at the University of Louisville (Norton Psychiatric Clinic) and University of Pittsburgh (Western Psychiatric Institute and Clinic) who played a fundamental role in developing the treatment programs described here. Our associates have been dedicated, creative, and stimulating. In difficult times, they have shouldered burdens with equanimity.

A team of highly skilled professionals assisted with manuscript preparation and editing. Word processing was handled in an expert and cheerful manner by Kathy Sinkhorn and Lisa Stupar. Additional help was provided by Colleen Newton. Mary Beth Zickel provided invaluable assistance in the editing process. Larry Trexler, Ph.D., and Laura Krome, A.C.S.W., read portions of the manuscript and made many useful suggestions. Administrators of the Alliant Health System and the Western Psychiatric Institute and Clinic have been consistent advocates for our cognitive therapy units. Also, funding from grants MH-41884-04 and MH-30915 (Mental Health Clinical Research Center) has supported the cognitive therapy research program at the University of Pittsburgh. The editors wish to express their deep appreciation to those who helped bring this project to fruition.

Contents

Part I
GENERAL PRINCIPLES OF INPATIENT COGNITIVE THERAPY

Part II
TREATMENT MODALITIES

Part V
EDUCATION AND RELAPSE PREVENTION

COGNITIVE THERAPY WITH INPATIENTS

Part I

GENERAL PRINCIPLES OF INPATIENT COGNITIVE THERAPY

Chapter 1

An Overview of Cognitive Therapy

Michael E. Thase, M.D.,
and Aaron T. Beck, M.D.

Over the past three decades, cognitive therapy (CT) has become one of the predominant forces in psychotherapeutic practice (e.g., Mahoney, 1974; Norcross, 1986; Arkowitz & Hannah, 1989). The publication of a book specifically devoted to inpatient applications of Beck's model of cognitive therapy is further evidence of the growth of this approach. Several groups of investigators have reported successful experiences in using the cognitive model with psychiatric inpatients (Schrodt & Wright, 1987; Scott, 1988; Miller, Norman, & Keitner, 1989; Bowers, 1990; Thase & Wright, 1991; Thase, Bowler, & Harden, 1991). Also, recent developments in CT applications for eating disorders, substance abuse, schizophrenia, and severe personality disorders have had particular relevance for inpatient treatment (e.g., Freeman, Simon, Beutler, & Arkowitz, 1989; Beck et al., 1990; Kingdon & Turkington, 1991).

In this chapter, we present an overview of the basic principles of cognitive therapy (Beck, 1976; Beck, Rush, Shaw, & Emery, 1979; Wright & Beck, 1983; Beck & Greenberg, 1988). Following a brief review of the historical background of the cognitive model, we discuss the various types of cognitive and behavioral changes seen in psychopathological states, the relationship of these disturbances to stressful life events, and the formation of underlying schemas or silent assumptions that may operate as vulnerability factors. Next, we describe key elements of the practice of CT. This discussion includes a consideration of the core psychotherapeutic skills, methods, and techniques utilized in cognitive therapy. Finally, we summarize relevant studies of treatment efficacy and review recent research on the application of CT to inpatient settings.

HISTORICAL BACKGROUND

The theoretical basis of CT has been derived from these three primary sources: (1) the phenomenological perspective, (2) the structural view of personality and psychopathology, and (3) contemporary work in cognitive and behavioral psychology (Beck, 1976; Beck et al., 1979). Cognitive therapy shares with the phenomenological approach an emphasis on concepts of self and the personal world as key determinants of behavior (Frankl, 1985). This contribution dates to the ancient Greek school of Stoic philosophy (Beck, 1976). The writings of the post-Freudian analysts such as Adler (1936), Horney (1950), and Sullivan (1953) stressed this viewpoint on personality and psychopathology.

Freud's structural theory that partitioned cognition (thought) into primary and secondary processes and recognitized the role of conscious, preconscious, and unconscious mental activity was a second major influence. The psychoanalytic model also postulated the existence of personality constructs and defense mechanisms that, at times of distress or conflict, are central to the etiology of psychopathological reactions. George Kelly's (1955) formulation of personal constructs and Jean Piaget's (1954) studies of schemas (i.e., internalized and hierarchical sets of rules used for problem solving) in the cognitive development of children and adolescents also helped to shape the cognitive model for psychotherapy.

The fundamental principles of cognitive therapy were outlined by Beck in a series of papers in the early 1960s (Beck, 1961, 1963, 1964). Subsequently, a number of research studies solidified the importance of cognitive distortions in various psychopathological states (e.g., Beck, 1967, 1976; Braff & Beck, 1974; Weissman, 1979; Nelson & Craighead, 1977; Rizley, 1978; Hollon & Kendall, 1980). Another influence was the introduction of Albert Ellis's (1962) system of rational–emotive therapy. Ellis (who, like Beck, had been trained as an analyst) also emphasized the significance of irrational or distorted beliefs in the origin and maintenance of "neurotic" psychopathology and similarly advocated active and direct interventions in psychotherapy of depressed patients.

Beck's model of cognitive therapy continued to evolve during the 1960s and '70s (Beck, 1967, 1970) and was first published in a fully developed form in the text *Cognitive Therapy and the Emotional Disorders* (Beck, 1976). The approach was elaborated further in a treatment manual, *Cognitive Therapy of Depression* (Beck et al., 1979), that also described use of behavioral methods such as activity scheduling (Lewinsohn, Sullivan, & Grosscup, 1982), self-reinforcement and self-monitoring (McLean, 1982), and social skills training (Hersen, Bellack, Himmelhoch, & Thase, 1984).

THE COGNITIVE MODEL OF PSYCHOPATHOLOGY

Depressive and anxiety syndromes are quite heterogeneous. Despite the availability of reliable diagnostic criteria for syndromes such as major depression, dysthymic disorder, and panic disorder, rarely are two patients encountered whose syndromes look exactly alike. Nevertheless, such persons usually have difficulties in at least one of two major areas of cognitive functioning: (1) negatively biased thoughts, attitudes, and assumptions and (2) impairment in learning and memory functioning. In this section, we review cognitive disturbances that are characteristic of psychopathological states, using depression as a general model.

Perhaps the most obvious examples of cognitive symptoms include mood-congruent delusions and ruminations. More commonly, individuals with depression are plagued by apprehensive, negative, or pessimistic thoughts about the self, world, and future. This set of negatively distorted ideations has been termed the negative cognitive triad (Beck, 1976). Anxious patients usually have negative thoughts in which the risk or danger of a situation, or the significance of bodily sensations, is exaggerated (Wright & Borden, 1991).

Automatic thoughts are a special type of cognitions that are of particular significance in depression and anxiety disorders (Beck, 1963, 1976). The term "automatic thought" is essentially synonymous with expressions such as self-statements, private thoughts, or internal dialogue. Automatic thoughts occur without deliberation and, unless challenged, may have unquestioned believability. Although automatic thoughts are a normal part of mental life, in psychopathological states they tend to have a repetitive, personalized, and dysfunctional content (Beck, 1976). Automatic thoughts have an interactive relationship with mood states. The level of emotional distress is amplified by the frequency and intensity of negative automatic thoughts (Beck, 1963, 1976), and the probability of having such thoughts is increased by a dysphoric or anxious mood. Some individuals may have almost instantaneous recognition of their automatic thoughts, but in other cases there may be difficulties in eliciting automatic thoughts during early therapeutic encounters. When automatic thoughts are not easily recognized, the therapist must explicitly teach the patient to identify and record these cognitions (Beck et al., 1979; Thase & Wright, 1991).

Both clinical experience and research utilizing self-report measures such as the Automatic Thoughts Questionnaire (Hollon & Kendall, 1980) and the Dysfunctional Attitude Scale (Weissman, 1979) have documented the high prevalence and relative specificity of negative automatic thoughts and dysfunctional attitudes during depressive and anxious states (Harrell, Chambless, & Calhoun, 1981; Clark, 1986; Hollon, Kendall, & Lumry, 1986). A moderate to high degree of correlation among measures of automatic thoughts, dysfunctional attitudes, and ratings of symptomatic severity suggests either (1) that such cognitions may have a primary role in "driving" the mood disturbance (e.g., Beck, 1976; Clark, 1986; Shaw & Segal, 1988) or (2) that negative cognitions are, more simply, mental symptoms of distress without special etiological significance (Beidel & Turner, 1986; Coyne & Gotlib, 1983, 1986). Nevertheless, CT methods designed to reduce negative automatic thoughts have been shown to be effective methods of reducing depression and anxiety (e.g., Rush, Beck, Kovacs, & Hollon, 1977; Barlow, Craske, Cerny, & Klosko, 1989). Most studies have shown substantial changes in cognitive functioning after a course of CT, but normalization of dysfunctional patterns of thinking does not always accompany response to treatment (Eaves & Rush, 1984; Miller & Norman, 1986; Thase et al., 1992). Thus, some types of cognitive dysfunction may persist as a "marker" of future vulnerability.

In nonpsychotic states, the content of a person's negative automatic thoughts typically corresponds to the perceived meaning of the event that precipitated the emotional upset. Stimuli that trigger automatic thoughts may include memories, daydreams, and anticipated or hypothetical events (Beck, 1976; Clark, 1986). Because the content and frequency of automatic thoughts are consistent with the severity of the mood disturbance, the dysphoric or anxious reaction might be justified *if* the negative thoughts were absolutely accurate. However, negative automatic thoughts are frequently associated with errors in informational processing, as summarized in Table 1.1. These cognitive errors provide one of the principal bases for psychotherapeutic intervention (Beck, 1976).

The content of a series of automatic thoughts may be sorted into themes or patterns that can be used by the therapist to infer deeper cognitive patterns and structures (Beck, 1976). Such constructs include a person's beliefs or attitudes as well as schemas. In more traditional approaches to psychopathology, beliefs and attitudes might be considered "preconscious" material, whereas schemas would be viewed as "unconscious." From the cognitive therapy viewpoint, both attitudes and schemas are considered to be directly accessible through questioning techniques (Beck et al., 1979). In psychopathological states, dysfunctional attitudes such as unrealistically demanding standards or the assumption that one must always be loved or respected are frequently observed. Examples of common dysfunctional attitudes are provided in Table 1.2.

Schemas are fundamental and enduring patterns that serve as our

TABLE 1.1. Common Patterns of Irrational Thinking

1. *Emotional reasoning*. A conclusion or inference is based on an emotional state, i.e., "I *feel* this way; therefore, I *am* this way."
2. *Overgeneralization*. Evidence is drawn from one experience or a small set of experiences to reach an unwarranted conclusion with far-reaching implications.
3. *Catastrophic thinking*. An extreme example of overgeneralization, in which the impact of a clearly negative event or experience is amplified to extreme proportions, e.g., "If I have a panic attack I will lose *all* control and go crazy (or die)."
4. *All-or-none (black-or-white; absolutistic) thinking*. An unnecessary division of complex or continuous outcomes into polarized extremes, e.g., "Either I am a success at this, or I'm a total failure."
5. *Shoulds and musts*. Imperative statements about self that dictate rigid standards or reflect an unrealistic degree of presumed control over external events.
6. *Negative predictions*. Use of pessimism or earlier experiences of failure to prematurely or inappropriately predict failure in a new situation. Also known as "fortune telling."
7. *Mind reading*. Negatively toned inferences about the thoughts, intentions, or motives of another person.
8. *Labeling*. An undesirable characteristic of a person or event is made definitive of that person or event, e.g., "Because I *failed* to be selected for ballet, I am a *failure*."
9. *Personalization*. Interpretation of an event, situation, or behavior as salient or personally indicative of a negative aspect of self.
10. *Selective negative focus (selective abstraction)*. Undesirable or negative events, memories, or implications are focused on at the expense of recalling or identifying other, more neutral or positive information. In fact, positive information may be ignored or disqualified as irrelevant, atypical, or trivial.
11. *Cognitive avoidance*. Unpleasant thoughts, feelings, or events are misperceived as overwhelming and/or insurmountable and are actively suppressed or avoided.
12. Somatic (mis)focus. The predisposition to interpret internal stimuli (e.g., heart rate, palpitations, shortness of breath, dizziness, or tingling) as *definite* indications of impending catastrophic events (i.e., heart attack, suffocation, collapse, etc.).

Adapted from Beck et al. (1979).

basic, yet unspoken, rules of life. These organizing principles are shaped through interactions with the environment, and although they may evolve over time (Guidano & Liotti, 1983), schemas tend to be derived early in development. Schemas serve as summary principles that permit the memories and recollections of multiple experiences to be stored and organized according to single themes or rules. When a particular schema is activated by a threatening or stressful event, it

TABLE 1.2. Common Dysfunctional Attitudes

To be happy, I must be accepted by all people at all times.
If I make a mistake, it means that I am inept.
I can't live without you.
If somebody disagrees with me, it means that person doesn't like me.
My value as a person is dependent on what others think of me.
I must avoid embarrassment at all cost.
If I lose control of my emotions, I may go crazy.
I must hide my inner weaknesses from others in all circumstances.

Adapted from Beck (1976).

serves as a template against which new experiences are processed (Beck et al., 1979). Schemas operate via information-processing mechanisms such as selective attention and selective recall. These mechanisms promote the "filtering" of new information, so that data are perceived as consistent with the overarching rule of the schema. Strong emotional states transiently affect this filtration process in all individuals, whereas more pronounced and persistent changes are seen in depression, generalized anxiety disorder, and panic disorder (Beck & Greenberg, 1988; Shaw & Segal, 1988).

It is useful to conceptualize a structural hierarchy of cognitive processes in which automatic negative thoughts may be organized with respect to attitudes or beliefs that in turn may point to schemas. Of greatest clinical relevance are the self-schemas that organize personally relevant information. Young (1987) has summarized 15 relatively common psychopathological schemas, subdividing these into four main themes: autonomy, connectedness, worthiness, and limits and standards (see Table 1.3).

The cognitive model posits a specific, interactive relationship between schemas and emotional responses to adverse life events. One research group recently found that a measure of excessive dependency was predictive of depressive relapse only following life events that matched the area of vulnerability, such as romantic rejection or divorce (Hammen, Ellicott, Gitlin, & Jamison, 1989). An example of a similarly matching schema and event in an individual with an anxiety disorder would be when a man with a silent assumption about threats to physical integrity begins to suffer panic attacks shortly after experiencing an episode of unexplained chest pain.

Difficulties with concentration and memory during states of emotional distress are so well established that, when taken together, they represent one of the eight core symptoms of depression in DSM-III-R

TABLE 1.3. Proposed Maladaptive Schemas

Autonomy
Dependence. The belief that one is unable to function without the constant support of others.
Subjugation/Lack of Individuation. The voluntary or involuntary sacrifice of one's own needs to satisfy others' needs.
Vulnerability to Harm or Illness. The fear that disaster (i.e., natural, criminal, medical, or financial) is about to strike at any time.
Fear of Losing Self-Control. The fear that one will involuntarily lose control of one's own impulses, behavior, emotions, mind, etc.

Connectedness
Emotional Deprivation. The expectation that one's needs for nurturance, empathy, or affection will never be adequately met by others.
Abandonment/Loss. Fear that one will imminently lose significant others and/or be emotionally isolated forever.
Mistrust. The expectation that others will hurt, abuse, cheat, lie, or manipulate.
Social Isolation/Alienation. The belief that one is isolated from the rest of the world, is different from other people, and/or doesn't belong to any group or community.

Worthiness
Defectiveness/Unlovability. The assumption that one is inwardly defective or that, if the flaw is exposed, one is fundamentally unlovable.
Social Undesirability. The belief that one is outwardly undesirable to others (e.g., ugly, sexually undesirable, low in status, dull, or boring).
Incompetence/Failure. The assumption that one cannot perform competently in areas of achievement, daily responsibilities, or decision making.
Guilt/Punishment. The conclusion that one is morally bad or irresponsible and deserving of criticism or punishment.
Shame/Embarrassment. Recurrent feelings of shame or self-consciousness experienced because one believes that one's inadequacies (as reflected in schemas 9–12) are totally unacceptable to others.

Limits and Standards
Unrelenting Standards. The relentless striving to meet extremely high expectation of oneself at all costs (i.e., at the expense of happiness, pleasure, health, or satisfying relationships).
Entitlement. Insistence that one should be able to do, say, or have whatever one wants immediately.

Adapted from Young (1987).

(American Psychiatric Association, 1987). Concentration disturbances also are commonly observed in the anxiety disorders (Clark, 1986). Much research on this topic has focused on the existence of specific types of cognitive deficits (e.g., Johnson & Magaro, 1987; Wright & Salmon, 1990). For example, in research protocols utilizing standardized psychological tests, clinically depressed patients generally have been found to perform more slowly than control subjects on timed tests

(Brand & Jolles, 1987; Glass, Uhlenhuth, Hartel, Matuzas, & Fischman, 1981; Breslow, Kocsis, & Belkin, 1980; Wright, 1986). Such slowing has been linked to both psychomotor retardation and decreased effortful processing (Johnson & Magaro, 1987; Wright & Salmon, 1990).

In a series of small but well-controlled studies conducted at the National Institute of Mental Health, Weingartner and associates (Weingartner, Cohen, Murphy, Martello, & Gerdt, 1981; Cohen, Weingartner, Smallberg, Pickar, & Murphy, 1982; Roy-Byrne, Weingartner, Bierer, Thompson, & Post, 1986) documented that severely depressed patients have greatest difficulty on semantic tasks that are either technically complex or that require a considerable effort. By contrast, depressed patients often perform reasonably well (i.e., nearly equivalent to controls) when the tasks are relatively easy or involve automatic processing. A relationship between the complexity of new material and impaired performance in depression has been confirmed in studies by Watts and Sharrock (1987) and Wolfe and associates (Wolfe, Granholm, Butters, Saunders, & Janosky, 1987). Such findings also are related to impairments in abstraction that have been documented in several studies of severe depression (Donnelly, Dent, & Murphy, 1972; Braff & Beck, 1974; Rubinow, Post, Savard, & Gold, 1984). Many of the procedures detailed in this chapter can help counter the effects of impaired learning and memory functioning.

GUIDING PRINCIPLES OF COGNITIVE THERAPY

Cognitive therapy is typically a short-term treatment in which the therapist helps the patient to learn more effective methods of dealing with troubling thoughts, feelings, and behavior. It also is a problem-oriented psychotherapy that both addresses the situational difficulties that may have provoked anxious or depressive episodes and the underlying cognitive problems that may relate to the pathogenesis of emotional disorders.

Although it is possible to train cognitive therapists *de novo*, such training must, from the beginning, include ample attention to development of general psychotherapeutic skills, such as genuineness, understanding, and accurate empathy (e.g., Traux & Mitchell, 1971). In milder cases of anxiety or depression, such nonspecific factors may supersede the technical contributions of any particular model of psychotherapy in obtaining symptomatic relief (e.g., Zeiss, Lewinsohn, & Munoz, 1979). Nevertheless, in one preliminary study of skilled therapists, an additive effect for both basic clinical skills and the technical interventions of CT was documented (Persons & Burns, 1985). It also is important for the therapist to be sufficiently experienced that the cognitive model of treatment can be adapted for use with individuals of diverse backgrounds and clinical presentations (Rush, 1982).

When selecting candidates for training in CT, we favor therapists who can be active within sessions while maintaining high levels of empathy and understanding. It is sometimes difficult to overcome the therapy habits instilled over years of training in more reflective, traditional models of therapy such as psychodynamic or client-centered therapy. Indeed, through the process of "active listening," the therapist may inadvertently shape or reinforce dysfunctional thoughts (i.e., through "parroting" statements, nodding, or other nonverbal communication). The therapist trainee thus needs to learn to blend accurate empathy with an active and problem-oriented focus. When working with psychiatric inpatients, it is important to demonstrate this skill during the initial visit (Thase & Wright, 1991).

The style of the therapeutic relationship in CT is referred to as collaborative empiricism (Beck et al., 1979). It is the therapist's responsibility to establish a working alliance in order to ensure compatible goals, reduce potential points of resistance or competition, and enhance the directness and clarity of communication. A solid therapeutic alliance is seen as a necessary, but not sufficient, ingredient of effective cognitive therapy (Beck et al., 1979).

One of the main collaborative methods employed to help patients learn to identify the relationships among thoughts, feelings, and behavior is Socratic questioning (Beck et al., 1979). In addition, the therapist emphasizes the importance of giving and receiving feedback in treatment sessions. This strengthens the explicit collaboration between therapist and patient and provides a concrete method to address the memory difficulties and the tendency to distort information that are so characteristic of severely depressed or anxious persons (Wright, 1988; Wright & Salmon, 1990).

There also is a strong empirical tone to the therapy. One of the goals of each therapeutic intervention is to identify and test a hypothesis relevant to a particular aspect of the patient's condition. In an effective CT dyad, the patient and therapist often address problems by designing experiments to support or refute hypotheses. These experiments may range from relatively uncomplicated behavioral tasks (e.g., an assignment to test the relationship between mood and participation in a particular type of activity) to more complex cognitive/emotional interactions (e.g., an assignment to test the associations among thoughts about rejection, feelings of sadness, and the urge to reactivate a recently terminated, dysfunctional relationship). During inpatient treatment, an experiment designed in a morning therapy session can be carried out that afternoon or evening, often with the help of a nurse or ancillary staff member. Such relatively immediate tests can have powerful therapeutic impact (Thase & Wright, 1991).

The high level of activity in therapy also extends to the patient, who is asked to begin completing homework assignments in the very first session (Beck et al., 1979; Thase & Wright, 1991). Homework or self-help assignments are considered an integral part of broadening and generalizing the impact of the therapy. The therapist needs to learn to make relevant and focused assignments and to review the homework near the beginning of each subsequent session. Vague or unattended assignments can lead to noncompliance (Persons, 1989). Nursing staff can facilitate completion of homework assignments by the use of individual or group "wrap-up" sessions.

As noted earlier, cognitive therapy usually is a short-term treatment approach, whether it is conducted in an outpatient or inpatient setting. A typical course of outpatient treatment involves sessions once or twice a week for a total of 12 to 20 sessions (Beck et al., 1979; Wright & Beck, 1983). In the inpatient setting, the frequency of individual sessions usually ranges from three to five times a week (Bowers, 1989; Schrodt & Wright, 1987; Scott, 1988; Shaw, 1981; Thase & Wright, 1991). Inpatient treatment is augmented by group and/or family sessions whenever possible, and subsequent outpatient therapy may prove invaluable in maintaining clinical improvement (Thase et al., 1991).

In the early stages of treatment, the therapist has several major goals. These include establishing a specific problem list and developing an initial case formulation. The therapist is responsible for achieving these goals by obtaining a comprehensive history of the patient's current situation, past difficulties, and syndromal presentation, including eliciting the patient's perception of the most pressing life problems and distressing symptoms (Beck et al., 1979; Persons, 1989). The problems encountered by therapists working on inpatient units typically are both more severe and more complicated than those seen in outpatient practice (Thase & Wright, 1991). As discussed in subsequent chapters, the therapist also must collaborate with the remainder of the multidisciplinary treatment team in order to integrate the cognitive interventions with the overall treatment plan (Thase & Wright, 1991).

The patient's problem list is used in both individual and group CT to set priorities collaboratively. Each session is structured around an agenda so that the most pertinent issues can be approached in an efficient manner. Normally, the decision is made to focus initially on the life problems, symptoms, or thought patterns that are both central to the patient's perception of his or her difficulties and more readily amenable to change. As an important part of this process, the therapist inquires about thoughts of pessimism about the therapy, hopelessness about the future, and suicidal ideation (Beck et al., 1979; Thase & Wright, 1991). Although assessment and treatment of suicidal ideation form an important component of any course of therapy, it is particularly salient in work with hospitalized patients. Even within the first session, the therapist should attempt to help the patient gain some symptomatic relief or resolution of at least one problem area in order to demonstrate that the patient's dilemma is not completely unsolvable (Beck et al., 1979; Freeman & White, 1989). When this goal is accomplished, most patients will experience a lift in mood and a reduction of hopelessness.

THE PROGRESS OF A TYPICAL COURSE OF THERAPY

After an agenda has been set and the homework from the previous session is reviewed, the therapist and the patient proceed to discuss the other issues on the agenda in order of importance. Generally, it is possible to make progress on one to three problem areas in a particular session.

In addressing a typical issue, the therapist usually begins by asking the patient a series of questions in order to clarify the nature of the difficulty. For example, is the patient misinterpreting events? To what extent is the problem "real"? Are the patient's expectations realistic? Are there alternative explanations or solutions? If the problem is symptomatic or behavioral (e.g., insomnia, appetite disturbance, anhedonia, or "overwhelming" chores or tasks), more specific history taking and behavioral analysis may be necessary. At the end of this questioning process, the therapist suggests focusing on one or two key thoughts, assumptions, images, or behaviors during the session. Once such targets are selected, the therapist recommends a cognitive or behavioral intervention and explains the rationale for use of the technique to the patient. These procedures may include actions such as setting up an experiment, role playing or cognitive rehearsal, generating alternatives, weighing advantages and disadvantages, and activity scheduling (Beck et al., 1979).

Toward the end of the session, the therapist again asks the patient for feedback. It is generally useful to encourage questions about potential areas of confusion and to ask the patient to summarize the major points of the session. Finally, the therapist suggests a relevant homework assignment. The homework is tailored to help the patient apply what is being learned in CT during the interval between sessions.

Although the structure of the cognitive therapy session illustrated above does not change substantially as treatment progresses, the content does. The initial sessions are generally concerned with setting priorities, building empathy and rapport, reducing hopelessness, demonstrating the relationship between thoughts and feelings, identifying errors in thinking, and making rapid progress on readily solvable problems. There tends to be an emphasis on behavioral methods early in therapy, especially with severely depressed inpatients (Thase & Wright, 1991).

In general, the middle phase of therapy (e.g., sessions 5–10) is likely to be spent in helping the patient to integrate and expand on cognitive concepts introduced in the first phase of treatment. This is accomplished through a variety of procedures including intensive use of Socratic questioning, application of the rational response technique to counter specific dysfunctional automatic thoughts, and completion of homework assignments that utilize a systematic approach to thought recording.

By the later part of therapy (e.g., sessions 10–20), usually the patient's symptoms lessen, and the work shifts to the modification of schemas or other long-standing problems. A schema such as "Unless I perform perfectly, I am a failure" might be identified, and a plan developed to work on progressive revision of this approach to life. As noted earlier, it is hypothesized that alteration of schemas is necessary before termination of therapy in order to reduce the risk of relapse (Beck et al., 1979; Persons, 1989). Many therapists begin to address schematic issues even earlier in a course of therapy once they have gained experience and comfort with the cognitive model of treatment.

The patient is encouraged to take an increasing amount of responsibility as the therapy proceeds to its conclusion. Ideally, the therapist serves more as a consultant than a provider of solutions during this stage of therapy. Nevertheless, the therapist must ensure that the patient has some opportunity to prepare for anticipated setbacks. Interventions at this phase include rehearsal of relapse-prevention strategies (see Chapter 14). Also, patients typically are asked to generate their own homework assignments and to apply cognitive therapy techniques without constant feedback or support. Prior to termination from outpatient therapy, the frequency of sessions usually is reduced to biweekly or even monthly. The University of Pittsburgh group recommends that patients achieve at least two stable months of remission before termination of CT (Thase et al., 1992).

COGNITIVE TECHNIQUES

Four major steps are involved in the cognitive approach to a particular problem: (1) eliciting automatic thoughts; (2) testing the accuracy of automatic thoughts; (3) developing rational alternatives; and (4) identifying and modifying maladaptive schemas. These processes are discussed below.

Identification of Dysfunctional Automatic Thoughts

One of the initial techniques is to teach the patient to identity negative automatic thoughts. As noted earlier, some patients are unaware of having these thoughts unless they are taught to recognize them. A variety of interventions are available to help patients identify dysfunctional ideation. Automatic thoughts can be described to patients in a didactic manner, and relevant reading material can be provided (see, for example, *Coping with Depression*, Beck & Greenberg, 1974). However, it is more important to engage the patient in a series of collaborative exercises designed to demonstrate the presence of negative automatic thoughts. In cognitive therapy, unlike rational emotive therapy (Ellis, 1962), the process for identifying and monitoring negative automatic thoughts is established before the therapist focuses intensively on modification of such thoughts.

Several techniques are useful in helping the patient to identify negative automatic thoughts. The therapist may make direct inquiries about what "passed through" the patient's mind during a strong emotional response. Asking the patient about thoughts that accompany visible mood shifts observed during the course of a session provides an especially potent way to illustrate the relationship between thoughts and feelings. Past events associated with dysphoric mood can be examined by asking patients to recall specific thoughts and feelings while imagining a troubling event taking place. For some individuals, the use of imagery comes easily, whereas others may need coaching in order to evoke intense images. In the latter case, the therapist may need to act much like a stage director to help the patient "set the scene." Detailed preparatory work (including asking questions about the antecedents of the event, timing of actions, visual cues in the image, etc.) may be needed in some instances to bring a scene alive. Role playing also may be utilized to facilitate recall of past events and associated thoughts and feelings.

Often, patients are more readily able to identify thoughts that appear to be mild or "sanitized" versions of markedly distorted cognitions. For example, a tearful patient may report the thought "My girlfriend dumped me." Although romantic breakups typically result in sadness, the patient's level of despair or dysphoria may appear to be in excess of normal expectation. In this case, the therapist can use a series of increasingly more incisive or revealing Socratic questions to uncover deeper layers of automatic thoughts and/or schemas (see Fig. 1.1). This procedure has been termed the "downward arrow" (or inference chain) technique. Each query should build on the information learned from previous questions.

Homework assignments are used to improve recognition of automatic thoughts and their relationship to emotional reactions. For example, the Daily Record of Dysfunctional Thoughts (DRDT; see Tables 1.4 and 1.5; Young & Beck, 1982) is particularly helpful in teaching patients to record variations in mood according to three components: the environmental situation, automatic thoughts, and rational thoughts. We usually recommend that patients keep their thought records as part of a journal or notebook containing all therapeutic materials. This helps reinforce learning and promotes the self-help nature of CT. Notebooks can be drawn on frequently during the course of therapy and can serve as a useful resource after completion of treatment. Another homework assignment, thought counting, may be utilized when patients have trouble recognizing certain types of automatic thoughts. A wrist counter or a golf stroke scorer can be used to facilitate counting targeted thoughts.

Testing the Accuracy of Automatic Negative Thoughts

After it has been demonstrated that negative automatic thoughts appear to correlate with or trigger dysphoric moods, the empirical approach is extended to testing the accuracy of the patient's thoughts. One goal of this step is to encourage the patient to learn to think like a scientist, so that his or her initial conclusions can be viewed as hypotheses that can be examined against all available evidence. This type of therapeutic intervention stands in contrast to the simpler method of persuasion, in which the therapist directly tries to convince the patient that his or her thoughts are irrational. The empirical nature of CT is a fundamental element of the "Beckian" approach and relies heavily on Socratic questioning and related methods of inquiry. The majority of therapist–patient interactions in CT are devoted to this process.

Negative automatic thoughts that occur during emotionally

Patient	Therapist
"I think the date went poorly *(chuckles with gallows humor)* . . . I'm so depressed!"	
↓	"Is it true that the date went that poorly? Could this be an example of how negative thinking is involved with feeling depressed?"
"No—it's true. He didn't mention another date and hasn't called me since."	
↓	"Okay . . . that sounds convincing enough. So, if the date went badly, what's that really say about you?"
"Stuff like this happens to me a lot!"	
↓	"And, if that's true?"
"There is something seriously wrong with me." *(There is a visible shift in affect.)*	
↓	"Such as . . ."
"I must be a reject . . . a social basket case . . . I'm so pathetic!" *(tearful)*	
↓	"And if that's true, which we still have to test out, what does that say about your world and future?"
"It says that no one will ever love me . . . I'll be lonely forever . . . an old maid. . . ." *(more tears).*	
↓	"I can see from your tears that these thought really hit you where it hurts. I've written down some of the more dramatic and hurtful statements. Do you feel up to taking a look at them and testing their accuracy?"

FIGURE 1.1. The downward arrow technique.

charged situations are examined closely to evaluate their accuracy and logic. One useful approach is to teach patients to ask themselves a series of questions regarding their negative automatic thoughts:

1. "What is the evidence to support this thought?" The therapist typically uses Socratic questioning to examine the logic on which conclusions are based and to uncover examples of cognitive distortion or irrational thinking. In addition, the patient may benefit from watching the therapist "model" more rational thinking processes.

TABLE 1.4. Daily Record of Dysfunctional Thoughts[a]

Situation	Automatic thought(s)	Emotion(s)	Rational response	Outcome
Describe: 1. Actual event leading to unpleasant emotion or 2. Stream of thoughts, daydreams, or recollection, leading to unpleasant emotion.	1. Write automatic thought(s) that preceded emotion(s) 2. Rate beliefs in automatic thought(s), 0–100%	1. Specify sad/anxious/angry, etc. 2. Rate degree of emotion, 1–100%	1. Write rational response to automatic thought(s). 2. Rate belief in rational response 0–100%	1. Rerate belief in automatic thought(s), 0–100% 2. Specify and rate subsequent emotions, 0–100%

[a]Explanation: When you experience an unpleasant emotion, note the situation associated with the emotion. (If the emotion occurred while you were thinking, daydreaming, etc., please note this.) Then note the automatic thought that stimulated the emotion. Record the degree to which you believe this thought: 0%, not at all; 100% completely. In rating degree of emotion: 1 = a trace; 100 = the most intense possible.

Adapted from Young and Beck (1982).

TABLE 1.5. Instructions for Completing the Daily Record of Dysfunctional Thoughts

The Daily Record of Dysfunctional Thoughts is designed to help you analyze and resolve situations that cause you to feel or act in a way that is not in your best interest.

Column 1: Situation. In this column you describe the actual events that were associated with an unpleasant emotion. In filling out this column you must be objective. That is, briefly describe what happened as a videotape would have recorded it. Sometimes there isn't a specific event that you can identify. Rather, unpleasant emotions often result from just daydreaming about something. In this case, briefly describe the daydream or stream of thought leading to the unpleasant emotion.

Column 2: Automatic Thought(s). Most people assume that it is the situation that causes the feeling. In actuality, it is our thoughts about the situation that lead to our feelings. In this column you are to write down the automatic thoughts that preceded the emotion. Sometimes it is easy for you to identify your automatic thoughts. Sometimes, they are harder to identify because they are so automatic. For these cases, you have to concentrate on what happened and your reaction to the event. Then, write down all your thoughts, exactly as they came to you. Then, rate how strongly you believe the automatic thoughts to be true using the 0–100 scale described on the bottom of the form.

Column 3: Emotion(s). Indicate how you felt (feel) at the time. Emotions are feelings, such as sad, angry, depressed, lonely, afraid, and anxious. These are your emotions, not your thoughts. Remember that thoughts are really words, phrases, or sentences that we say to ourselves. It may take some practice to be able to distinguish between thoughts and emotions, but you will be able to do so. Also, indicate the degree that you felt these emotions using the 0–100 scale described on the bottom of the form.

Column 4: Rational Response. After you have written down your automatic thoughts, you need to examine the reasonableness of each thought. Is the thought accurate? What is the evidence to support it? Is there another interpretation of the event? Is there another way of looking at the situation that would not make you feel so bad? Work hard at these rational responses. It may help to ask someone who may be more objective and rational about an event. Also, rate the degree to which you believe the rational response to be true using the 0–100 scale described on the bottom of the form.

Column 5: Outcome. After you have completed columns 1–4, rate how strongly you now believe the automatic thoughts. In addition, indicate how your emotions have changed.

Adapted from Young and Beck (1982) and Sacco and Beck (1985).

2. "Are there any alternative interpretations?" Depressed patients are likely to have negative interpretations of ambiguous situations for which, in actuality, numerous alternatives are possible, and individuals with panic disorder may have catastrophic thoughts about normal bodily sensations. The therapist encourages the patient to search for other explanations and then to order them from the most to least believable.

This process helps the patient to assume a more neutral or objective role in evaluating the veracity of negative automatic thoughts.

3. "Am I totally to blame for this negative event, and can I do anything about it?" The tendency toward self-blame and passive acceptance of problems needs to be countered actively. Misattributions regarding the perceived causality, globality, and permanence of the problem (Abramson et al., 1978) also are recognized and challenged.

4. "What if my interpretation is true? How will I manage then?" Patients need to learn to use a process analogous to "damage control" if they have realistic problems or actual skill deficits. The "worst case scenario" strategy may be particularly helpful in such situations. When patients confront the worst possibility, they often begin to gain a sense of mastery over their destiny. They can move from being terrified or defeated by a stressful event or personal liability to developing an active, problem-oriented method for managing adversity.

Developing Rational Alternatives

Learning to identify more rational responses to dysfunctional automatic thoughts occurs as a direct result of the questioning process described above. Patients are taught to identify and test alternative self-statements that are consistent with available evidence. Initially, patients are encouraged to write down their dysfunctional thoughts and the possible rational responses during therapy sessions. This is then followed by written homework. The explicit, written approach to coping with affectively laden or "hot" automatic thoughts is an important part of this learning process. Often, patients who are just beginning to use the rational response technique may not be able to think of particularly effective alternative responses, especially at times of marked emotional arousal. In such cases, "on the spot" recording of the automatic thoughts may be recommended, and work on the rational response portion of the DRDT may be delayed until a therapist is available to help. Selection and timing of interventions to match the patient's learning capacity are particularly important for inpatient CT because patients may be both more markedly distressed and less able to use self-help interventions than most outpatients (Thase & Wright, 1991).

The therapist also needs to be sensitive to the patient's unstated reservations about the accuracy of the rational response. This phenomenon typically is perceived by the therapist on the basis of changes in affect, posture, or facial expression. Many patients find that their initial efforts to develop rational responses may elicit additional negative automatic thoughts that, in turn, undercut the mood-altering effect of the intervention. These "second-order" automatic thoughts also must be identified, tested, and countered if the patient is to benefit from the rational response. As therapy progresses, patients usually begin to answer their dysfunctional automatic thoughts *in vivo*, that is, using an unwritten "mental" variation of the DRDT.

Identification of Schemas and Dysfunctional Silent Assumptions

The therapist and patient may begin to focus on identifying basic schemas as soon as the collaborative alliance is solidified and the basic framework of therapy is in place. In relatively straightforward cases, such work may begin within the first few meetings, whereas some patients may require a number of sessions before they can make use of this aspect of CT. One useful method to elicit schemas involves having patients review their therapy notebooks for particular patterns or themes revealed in the Daily Record of Dysfunctional Thoughts. However, most schemas are identified in therapy sessions through Socratic questioning, imagery, role-play exercises, or other cognitive procedures. In some cases, the Dysfunctional Attitude Scale (Weissman, 1979) may be useful in helping the patient recognize underlying assumptions. The patient also may be asked to write an autobiography to trace the historical development of schemas (Beck et al., 1979; Thase & Wright, 1991).

Generally, modification of schemas is based on procedures similar to those employed in testing and modifying negative automatic thoughts (see, for example, Beck et al., 1979; Persons, 1989). In one common exercise, the patient is asked to list the advantages and disadvantages of retaining a problematic attitude, belief, or schema. The patient also may write alternate schemas and begin to "try them out," even if the behaviors directed by the new schemas are not "natural" or the new attitude seems foreign. A skillful cognitive therapist can enhance the value of the exercise by eliciting pertinent automatic thoughts (e.g., "this is phony—it won't work") and helping the patient identify more rational alternatives (e.g., "All new skills and patterns of behavior feel unnatural at first. . . . Labeling my revised schema as phony is just another example of my self-critical bias."). Another technique designed to modify schemas involves having the patient perform an experiment in which he or she agrees to behave in a manner contrary to that dictated by the silent assumption. For example, a patient with perfectionistic attitudes might be asked to perform a task in an "only satisfactory" manner. With inpatients, relevant assignments could include performing "average" work in an occupational therapy project, withholding explicit support from an overly dependent peer during a group therapy session, or purposively *not* trying to be a dominant force in a unit-community meeting.

BEHAVIORAL TECHNIQUES

A variety of behavioral techniques also are used to help the patient cope with symptoms or situational and interpersonal problems. These behavioral procedures tend to be more active and less abstract than cognitive interventions and, thus, are important components of treatment of severely impaired inpatients (Scott, 1988; Thase & Wright, 1991; also see Chapter 4). Behavioral interventions usually have the additional benefit of aiding in the ultimate goal of modifying dysfunctional cognitions. For example, patients who complain of marked anhedonia often will note a change in the believability of the absolutistic thought "I can't enjoy anything" after completing a series of behavioral assignments designed to increase the number and variety of potentially pleasurable activities. Thus, behavioral change can be used to bring about cognitive change. The most commonly used behavioral techniques are described below.

Scheduling Activities

The therapist and ward staff use an activity schedule to help the patient plan activities hour by hour during the day (see Beck & Greenberg, 1974, for a useful template). The patient then keeps a record of the activities that are actually performed. Mood ratings may be added, either retrospectively or concurrently. Scheduling activities is usually one of the first techniques used with a depressed patient. This procedure helps to counteract loss of motivation, hopelessness, and excessive rumination and points out the relationship between inactivity and worsening of mood.

Goals of activity scheduling include deriving more pleasure from events, using more adaptive methods of distraction, and increasing the "output" of functional activity on a day-to-day basis. To do this, the patient rates each completed activity for both mastery and pleasure on a scale from 0 to 10. These ratings may be used to challenge patients' beliefs that they cannot obtain a sense of accomplishment or enjoy anything or that all activities result in increased nervousness. Moreover, this technique may be used to identify areas of pleasure or mastery deficits that can be addressed with specific behavioral assignments.

Graded Task Assignments

In order to help some patients accomplish goals, the therapist may need to break down an activity into "chunks" or subtasks ranging from the simplest part to the most complex and demanding. This step-by-step approach permits patients to manage tasks that originally seem impossible or overwhelming. Graded task assignments teach the utility of a step-wise approach to problem solving and are particularly useful for reducing procrastination. In the early phases of treatment, graded task assignments also may help a severely ill patient realize that accommodations need to be made in order to cope with the symptoms of the disorder.

Behavioral and Cognitive Rehearsal

Some patients have difficulty carrying out tasks requiring successive steps for completion. This can be a result of problems in concentration, motivation, predictions of failure, and/or skill deficits. Rehearsal strategies can be used to help the patient practice and master each step leading to completion of the task. Also, by monitoring automatic thoughts during a rehearsal exercise, the patient can identify potential cognitive obstacles. Modeling and coaching procedures may then be used to teach methods of managing difficult situations. This enables the patient to develop new patterns of behavior, such as more effective ways of handling anger or enhanced assertiveness skills.

Diversion Techniques

Diversion is a commonly used strategy that may temporarily reduce most forms of painful affect, including dysphoria, anxiety, and anger. This may be accomplished through physical activity, social contact, work, play, or visual imagery. A regular exercise schedule also may have additive antidepressant effects (Simons, Epstein, McGowan, Kupfer, & Robertson, 1985).

STUDIES OF EFFECTIVENESS OF COGNITIVE THERAPY

Cognitive therapy is the most intensely studied psychotherapeutic treatment of depression. Several comprehensive reviews have documented the utility of this approach in a variety of populations and settings (see, for example, Dobson, 1989; Hollon & Najavitis, 1988). Of greatest relevance, five published studies have compared Beck's model of therapy with standard antidepressant medications. In the first such investigation, Rush et al. (1977) found CT to be superior to imipramine hydrochloride in the treatment of depressed outpatients. Subsequently, Blackburn, Bishop, Glen, Whalley, and Christie (1981) and Teasdale, Fennell, Hibbert, and Amies (1984) found CT to be more effective than standard pharmacological treatments when provided in family practice settings. In the Blackburn et al. (1981) study, CT and pharmacotherapy appeared comparably effective in patients treated in a psychiatric specialty clinic, a finding subsequently replicated by Murphy, Simons, Wetzel, and Lustman (1984), Hollon and associates (cited in Hollon & Najavitis, 1988), and Elkin et al. (1989). In the latter study, CT was somewhat less rapidly effective than imipramine and, also, was less effective than pharmacotherapy in a subgroup of patients with higher initial depression severity scores. However, the existence of a treatment-site-by-treatment-type interaction may limit the interpretation of this otherwise carefully designed and well-executed study (Elkin et al., 1989).

The efficacy of cognitive therapy in markedly severe or "endogenous" depressions is not yet as well established. Most studies have failed to find any relationship between the presence of endogenous features of depression and responsivity to cognitive therapy (Blackburn et al., 1981; Jarrett, Rush, Khatami, & Roffwarg, 1990; Kovacs, Rush, Beck, & Hollon, 1981; Teasdale et al., 1984; Thase, Simons, Cahalane, & McGeary, 1991b). However, Thase, Simons, Cahalane, and McGeary (1991a) found a slightly less robust ultimate response to CT in more severely depressed patients (dividing the sample according to the Hamilton depression score criteria of Elkin et al., 1989). Both the milder and the more severe patent groups in this study generally had excellent outcomes by the end of therapy, but more severely depressed patients were subsequently found to have a higher risk of relapse (Thase et al., 1992).

Neither Thase and Simons (1992) nor Jarrett et al. (1990) found a predictive negative relationship between response to CT and the presence of reduced latency to the onset of the first episode of rapid eye movement sleep (i.e., REM latency), an objective, biological correlate of endogenous depression (see, for example, Thase, Frank, & Kupfer, 1985). Indeed, in the Pittsburgh study there was a tendency, on some measures of outcome, for patients with reduced REM latency to respond more rapidly to CT than patients with nonreduced (i.e., normal) values (Thase et al., 1991b).

As Hollon and Najavitis (1988) have noted, CT may offer a unique advantage relative to pharmacotherapy with respect to relapse prevention. Cognitive therapy teaches an approach to recognizing and managing depressive symptomatology that can be continued long after therapy is formally terminated. To date, four studies have documented significantly reduced risk of relapse of depression following CT compared to pharmacotherapy of depression (Blackburn, Eunson, & Bishop, 1987; Hollon et al., cited in Hollon & Najavitis, 1988; Simons, Murphy, Levine, & Wetzel, 1986; Shea et al., in press), with a similar trend reported in a fifth study (Kovacs et al., 1981). These most promising and consistent findings provide the strongest justification to date that cognitive therapy may have a truly unique impact on the course of depressive disorder. Nevertheless, hospitalized patients are at significantly greater risk for relapse and recurrence (Thase, in press), and the benefit of continued outpatient CT following discharge has already been demonstrated (Miller et al., 1989; Thase, Bowler, & Harden, 1991). It thus seems virtually certain that continued outpatient therapy is indicated when CT is used in lieu of pharmacotherapy (Thase, Bowler, & Harden, 1991). Specific therapeutic techniques used to help prevent or lower the risk of relapse are reviewed in Chapter 14.

There are, as yet, no published studies that test the efficacy of CT alone compared to pharmacotherapy or standard inpatient treatment for hospitalized patients. The development and implementation of inpatient CT programs that exclude the use of pharmacotherapy are not likely to be of major public health significance. However, the availability of such treatment is of considerable importance for those patients who cannot or will not take antidepressant medications because of side effects, nonresponse, health concerns, or pregnancy (Wright, 1988; Wright & Schrodt, 1989; Thase & Wright, 1991).

Preliminary experiences adapting this therapy to the psychiatric inpatient setting have been described by Shaw (1981), Schrodt and Wright (1987), Scott (1988), and Bowers (1989). Results of an intensive (five sessions per week) CT protocol, used with 16 nonpsychotically depressed, unmedicated inpatients, were reported by Thase, Bowler, and Harden. (1991). In this "open-label" trial, 13 patients (81%) responded to treatment following an average of 13 sessions (i.e., about 3 weeks of treatment). Three of four responders to this program who did not receive outpatient cognitive therapy subsequently relapsed within 4 months following discharge, as compared to only one of nine responders who received CT aftercare (Thase, Bowler, & Harden, 1991).

Cognitive therapy in combination with pharmacotherapy may be especially useful in the hospital setting (Wright, 1987; Wright & Schrodt, 1989; Wright & Thase, in press). In two studies, Bowers (1990) and Miller, Norman, and Keitner (1989) found that both Beck's model of CT and alternative behavioral treatment strategies improved response to tricyclic antidepressants in hospitalized depressed patients. Wright (1986) similarly found a high response rate in depressed inpatients treated with CT and nortriptyline. Miller, Norman, Keitner, Bishop, and Dow (1989) reported that the additive effect of cognitive and behavioral treatment was more clinically significant after 1 year of follow-up than was apparent at the time of discharge. In a subsequent analysis, Whisman, Miller, Norman, and Keitner (1991) found that such improvements were particularly apparent on measures of dysfunctional attitudes and cognitive distortions. These findings indicate that an integrated cognitive and biological approach has considerable promise for the treatment of depressed inpatients (also, see Chapter 7).

A number of controlled studies of cognitive–behavioral therapies of anxiety disorders also have been completed. In open series of cases (Clark, 1986; Beck & Greenberg, 1988; Sokol, Beck, Greenberg, Berchick, & Wright, 1989) and controlled treatment trials (Barlow et al., 1989; Power et al., 1990; Butler, Fennell, Robson, & Gelder, 1991; Beck, Sokol, Clark, Berchick, & Wright, 1992), the combination of behavioral exposure to feared situations and use of cognitive strategies to cope with ruminative, catastrophic, or somatically focused automatic negative thoughts have been effective in reducing levels of generalized anxiety, decreasing the frequency of panic attacks, and lessening avoidance behavior. Of interest, CT techniques have been found to be useful in aiding patients to discontinue potentially habit-forming antipanic medications such as alprazolam and clonazepam (Otto, Pollock, & Rosenbaum, 1992). Inpatients with anxiety disorders also typically suffer from a comorbid depressive syndrome (including suicidal intent or behavior) and/or marked incapacity. Thus, CT approaches for anxious and depressive symptoms are blended together commonly in hospital settings.

SUMMARY

Cognitive therapy is grounded in a clearly formulated theoretical model and an extensive amount of research documenting the relationship between disordered information processing and psychopathology. In treatment sessions, the therapist and patient work collaboratively to elucidate relationships among dysfunctional cognitions, emotional distress, and problematic patterns of behavior. Interventions move progressively from surface (i.e., behavioral disturbances and recognition of automatic negative thoughts) to deeper levels (i.e., maladaptive schemas) of psychopathology. Selected behavioral techniques are used to address specific symptoms and to facilitate the cognitive aspects of therapy. Procedures for structuring and pacing sessions include identification of well-defined goals, the systematic use of an agenda, the provision and receipt of feedback, and the regular use of homework assignments. Hypotheses are explicitly stated and tested in order to enhance collaboration and establish an empirical basis for therapeutic change. The cognitive approach can readily be used in concert with pharmacotherapy when a combined treatment plan is indicated, and available evidence suggests that this strategy may have additive effects.

Cognitive therapy is the most intensively studied psychological treatment of major depression. A growing literature suggests that it has similar value for anxiety disorders. In the case of severely disturbed hospitalized patients, this form of therapy provides specific strategies for addressing commonly encountered symptoms such as suicidal ideation, hopelessness, guilty ruminations, functional incapacity, intense anxiety, pathological avoidance, and moribund inactivity. As discussed in subsequent chapters, recent work also supports a broader application of CT in the treatment of substance abuse, eating disorders, personality disturbances, and chronic mental illness. In addition, cognitive therapy procedures exert a significant relapse prevention effect. These positive features suggest that cognitive therapy has considerable potential for adding to the effectiveness and durability of inpatient treatment.

REFERENCES

Abramson, L. Y., Seligman, M. E. P., & Teasdale, J. D. (1978). Learned helplessness in humans: Critique and reformulation. *Abnormal Psychology, 89,* 49–74.

Adler, A. (1936). The neurotic's picture of the world. *International Journal of Individual Psychology, 2,* 3–10.

American Psychiatric Association. (1987). *Diagnostic and statistical manual of mental disorders* (3rd ed., revised). Washington, DC: American Psychiatric Association.

Arkowitz, H., & Hannah, M. T. (1989). Cognitive, behavioral, and psychodynamic therapies. In A. Freeman, K. M. Simon, L. E. Beutler, & H. Arkowitz (Eds.), *Comprehensive handbook of cognitive therapy* (pp. 143–167). New York: Plenum Press.

Barlow, D. H., Craske, M. G., Cerny, J. A., & Klosko, J. S. (1989). Behavioral treatment of panic disorder. *Behavior Therapy, 20,* 261–282.

Beck, A. T. (1961). A systematic investigation of depression. *Comprehensive Psychiatry, 2,* 163–.

Beck, A. T. (1963). Thinking and depression. *Archives of General Psychiatry, 9,* 324–333.

Beck, A. T. (1964). Thinking and depression, 2: Theory and therapy. *Archives of General Psychiatry, 10,* 561–571.

Beck, A. T. (1967). *Depression: Clinical, experimental, and theoretical aspects.* New

York: Harper & Row. Republished as: *Depression: Causes and treatment.* Philadelphia: University of Pennsylvania Press, 1972.

Beck, A. T. (1970). Cognitive therapy: Nature and relation to behavior therapy. *Behavior Therapy, 1,* 184–200.

Beck, A. T. (1976). *Cognitive therapy and the emotional disorders.* New York: International Universities Press.

Beck, A. T., Freeman, A., & Associates. (1990). *Cognitive therapy of personality disorders.* New York: Guilford Press.

Beck, A. T., & Greenberg, R. L. (1974). *Coping with depression (a booklet).* New York: Institute for Rational Living.

Beck, A. T., & Greenberg, R. L. (1988). Cognitive therapy of panic disorder. In A. J. Frances & R. E. Hales (Eds.), *American Psychiatric Press review of psychiatry,* Vol. 7 (pp. 571–584). Washington, DC: American Psychiatric Press.

Beck, A. T., Rush, A. J., Shaw, B. F., & Emery, B. (1979). *Cognitive therapy of depression.* New York: Guilford Press.

Beck, A. T., Sokol, L., Clark, D. A., Berchick, R. J., & Wright, F. D. (1992). A cross-over study of focused cognitive therapy for panic disorder. *American Journal of Psychiatry, 149,* 778–783.

Beidel, D. C., & Turner, S. M. (1986). A critique of the theoretical bases of cognitive behavioral theories and therapy. *Clinical Psychology Review, 6,* 177–197.

Blackburn, I. M., Bishop, S., Glen, A. I. M., Whalley, L. J., & Christie, J. E. (1981). The efficacy of cognitive therapy in depression. A treatment trial using cognitive therapy and pharmacotherapy, each alone and in combination. *British Journal of Psychiatry, 139,* 181–189.

Blackburn, I. M., Eunson, K. M., & Bishop, S. (1987). A two-year naturalistic follow-up of depressed patients treated with cognitive therapy, pharmacotherapy, and a combination of both. *Journal of Affective Disorders, 10,* 67–75.

Bowers, W. A. (1989). Cognitive therapy with inpatients. In A. Freeman, K. M. Simon, L. E. Beutler, & H. Arkowitz (Eds.), *Comprehensive handbook of cognitive therapy* (pp. 583–596). New York: Plenum Press.

Bowers, W. A. (1990). Treatment of depressed inpatients. Cognitive therapy plus medication, relaxation plus medication, and medication alone. *British Journal of Psychiatry, 156,* 73–78.

Braff, D. L., & Beck, A. T. (1974). Thinking disorder in depression. *Archives of General Psychiatry, 31,* 456–459.

Brand, N., & Jolles, J. (1987). Information processing in depression and anxiety. *Psychological Medicine, 17,* 145–153.

Breslow, R., Kocsis, J., & Belkin, B. (1980). Memory deficits in depression. Evidence utilizing the Wechsler Memory Scale. *Perceptual and Motor Skills, 51,* 541–542.

Butler, G., Fennell, M., Robson, P., & Gelder, M. (1991). Comparison of behavior therapy and cognitive behavior therapy in the treatment of generalized anxiety disorder. *Journal of Consulting and Clinical Psychology, 59,* 167–175.

Clark, D. M. (1986). A cognitive approach to panic. *Behavior Research and Therapy, 24,* 461–470.

Cohen, R. M., Weingartner, H., Smallberg, S. A., Pickar, D., & Murphy, D. L. (1982). Effort and cognition in depression. *Archives of General Psychiatry, 39,* 593–597.

Coyne, J. C., & Gotlib, I. H. (1983). The role of cognition in depression: A critical appraisal. *Psychological Bulletin, 94,* 472–505.

Coyne, J. C., & Gotlib, I. H. (1986). Studying the role of cognition in depression: Well-trodden paths and cul-de-sacs. *Cognitive Therapy and Research, 10,* 695–705.

Dobson, K. (1989). A meta-analysis of the efficacy of cognitive therapy of depression. *Journal of Consulting and Clinical Psychology, 57,* 414–419.

Donnelly, E. F., Dent, J. K., & Murphy, D. L. (1972). Comparison of temporal lobe epileptics and affective disorders on the Halstead-Reitan test battery. *Journal of Clinical Psychology, 28,* 61–62.

Eaves, G., & Rush, A. J. (1984). Cognitive patterns in symptomatic and remitted unipolar major depression. *Journal of Abnormal Psychology, 93,* 31–40.

Elkin, I., Shea, M. T., Watkins, J. T., Imber, S. D., Sotsky, S. M., Collins, J. F., Glass, D. R., Pilkonis, P. A., Leber, W. R., Docherty, J. P., Fiester, S. J., & Parloff, M. B. (1989). National Institute of Mental Health Treatment of Depression Collaborative Research Program: General effectiveness of treatments. *Archives of General Psychiatry, 46,* 971–982.

Ellis, A. (1962). *Reason and emotion in psychotherapy.* New York: Lyle Stuart.

Frankl, V. E. (1985). Logos, paradox, and the search for meaning. In M. J. Mahoney, & A. Freeman (Eds.), *Cognition and psychotherapy* (pp. 3–49). New York: Plenum Press.

Freeman, A., Simon, K. M., Beutler, L. E., & Arkowitz, H. (1989). *Comprehensive handbook of cognitive therapy.* New York: Plenum Press.

Freeman, A., & White, D. M. (1989). The treatment of suicidal behavior. In A. Freeman, K. M. Simon, L. E. Beutler, & H. Arkowitz (Eds.), *Comprehensive handbook of cognitive therapy* (pp. 321–346). New York: Plenum Press.

Glass, R. M., Uhlenhuth, E. H., Hartel, F. W., Matuzas, W., & Fischman, M. W. (1981). Cognitive dysfunction and imipramine in outpatient depressives. *Archives of General Psychiatry, 38,* 1048–1051.

Guidano, V. F., & Liotti, G. (1983). *Cognitive processes and emotional disorders.* New York: Guilford Press.

Hammen, C., Ellicott, A., Gitlin, M., & Jamison, K. R. (1989). Sociotropy/autonomy and vulnerability to specific life events in patients with unipolar depression and bipolar disorders. *Journal of Abnormal Psychology, 98,* 154–160.

Harrell, T., Chambless, D., & Calhoun, J. (1981). Correlational relationships between self-statements and affective statements. *Cognitive Therapy and Research, 5,* 159–173.

Hersen, M., Bellack, A. S., Himmelhoch, J. M., & Thase, M. E. (1984). Effects of social skill training, amitriptyline, and psychotherapy in unipolar depressed women. *Behavior Therapy, 15,* 21–40.

Hollon, S. D., & Kendall, P. C. (1980). Cognitive self-statements in depression: Clinical validation of an automatic thoughts questionnaire. *Cognitive Therapy and Research, 4*, 383–395.

Hollon, S. D., Kendall, P. C., & Lumry, A. (1986). Specificity of depressotypic cognitions in clinical depression. *Journal of Abnormal Psychology, 95*, 52–59.

Hollon, S. D., & Najavitis, L. (1988). Review of empirical studies on cognitive therapy. In A. J. Frances & R. E. Hales (Eds.), *American Psychiatric Press review of psychiatry,* Vol. 7 (pp. 643–666). Washington, DC, American Psychiatric Press.

Horney, K. (1950). *Neurosis and human growth: The struggle toward self-realization.* New York: W. W. Norton.

Jarrett, R. B., Rush, A. J., Khatami, M., & Roffwarg, H. P. (1990). Does the pretreatment polysomnogram predict response to cognitive therapy in depression outpatients? A preliminary report. *Psychiatry Research, 33*, 285–299.

Johnson, M. H., & Magaro, P. A. (1987). Effects of mood and severity on memory processes in depression and mania. *Psychological Bulletin, 101*, 28–40.

Kelly, G. (1955). *The psychology of personal constructs.* New York, W. W. Norton.

Kingdon, D. G., & Turkington, D. (1991). A role for cognitive–behavioral strategies in schizophrenia? *Social Psychiatry and Psychiatric Epidemiology, 26,* 101–103.

Kovacs, M., Rush, A. J., Beck, A. T., & Hollon, S. D. (1981). Depressed outpatients treated with cognitive therapy or pharmacotherapy. *Archives of General Psychiatry, 38*, 33–39.

Lewinsohn, P. M., Sullivan, J. M., & Grosscup, S. J. (1982). Behavioral therapy: Clinical applications. In A. J. Rush (Ed.), *Short-term psychotherapies for depression* (pp. 50–87). New York: Guilford Press.

Mahoney, M. J. (1974). *Cognition and behavior modification.* Cambridge, MA: Ballinger.

McLean, P. D. (1982). Behavior theory and research. In A. J. Rush (Ed.), *Short-term psychotherapies for depression* (pp. 19–49). New York: Guilford Press.

Miller, I. W., & Norman, W. H. (1986). Persistence of depressive cognitions within a subgroup of depressed inpatients. *Cognitive Therapy and Research, 10,* 211–224.

Miller, I. W., Norman, W. H., & Keitner, G. I. (1989). Cognitive-behavioral treatment of depressed inpatients: Six- and twelve-month follow-ups. *American Journal of Psychiatry, 146*, 1274–1279.

Miller, I. W., Norman, W. H., Keitner, G. I., Bishop, S. T., & Dow, M. G. (1989). Cognitive behavioral treatment of depressed inpatients. *Behavior Therapy, 20*, 25–47.

Murphy, G. E., Simons, A. D., Wetzel, R. D., & Lustman, P. J. (1984). Cognitive therapy and pharmacotherapy, singly and together, in the treatment of depression. *Archives of General Psychiatry, 41*, 33–41.

Nelson, R. E., & Craighead, W. E., (1977). Selective recall of positive and negative feedback, self-control behaviors, and depression. *Journal of Abnormal Psychology, 86,* 378–388.

Norcross, J. C. (1986). *Handbook of eclectic psychotherapy*. New York: Brunner/Mazel.

Otto, M. W., Pollock, M. H., & Rosenbaum, J. F. (1992). Cognitive-behavioral therapy for benzodiazepine discontinuation in panic disorder patients. *Psychopharmacology Bulletin, 28,* 123–130.

Persons, J. B. (1989). *Cognitive therapy in practice: A case formulation approach*. New York: W. W. Norton.

Persons, J. B., & Burns, D. D. (1985). Mechanisms of action of cognitive therapy: The relative contributions of technical and interpersonal interventions. *Cognitive Therapy and Research, 9,* 539–551.

Piaget, J. (1954). *The construction of reality in the child*. New York: Basic Books.

Power, K. G., Simpson, R. J., Swanson, V., Wallace, L. A., Feistner, A. T. C., & Sharp, D. (1990). A controlled comparison of cognitive–behaviour therapy, diazepam, and placebo, alone and in combination, for the treatment of generalized anxiety disorder. *Journal of Anxiety Disorders, 4,* 267–292.

Rizley, R. (1978). Depression and distortion in the attribution of causality. *Journal of Abnormal Psychology, 87,* 32–48.

Roy-Byrne, P. P., Weingartner, H., Bierer, L. M., Thompson, K., & Post, R. M. (1986). Effortful and automatic cognitive processes in depression. *Archives of General Psychiatry, 43,* 265–267.

Rubinow, D. R., Post, R. M., Savard, R., & Gold, P. W. (1984). Cortisol hypersection and cognitive impairment in depression. *Archives of General Psychiatry, 41,* 279–283.

Rush, A. J. (1982). Diagnosing depressions. In A. J. Rush (Ed.), *Short-term psychotherapies for depression* (pp. 1–18). New York: Guilford Press.

Rush, A. J., Beck, A. T., Kovacs, M., & Hollon, S. D. (1977). Comparative efficacy of cognitive therapy and pharmacotherapy in the treatment of depressed outpatients. *Cognitive Therapy and Research, 1,* 17–37.

Sacco, W. P., & Beck, A. T. (1985). Cognitive therapy of depression. In E. E. Beckham & W. R. Leber (Eds), *Handbook of depression, treatment, assessment, and research* (pp. 3–38). Homewood, IL: Dorsey Press.

Schrodt, G. R., & Wright, J. H. (1987). Inpatient treatment of adolescents. In A. Freeman & V. Greenwood (Eds.), *Cognitive therapy: Applications in psychiatric and medical settings* (pp. 36–50). New York: Human Sciences Press.

Scott, J. (1988). Cognitive therapy with depressed inpatients. In W. Dryden & P. Trower (Eds.), *Developments in cognitive psychotherapy* (pp. 177–189). London: Sage Publications.

Shaw, B. F. (1981). Cognitive therapy with an inpatient population. In G. Emery, S. D. Hollon, & R. C. Bedrosian (Eds.), *New directions in cognitive therapy* (pp. 29–49). New York: Guilford Press.

Shaw, B. F., & Segal, Z. V. (1988). Introduction to cognitive theory and therapy. In A. J. Frances & R. E. Hales (Eds.), *American Psychiatric Press review of psychiatry,* Vol. 7 (pp. 538–553). Washington, DC: America Psychiatric Press.

Shea, M. T., Elkin, I., Imber, S. D., Sotsky, S. M., Watkins, J. T., Collins, J. F., Pilkonis, P. A., Leber, W. R., Krupnick, J., Dolan, R. T., & Parloff, M. B. (in press). Course of depressive symptoms over follow-up: Findings from the National Institute of Mental Health Treatment of Depression Collaborative Research Program. *Archives of General Psychiatry.*

Simons, A. D., Epstein, L. H., McGowan, C. R., Kupfer, D. J., & Robertson, R. J. (1985). Exercise as a treatment for depression: An update. *Clinical Psychology Review, 5,* 553–568.

Simons, A. D., Murphy, G. E., Levine, J. L., & Wetzel, R. D. (1986). Cognitive therapy and pharmacotherapy of depression: Sustained improvement over one year. *Archives of General Psychiatry, 43,* 43–48.

Sokol, L., Beck, A. T., Greenberg, R. L., Berchick, R. J., & Wright, F. D. (1989). Cognitive therapy of panic disorder: A nonpharmacological alternative. *Journal of Nervous and Mental Disease, 177,* 711–716.

Sullivan, H. S. (1953). *The interpersonal theory of psychiatry.* New York: W. W. Norton.

Teasdale, J. D., Fennell, M. J. V., Hibbert, G. A., & Amies, P. L. (1984). Cognitive therapy for major depressive disorder in primary care. *British Journal of Psychiatry, 144,* 400–406.

Thase, M. E. (in press). Cognitive behavior therapy of severe unipolar depression. In: L. Grunhaus & J. Greden (Eds.), *Severe depressive disorders.* Washington DC: American Psychiatric Press.

Thase, M. E., Bowler, K., & Harden, T. (1991). Cognitive behavior therapy of endogenous depression: Part 2. Preliminary findings in 16 unmedicated patients. *Behavior Therapy, 22,* 469–477.

Thase, M. E., Frank, E., & Kupfer, D. J. (1985). Biological processes of major depression. In E. E. Beckham & W. R. Leber (Eds.), *Handbook of depression: Treatment, assessment, and research* (pp. 816–913). Homewood, IL: Dorsey Press.

Thase, M. E., & Simons, A. D. (1992). The applied use of psychotherapy in the study of the psychobiology of depression. *Journal of Psychotherapy Practice and Research, 1,* 72–80.

Thase, M. E., Simons, A. D., Cahalane, J., & McGeary, J. (1991a). Severity of depression and response to cognitive behavior therapy. *The American Journal of Psychiatry, 148,* 784–789.

Thase, M. E., Simons, A. D., Cahalane, J., & McGeary, J. (1991b). Cognitive behavior therapy of endogenous depression: Part 1. An outpatient clinical replication series. *Behavior Therapy, 22,* 579–595.

Thase, M. E., Simons, A. D., McGeary, J., Cahalane, J. F., Hughes, C., Harden, T., & Friedman, E. (1992). Relapse after cognitive behavior therapy of depression: Potential implications of longer-term courses of treatment. *American Journal of Psychiatry, 149,* 1046–1052.

Thase, M. E., & Wright, J. H. (1991). Cognitive behavior therapy with depressed inpatients: An abridged treatment manual. *Behavior Therapy, 22,* 579–579.

Traux, C. B., & Mitchell, K. M. (1971). Research on certain therapist interpersonal skills in relation to process and outcome. In A. E. Bergin & S. L. Garfield (Eds.), *Handbook of psychotherapy and behavior change: An empirical analysis*. New York: John Wiley & Sons..

Watts, F. N., & Sharrock, R. (1987). Cued recall in depression. *British Journal of Clinical Psychology*, *26*(2), 149–150.

Weingartner, H., Cohen, R. M., Murphy, D. K., Martello, J., & Gerdt, C. (1981). Cognitive processes in depression. *Archives of General Psychiatry*, *38*, 42–47.

Weissman, A. N. (1979). *The Dysfunctional Attitude Scale: A validation study*. Unpublished doctoral dissertation. Philadelphia: University of Pennsylvania.

Whisman, M. A., Miller, I. W., Norman, W. H., & Keitner, G. A. (1991). Cognitive therapy with depressed inpatients: Side effects on dysfunctional cognitions. *Journal of Consulting and Clinical Psychology*, *59*, 282–288.

Wolfe, J., Granholm, E., Butters, N., Saunders, E., & Janosky, D. (1987). Variable memory deficits associated with major affective disorders. A comparison of unipolar and bipolar patients. *Journal of Affective Disorders, 13*, 83–92.

Wright, J. H. (1986). Nortriptyline effects on cognition in depression. *Dissertation Abstracts International*, *47* (Section B), 2667.

Wright, J. H. (1987). Cognitive therapy and medication as combined treatment. In A. Freeman & V. Greenwood (Eds.), *Cognitive therapy: Applications in psychiatric and medical settings* (pp. 36–50). New York: Human Sciences Press.

Wright, J. H. (1988). Cognitive therapy of depression. In A. J. Frances & R. E. Hales (Eds.), *American Psychiatric Press review of psychiatry,* Vol. 7 (pp. 554–570). Washington, DC: American Psychiatric Press.

Wright, J. H., & Beck, A. T. (1983). Cognitive therapy of depression: Theory and practice. *Hospital and Community Psychiatry*, *34*(12), 1119–1127.

Wright, J. H., & Borden, J. (1991). Cognitive therapy of depression and anxiety. *Psychiatric Annals, 21*(7), 424–428.

Wright, J. H., & Salmon, P. G. (1990). Learning and memory in process. In C. D. McCann & N. S. Endler (Eds.), *Depression: New directions in theory, research, and practice* (pp. 211–236). Toronto: Wall & Emerson.

Wright, J. H., & Schrodt, G. R. (1989). Combined cognitive therapy and pharmacotherapy. In A. Freeman, K. M. Simon, L. E. Beutler, & H. Arkowitz (Eds.), *Comprehensive handbook of cognitive therapy* (pp. 267–282). New York: Plenum Press.

Wright, J. H., & Thase, M. E. (in press). Cognitive and biological therapies: A synthesis. *Psychiatric Annals.*

Young, J. (1987). *Schema-focused cognitive therapy for personality disorders*. Unpublished manuscript, Cognitive Therapy Center of New York, 111 W. 88th Street, New York, NY 10024.

Young, J. E., & Beck, A. T. (1982). Cognitive therapy: Clinical applications. In

A. J. Rush (Ed.), *Short-term psychotherapies for depression* (pp. 182–214). New York: Guilford Press.

Zeiss, A. M., Lewinsohn, P. M., & Munoz, R. F. (1979). Nonspecific improvement effects in depression using interpersonal skills training, pleasant activity schedules, or cognitive training. *Journal of Consulting and Clinical Psychology*, *47*, 427–439.

Chapter 2

Hospital Psychiatry in Transition

Jesse H. Wright, M.D., Ph.D.,
and Mary Helen Davis, M.D.

Cognitive therapy inpatient programs represent a new direction for hospital psychiatry. However, a portion of the theory and practice of inpatient cognitive therapy is based on elements of earlier treatment models. This chapter traces the development of hospital psychiatry in order to understand how the influences of other approaches have been blended with the unique contributions of cognitive therapy. The distinguishing features of cognitively oriented milieus are highlighted. General treatment issues and procedures for hospital psychiatry also are described.

MODELS OF HOSPITAL PSYCHIATRY

Early Treatment Approaches

From the time the first asylums for the mentally ill were established, hospital conditions and practices have been shaped by prevailing philosophical beliefs, political forces, economic pressures, and societal concerns. For example, treatment in England and Spain during the 14th and 15th centuries was based on widely accepted punitive religious concepts. Patients were treated with floggings, chains, and exorcism because they were viewed as evil or possessed by demons (Deutsch, 1949). These practices remained virtually unchanged until the 18th century, when democratic revolutions in France and the United States kindled an increased respect for personal freedom and dignity. Political and social upheaval was associated with dramatic experiments in treatment of the mentally ill. Chains were removed from patients at the

Bicetre and Salpêtrière in Paris, and new humanitarian approaches to treatment were introduced by the Quakers at the Pennsylvania Hospital in Philadelphia (Deutsch, 1949).

Conditions improved further during the early 19th century, a time of increased social awareness. A new form of treatment, moral therapy, was advocated at institutions such as the Hartford Retreat, Worcester State Hospital, and the Bloomingdale Asylum. Patients were treated kindly but were exhorted to behave in a rational and acceptable manner. The treatment program included history taking and involvement in structured activities. Restraint was used infrequently. Reports of astounding success rates (75–100%) at these hospitals generated considerable optimism about the curability of mental illness (Maxmen, Tucker, & LeBow, 1974).

During the middle of the 19th century, Dorothea Dix led a crusade to extend treatment opportunities to all individuals in need. Her efforts contributed to the building of over 30 state hospitals, including St. Elizabeth's in Washington, D.C. (Goshen, 1967). Unfortunately, by the end of the century, hospitals had become severely overcrowded, the quality of care had eroded, and staff morale was low. These problems were caused in part by declining resources after the Civil War and a flood of new immigrants who required psychiatric treatment.

Institutionalization was the predominant mode of treatment for most patients during the first half of the 20th century. Conditions deteriorated in the 1930s to the point that only 5% of patients were markedly improved on discharge (Clark, 1973). However, there were several more positive developments. The noted physician S. Weir Mitchell became an outspoken critic of hospital psychiatric practices. He was particularly concerned with the estrangement of psychiatrists from other branches of medicine and the isolation of psychiatric hospitals in rural areas (Clark, 1973). Mitchell's contributions were followed by the publication of Clifford Beers's *A Mind That Found Itself* (Beers, 1908). This expose of hospital psychiatry led to the founding of a reform movement, "The National Mental Hygiene Association."

Hospital programs initiated at major universities were the most notable exceptions to the general trend for institutionalization (Schneck, 1975). The Neuropsychiatric Institute at the University of Michigan and the Phipps Clinic at Johns Hopkins provided alternatives to the large state hospital. Programs were also established in Boston, Iowa, and other academic centers. These units became models for the reintroduction of psychiatry into medicine and the development of inpatient units in general hospitals.

Biological therapies such as sedatives, bromides, and insulin coma became an important part of inpatient psychiatry in the 1930s. The first clearly effective somatic treatment, electroconvulsive therapy, was introduced by Cerletti and Bini in 1938 (Cerletti, 1950). Subsequently, many hospitals utilized this technique as the primary approach to psychiatric illnesses of all types. Some patients, especially those with severe depression, had excellent responses, but the psychological milieu of most hospitals changed very little until the advent of psychoanalytically oriented programs and the therapeutic community.

Psychoanalytically Oriented Inpatient Treatment

At about the same time that electroconvulsive therapy was discovered, Harry Stack Sullivan, Freida Fromm-Reichman, and Karl Menninger began to apply psychoanalytic concepts to inpatient treatment at Chestnut Lodge and the Menninger Clinic (Maxmen et al., 1974). Patients were treated with psychoanalytically oriented therapy or, at times, full psychoanalysis, and the hospital milieu was constructed to support this activity. Often a ward administrator would be appointed to manage clinical decisions, so that transference would not be contaminated by the daily activities of the ward. Generally, length of stay was quite prolonged because the treatment model required an intensive and extended course of therapy.

During the middle years of this century, psychoanalytically oriented inpatient programs were regarded by many as the premier form of hospital treatment. Although relatively few patients could be treated, and the cost of therapy was high, it was thought that psychoanalysis offered the best hope for recovery. By the 1980s this treatment model had been eclipsed by several alternate approaches that were more cost effective and were grounded in empirical evidence for effectiveness.

Although psychoanalytic concepts no longer dominate inpatient treatment, their heritage can be seen in most modern hospital programs. Transference and countertransference are particularly important in the inpatient setting. The reactions of patients to staff or other patients are frequently influenced by earlier relationships. Similarly, staff members may have either effective or dysfunctional responses to others based upon their previous experiences. Psychoanalytic treatment programs also recognized the importance of arranging the daily ward schedule to complement the overall treatment model.

The Therapeutic Community

The first therapeutic community was developed in England by Maxwell Jones during World War II (Jones, 1953). He initially decided to use group process and teamwork because of the limited resources available during wartime. Jones later recognized that all of the activities and interactions in the milieu could have a powerful effect on outcome. Although therapeutic communities vary widely, they share several common operational principles: (1) patients are regarded as responsible persons and are asked to share in ward decision making; (2) multiple therapists and therapeutic activities are utilized; (3) the daily program is structured; (4) therapists monitor and attempt to influence the ward culture through community meetings, group therapy, and staff conferences; (5) social interchanges are viewed as important learning experiences that will help the patient manage situations in the outside world; and (6) communication problems between staff and patients can serve as opportunities for therapeutic intervention (Jones, 1953; Wilmer, 1958; Abroms, 1969; Almond, 1971).

Early reports usually extolled the virtues of therapeutic communities (Denber, Turns, & Seeman, 1959, 1968; Gralnick & D'Elia, 1969; Almond, 1971). For example, it was claimed that sharing power in the therapeutic community decreased isolation and acting out while increasing adaptive behavior (Greenley, 1973). However, attempts to study treatment outcome were marked by significant methodological problems. Little evidence was collected that the therapeutic community improved hospital effectiveness (Myers & Clark, 1972; Lehman & Ritzler, 1976).

A series of reports in the 1970s questioned the widespread belief that therapeutic communities offered the best approach to hospital psychiatry. Lehman and Ritzler (1976) noted that the therapeutic community was superior in ward atmosphere and patient and staff satisfaction as compared to a unit run according to a more traditional medical model. Yet, readmission rates were twice as high for the therapeutic community. This raised concerns that patients may wish to return to a place where they were comfortable and could get along with others. Perhaps the therapeutic community created an ideal society that could not be reconstructed outside the hospital.

Other negative reports on the therapeutic community included observations that schizophrenics may be harmed by intense involvement and sensory overload (Van Putten, 1973), that manic patients can do poorly because of their disruptive force on patient and staff communication (Bjork, Steinberg, Lindenmayer, & Pardes, 1977), and that those with severe character disorders are usually not helped (Whitely, 1970). However, the major forces that led to the decline of the therapeutic community were the economics of health care and the development of effective biological interventions and short-term psychotherapeutic procedures. The therapeutic community was designed for long-term care. Patients often remained in therapeutic communities for 6 months to 4 years, a length of stay that is incompatible with current practices in most countries.

Many contemporary inpatient programs, including those that use cognitive therapy, have adopted and modified therapeutic community principles for their use. The major differences from a "pure" therapeutic community are shorter lengths of stay, less reliance on social learning as an ingredient of change, greater emphasis on structure, and implementation of more recently developed treatment procedures from biological psychiatry, cognitive therapy, or other disciplines.

Crisis Intervention Units

Crisis intervention is another inpatient treatment model that was influenced by experiences during and shortly after World War II (Lieb, Libsitch, & Saby, 1973). It was found that treating soldiers near the front lines and returning them to action as rapidly as possible reduced psychological morbidity. Lindemann's classic study of the reactions of Coconut Grove fire victims also focused attention on responses to crises (Lindemann, 1944). These findings, coupled with a growing awareness that long-term hospitalization could promote social breakdown through institutionalization, encouraged the establishment of crisis therapy units in the late 1960s and 1970s. The discovery of effective psychopharmacological treatments also influenced the development of crisis intervention models. Because drugs could rapidly suppress symptoms, patients could be discharged much earlier than was possible in previous eras. The growing availability of third-party insurance reimbursement for acute care was an additional factor in the proliferation of short-term psychiatric inpatient units.

Crisis intervention programs have utilized very short stays of 3 to 4 days up to longer hospitalizations of 3 to 4 weeks (Weisman, Feirstein, & Thomas, 1969; Herz, Endicott, & Spitzer, 1975; Glick, Hargreaves, Drues, & Showstack, 1976a, 1976b). Several comparative studies have been completed, but there have been problems with nonspecific therapy effects and randomization of assignment to treatment units that make interpretation of results difficult (Swartzberg & Schwartz, 1976; Glick, Hargreaves, Raskin, & Kutner, 1975; Glick et al., 1976a, 1976b; Herz, Endicott, & Spitzer, 1975, 1977). The basic principles underlying the crisis intervention model are: (1) crises can be treated without going into psychodynamics or early childhood experiences; (2) crisis is a time for growth; and (3) rapid intervention discourages regression.

Therapeutic procedures in crisis therapy are not widely different from those used in eclectic milieus such as the "reactive environment" described by Maxmen et al. (1974). The major variations are in the rapidity of staff response and in the reduced scope of goals for hospitalization. Time-limited treatment contracts may be utilized. The therapeutic focus is on the "here and now." Treatment goals are quickly established, and the patient is discharged when the goals are met or it is obvious that they cannot be achieved. Effective teamwork is essential in the crisis unit. There is insufficient time to work through staff–staff or staff–patient conflicts or to use this process as a therapeutic tool.

The original crisis intervention units of 20 years ago were a radical departure from standard treatment. Today, hospitalizations in the United States are predominantly in the brief or short-term range. Other countries, such as England and Sweden, with different health care financing systems, can offer long-term treatment for selected patients who may benefit from this form of therapy (see Chapter 14). The implications of relying on crisis intervention or short-term hospitalization are not fully understood. There is some concern about increased relapse rates in patients treated with short stays, but there appears to be no disadvantage to treating most patients with short-term care (14–30 days) as opposed to long-term hospitalization (Glick et al., 1976a, 1976b). Of course, some individual patients may require longer stays because of persistent suicidal risk, unremitting psychosis, or other severe pathology.

The Token Economy

Unlike earlier approaches, the origins of the token economy are based largely on scientific research. Fundamental behavioral studies suggested that the actions of psychiatric inpatients could be shaped by positive and negative reinforcers (Ayllon & Azrin, 1965). The first token economy unit was developed at Anna State Hospital by Ayllon and Azrin (1965). Behavior was very carefully observed, recorded, and quantified. Tokens were then rewarded for behavior desired by staff. These tokens could be exchanged for activities desired by patients. Several investigators reported changes in the behavior of regressed, chronic patients treated in token economies (Ayllon & Azrin, 1965; Hersen, Eisler, Smith, & Agras, 1972; Lloyd & Abel, 1970).

After an initial flush of success, token economies quickly came under fire. Two major issues led to the demise of this paradigm. First, there were ethical questions raised because deprivation was required in withholding reinforcers or using negative reinforcement. The staff assumed a position of powerful control that inhibited a personalized and benevolent approach to treatment (Miron, 1968; Lucero, Vail, & Scherbert, 1968; Zeldow, 1976). Secondly, token economies were ineffective in treating primary symptoms of mental disorders (Carlson, Hersen, & Eisler, 1972), and the effects on secondary symptoms (e.g., regression, isolation) did not persist after the tokens were removed or the patient was discharged (Kazdin, 1972; Hersen, 1976).

Despite major difficulties, the token economy model demonstrated that behavioral treatment could lead to clinical improvement. Behavioral procedures for inpatients were later refined (see, for example, Liberman, McCann, & Wallace, 1976) into treatment methods that were more individualized and collaborative. Behavioral theory and techniques are used widely as a component of contemporary inpatient treatment programs, including cognitively oriented milieus (Thase & Wright, 1991). However, fully developed token economies now are rarely seen.

Rational Eclecticism

As the influence of the therapeutic community and the token economy began to ebb, efforts were directed at developing eclectic models for hospital psychiatry. The most extensive description of the eclectic approach to inpatient treatment is contained in Maxmen, Tucker, and Lebow's book, *Rational Hospital Psychiatry* (1974). The authors suggested that treatment should not be based on a singular etiological theory because this can prevent the patient from receiving a full range of potentially useful treatment procedures. Instead, they recommended that multiple theories and intervention strategies be used to reach the goal of rapidly eliminating the problems that led to hospitalization.

Maxmen et al. (1974) have called their treatment system "the reactive environment," presumably because of an emphasis on the therapeutic milieu's reaction to the individual needs of each patient. Moline (1976) used the term "rational eclecticism" to describe this form of treatment. Although eclecticism is probably the most widely used model in contemporary inpatient psychiatry, neither of the terms "reactive environment" nor "rational eclecticism" is commonly employed. Generally, milieus that do not have a stated theoretical orientation are not given a designated name (e.g., Gunderson, 1978; Friis, 1986a, 1986b, 1986c; Kleespies, 1986). We prefer Moline's terminology, rational eclecticism, because it best describes the pragmatic and broadly based nature of the therapy performed in these units. The Adult Psychiatry Service of the Norton Psychiatric Clinic, University of Louisville, described in detail later in this volume, and most of the other cognitive therapy units (CTUs) listed in the Appendix, were based on an eclectic model prior to their transition to cognitively oriented milieus. All of these CTUs still utilize components of rational eclectism because cognitive therapy is used in combination with other treatments such as biological psychiatry and family systems approaches (Wright, Thase, & Beck, 1992).

One of the advantages of rational eclecticism is that it gives a framework for incorporation of findings from different fields of study. In many ways, this treatment model is a logical outgrowth of the current environment. Clinicians are confronted with multiple lines of scientific investigation that have uncovered effective treatment strategies (e.g., biological, cognitive, behavioral, interpersonal, family). Ready access to these data (through journals, computer searches, lay publications, and television) undercuts provincialism. Also, patients are becoming informed consumers. They may come to treatment forearmed with knowledge about psychotherapeutic approaches or new medications. Thus, both clinicians and patients may be aware of a wide variety of therapeutic tools that can be used in the treatment process.

As might be expected, rational eclecticism has encouraged the development of multidisciplinary teams. When this treatment model is working well, the various professional disciplines function in a highly integrated and cooperative manner. They are able to direct their special skills toward symptom relief and rehabilitation. Individual therapies, biological interventions, group treatments, and activities programs are well coordinated and are individualized (as much as possible) to match the specific problems and assets of each patient.

The major liability of the rational eclecticism model is the lack of a specific underlying theory. It is often hard to understand how the broad collection of therapies is integrated or how specific measures are chosen for individual patients. This model may vary widely from site to site depending on the particular blend of theoretical biases and training experiences of staff members. Professional rivalries, theoretical disputes, and staff conflicts can significantly diminish the effectiveness of this form of inpatient treatment. Also, the eclectic milieu can be a confusing experience for the patient if, for example, the psychiatrist, the group therapist, and the family therapist all present different and competing views of how therapy should proceed. Finally, the diffuse nature of these inpatient programs has made outcome research virtually impossible. It is unlikely that the major treatment dimension, eclecticism, can be adequately defined in operational terms (as in a treatment manual) or experimentally controlled to the extent that meaningful outcome research can be accomplished.

The Cognitive Milieu

Cognitive therapy was introduced to the inpatient setting in the early 1980s. The inpatient cognitive therapy program at the Norton Psychiatric Clinic in Louisville, Kentucky was established in 1980, and an inpatient cognitive therapy unit was opened at Mesa Vista Hospital in San Diego, California in 1985. The first report on the usefulness of inpatient cognitive therapy appeared in 1981 (Shaw, 1981). Subsequently, a number of cognitive therapy units have been developed throughout the United States and Europe (Schrodt & Wright, 1987; Perris et al., 1987; Davis & Casey, 1990; see Appendix), and several groups have reported on the effectiveness of inpatient cognitive therapy (Scott, 1988; Miller, Norman, Keitner, Bishop, & Dow, 1989; Miller, Norman, & Keitner, 1989; Bowers, 1989, 1990; Thase, Bowler, & Harden, 1991).

We have chosen to use the term "cognitive milieu" to describe cognitively oriented treatment units because (1) the theories and procedures of cognitive therapy are used as the primary organizing theme for clinical practice; (2) the entire milieu (including the hospital environment and structure, actions of staff members, sociocultural influences, group interactions, and the family system) is involved in the treatment process; and (3) cognitive therapy is integrated theoretically and pragmatically with other major therapies used in contemporary hospital psychiatry (e.g., biological psychiatry, family therapy, behavior therapy).

Different forms of the cognitive milieu are described in Chapter 3. Some units, particularly in the early phase of development, may employ cognitive therapy as an "add-on" module to an eclectic milieu. Such hospital programs would not fully meet the requirements noted above for a cognitive milieu. Several other types of units that incorporate cognitive therapy principles throughout the milieu have been designed and implemented (Wright et al., 1992).

Cognitive therapy inpatient programs are based not only on the cognitive model for psychotherapy but also on the long tradition of milieu therapy described earlier in this chapter. The cognitive approach adds several important dimensions to previous models for inpatient milieu treatment. First, there is a specific theory that is grounded in extensive empirical research (Beck, Rush, Shaw, & Emery, 1979; Wright & Beck, 1983; Dobson & Shaw, 1986). The theory is pragmatic and understandable to therapists, patients, and staff. Second, the treatment approach is highly collaborative and promotes good working relationships among therapists, patients, and families. The inpatients and their family members are encouraged to become active and knowledgeable participants in treatment. Third, the structured nature of cognitive therapy helps promote a clear, well-organized, and efficient inpatient environment. Procedures such as agenda setting, feedback, activity scheduling, graded task assignments, and homework can add needed structure throughout the milieu (Thase & Wright, 1991).

Fourth, cognitive therapy is problem oriented and short term. Thus, it is particularly well suited to the treatment of inpatients who must learn rapidly how to cope with or manage the problems that led to hospitalization (Thase & Wright, 1991). Fifth, cognitive therapy has been proven to be effective (see Chapter 1). Therefore, patients can enter a cognitively oriented program with a reasonable expectation of receiving considerable benefit. Sixth, cognitive therapy has been integrated theoretically with biological psychiatry, and treatment methods for combining the two approaches have been outlined (Wright, 1987; Wright & Schrodt, 1989; Wright & Thase, in press; Chapter 7, this volume). Inpatient cognitive therapy programs use a mixture of cognitive and biological therapies for most patients (Wright et al., 1992). Seventh, there is considerable emphasis on psychoeducational activities in cognitively oriented inpatient programs. The principles of cognitive therapy, self-help procedures, information about medication, communication skills, and other topics are taught in therapy sessions and group meetings. Pamphlets, books, and audio and videotapes are also used widely (see Chapter 15). Finally, relapse prevention is an integral part of the cognitive therapy approach. One of the goals of treatment is to help the patient acquire skills that will reduce the chances of symptom recurrence or rehospitalization. Several outcome studies have documented the lasting effect of cognitive therapy (Blackburn, Eunson, & Bishop, 1987; Hollon & Najavitis, 1988; Simons, Murphy, Levine, & Wetzel, 1986; Shea et al., in press; Thase et al., 1992).

Cognitive therapy inpatient treatment programs also utilize significant contributions from earlier models for hospital psychiatry, particularly the therapeutic community, crisis intervention units, and rational eclecticism. Group therapies are used extensively, and many CTUs employ a modified version of the unit-community meeting. However, collaboration is emphasized instead of a democratic sharing of decision-making power (e.g., community votes on medication decisions), which was an important component of the therapeutic community. The most significant derivative of the therapeutic community is the concept that most, if not all, of the activities in the patient's day can be arranged to exert a therapeutic effect. Thus, group meetings, nursing rounds, family visits, and even the actions of other patients are considered in developing a cognitive milieu. For example, we have found that patients who are experienced in cognitive therapy can be an extremely beneficial source of information and support for the newly admitted individual. Efforts are made, therefore, to facilitate this process in unit-community meetings, group therapies, and other daily hospital activities.

Crisis intervention units and rational eclectic milieus made contributions in focusing the treatment team's efforts directly at resolution of the presenting problems. This approach is consistent with cognitive therapy in general and is particularly important in current hospital psychiatric practice because of economic pressures to reduce lengths of stay and cut the total cost of care. Unfortunately, the trend for brief hospitalization has in many cases led to an abandonment of any attempt at the development of an intensive therapeutic milieu (Kleespies, 1986). Cognitively oriented inpatient programs have reversed this trend by offering a meaningful psychotherapeutic, sociocultural, and educational experience that is designed to be more productive in the long run than simply admitting the patient, starting medication, providing supportive care (or a variety of therapies without clear organization), and discharging as soon as possible.

Most cognitive milieus in the United States have short lengths of stay. A recent survey of inpatient cognitive therapy programs found an average length of stay of 18.1 days (range 10 to 29; Wright et al., 1992). The CTU described in Chapters 2 and 3 (Norton Psychiatric Clinic Adult Service, University of Louisville) has an average hospital stay of 12.1 days. Because of short inpatient stays, cognitive therapy is continued after discharge, if possible, so that gains can be consolidated, and the patient is able to benefit from a full course of CT (Thase et al., 1992).

Some of the possible disadvantages of inpatient cognitive therapy are that it requires a significant initial investment in staff training and/or supervision and that an ongoing educational effort is required to maintain the proficiency of the therapists and the consistency of the program. Also, some patients may not be suitable for cognitive therapy (see Chapter 4 for indications). Units that admit a wide variety of patients must devise methods for selecting and customizing the treatment to match each individual's presenting problems, level of pathology, and ability to participate in treatment. It has been well documented than an overly stimulating milieu may actually be harmful to some psychotic patients (Van Putten, 1973; Friis, 1986b, 1986c; Cohen & Khan, 1990). Cognitively oriented inpatient units need to be mindful of the experiences of the therapeutic community and thus not indiscriminately assign all patients to an intensive cognitive therapy program. Alternative treatment sessions and even seclusion (if necessary) need to be provided for those with acute psychotic illnesses who are unable to benefit from cognitive therapy. Chapter 14 describes treatment methods for psychotic patients who are candidates for cognitively oriented therapy.

Procedures for developing a cognitive milieu are outlined in Chapter 3. The remaining part of this chapter considers general treatment issues in contemporary hospital psychiatry. These include the nature of the inpatient setting, goals for hospitalization, the therapeutic alliance, and formation of multidisciplinary teams. Although each cognitive milieu develops a somewhat unique approach to these issues, there are several common themes that are encountered by all inpatient programs that attempt to construct a therapeutic milieu.

GENERAL TREATMENT ISSUES

The Inpatient Setting

Inpatient treatment differs from outpatient work in a number of ways. Most outpatients have only one therapist, but inpatients are exposed to a diverse set of treatment procedures delivered by a multidisciplinary team. The intensity of treatment escalates dramatically. In many programs, observation and therapeutic activity continue 24 hours a day. Psychopathology is usually more severe in hospitalized patients than outpatients. Individuals who require hospitalization commonly have high degrees of demoralization, hopelessness, and functional impairment. They are also likely to have experienced severe stress such as interpersonal loss, physical illness, unemployment, or collapse of support systems. The high level of symptomatology, combined with diminished resources, calls for a vigorous and incisive response from the inpatient treatment team (Thase & Wright, 1991).

Although there has been no consensus on required ingredients for the hospital milieu, Gunderson (1978) has suggested that all inpatient settings need to provide five types of therapeutic functions: containment, support, structure, involvement, and validation. After reviewing the literature on milieu therapy, he concluded that variables such as patient–staff ratio, differences in patient behavior, or attitudes of patients and staff were not strongly related to treatment outcome. Nevertheless, Gunderson argued that milieu treatment, defined as "a specialized environment which is designed to fulfill the general purposes of preventing 'bad' things from happening and allowing 'good' things to occur," can have powerful therapeutic effects.

The first three of the essential therapeutic elements for inpatient milieus (e.g., containment, support, and structure) defined by Gunderson have a long history. Containment was the first function of psychiatric hospitals and was essentially the only intervention offered until humanitarian movements in the mid- to late 18th century and moral therapy in the early 19th century added a supportive component to the inpatient experience. Today, psychiatric hospitals continue to provide for containment, although the emphasis is on establishing a safe and secure environment that will protect the patient from self-harm or from intolerable environmental stresses. Practitioners in cognitively oriented milieus must be keenly aware of the importance of guarding the patient's safety. Suicide precautions should be used when there is significant risk of self-harm, and a safety committee should be charged with minimizing risks in the physical and psychosocial environment of the unit.

The therapeutic community devoted much attention to providing support. Current inpatient treatment models, including cognitive therapy, also are supportive in nature. Staff and patients are encouraged to have a generally hopeful attitude and to provide assistance to others in coping with problems, managing everyday tasks, and building self-esteem. However, in a cognitively oriented milieu, the provision of support is tempered by the expectation that patients will be active participants in therapy. Collaborative empiricism, self-help exercises, and homework assignments are utilized in an effort to avoid the excessive dependency or regression that can occur in overly supportive milieus (Thase & Wright, 1991). The short-term format of therapy also helps to prevent the formation of pathological dependency on the inpatient unit.

Structure, another basic feature of hospital milieus, is an important part of all of the treatment models described in this chapter. The most structured environment occurred with the classic token economies. In some cases, these units used a structured approach that interfered with other critical features of hospital psychiatry. The patient was forced to fit into the mold of the behavioral reward system. A supportive approach to meeting the individual needs of patients was given little importance. Generally, the structure of inpatient units has been consistent with the theories and practices of each treatment model. Thus, the therapeutic community was organized around community meetings, shared decision making, and other group interactions. Psychoanalytically oriented units were designed to complement the major treatment focus—intensive, individual psychotherapy. As noted earlier, cognitive milieus incorporate many structuring activities. A detailed description of the structure of inpatient cognitive therapy programs is contained in Chapter 3.

The last two of Gunderson's essential components for inpatient milieus are involvement and validation. Patient-led groups, shared decision making, and blurring of roles were recommended as measures to increase patient involvement, whereas open expression of feelings, individualized treatment planning, and respect for the patient's rights were suggested as measures for promoting a sense of validation (Gunderson, 1978). Cognitively oriented units also encourage involvement and validation. However, roles of staff and patients are clearly demarcated, and decisions are rarely delegated to the entire inpatient community. Patients become involved in multiple collaborative relationships that stimulate participation in psychotherapy, group meetings, social skill building, family interchanges, planning exercises, recreational pursuits, and other therapeutic activities.

A sense of personal validation is an important antidote to hopelessness, helplessness, and demoralization. Validation is accomplished in cognitively oriented programs by respecting the patient's basic rights and by developing an individualized treatment program to match each person's specific problem set. Further, the patient's assets are identified and used actively in the treatment process. In addition, group interactions in the cognitive milieu help develop a sense of universality. The patient recognizes that he or she is not alone in suffering a psychiatric disorder, and also that each person deserves a full opportunity to recover.

Goals for Hospitalization

The most obvious goal for short-term care is to discharge to outpatient status. This usually requires at least partial resolution of the symptoms that led to hospitalization. Development of new problem-solving strategies is also desirable. The specific goals for hospitalization are usually conceptualized within this general framework of symptom reduction and resource building (Maxmen et al., 1974).

Each treatment setting develops its own set of goals for a typical hospitalization. These are often based on the theoretical orientation of the unit. For example, a psychoanalytically oriented program may wish to develop insight, whereas the primary goals for a crisis unit may be rapid stabilization and discharge. Leeman and Autio (1978) described eight goals including limit setting, orientation, and provision of nurturance, among others. There also are standard goals for treatment in the cognitive milieu, such as targeting specific problems, developing collaborative therapeutic relationships, learning the basic cognitive model, identifying and modifying dysfunctional cognitions and behavior, utilizing self-help exercises, and learning relapse prevention strategies. However, with an emphasis on collaborative empiricism, the main objective is to help the patient articulate his or her own goals and then to work together to reach them (Schrodt & Wright, 1987).

The Therapeutic Alliance

One of the first tasks of inpatient treatment is the establishment of a therapeutic alliance (Allen, Deering, & Buskirk, 1988). The inpatient setting presents several challenges to the development of good working relationships. However, it also offers opportunities to form particularly strong collaborations between patients and therapists. Patients usually come to outpatient treatment as willing participants, but hospitalized patients may be highly ambivalent about getting help, confused about their intentions, or so profoundly ill that they have given up hope and have little interest in psychotherapy. Those who are committed to the hospital on an involuntary basis may actively resist therapeutic interventions. Even patients who are highly motivated for treatment must deal with the lingering problems of societal stigma and ignorance about psychiatric disorders (Thase & Wright, 1991).

There also can be difficulties in making the transition from an outpatient therapy relationship to the more complex inpatient scene. The nature of outpatient therapy is highly individualized, leading the patient to expect a private therapeutic relationship with clearly defined limits and strict confidentiality. In contrast, the hospital setting usually requires an extension of responsibility and confidentiality to various members of the treatment team.

Despite these obstacles, most patients are able to form strong therapeutic relationships in the hospital setting. The process of collaboration between the patient and his or her therapist can be enhanced by utilizing cognitive therapy procedures (see Chapter 4). Nevertheless, other "nonspecific" features of the inpatient program are also important. In our experience, the two most significant factors are equanimity and empathy. Inpatient therapists who can maintain an objective calm while responding sensitively to the patient's plight are much more likely to form good working relationships than those who react hastily or defensively to the patient's resistance.

Benjamin Rush's adage, "Never resent an affront offered to you by a sick man," holds particularly true in the inpatient setting. Patients with psychotic illnesses, hypomania, personality disorders, or substance abuse are especially prone to problems in forming therapeutic relationships.

The chances of destructive countertransference reactions can be minimized if personal reactions to patients are discussed in team meetings, therapeutic conferences, and therapy supervision. Involving the entire team in monitoring therapeutic relationships is one of the advantages of the inpatient setting. This process helps therapists identify their maladaptive reactions and offers support for managing difficult treatment situations.

Features of the broader milieu can also foster productive treatment alliances. A unit-community meeting, a component of the therapeutic community model, can be used to greet and orient new patients, thereby reducing confusion and anxiety (Margolis, Daniels, Carson, &

Meyer, 1963). Another feature of the hospital setting that can promote alliances is the capacity for frequent meetings with the patient. A case vignette will be used to illustrate how relationships can be strengthened in the hospital milieu. Mr. A. was a 50-year-old man who was admitted to the hospital on an involuntary basis after he had threatened his wife and had fired a gun in the house because he thought that giant rodents were attacking him. He had been drinking heavily (2 pints of whiskey per day) since being laid off from his job about 3 years earlier. In the first few days of hospitalization he was belligerent and demanded to be released immediately. He claimed to have no problems other than drinking "a bit too much."

Individuals like Mr. A. can stimulate intense reactions in staff members and other patients. However, in this case, the treatment team was highly experienced in working with alcoholics and knew that persistence often paid off. Mr. A. was seen daily by the attending psychiatrist, the psychologist who directed the Addictions Treatment Program, the chemical dependency counselor, a resident psychiatrist, a social worker, and a psychiatric nurse. A court hearing was held on the seventh day of hospitalization, and, on the advice of the treatment team, the patient was ordered by the judge to remain in treatment. By the 14th day of hospitalization, Mr. A. had openly admitted his alcoholism and had recognized that an underlying depression fueled his drinking. Numerous contacts with team members and an intense psychoeducational effort (e.g., videotapes, visits from Alcoholics Anonymous sponsors, and briefings from his physician) also played a role in forging a commitment to therapy and a bonding with the treatment team.

Pharmacotherapy is another tool that can be used to promote good working relationships. Mr. B., a 65-year-old man, was admitted to the hospital after developing a deep depression with psychotic features. He believed that his wife wanted him "out of the way" and that he would be "better off dead." He asked his doctor to leave him alone because "it was no use." Mr. B. refused initial efforts at cognitive therapy. Treatment with combined doxepin and trifluoperazine (i.e., tricyclic antidepressant and antipsychotic medication) was begun immediately, and the dosage was raised as rapidly as possible. Close monitoring of vital signs, clinical condition, side effects, and tricyclic antidepressant plasma levels helped reduce the risks of an accelerated approach to pharmacotherapy. Within 3 days, the delusions were beginning to fade. Mr. B. was somewhat more hopeful, and he was starting to engage in psychotherapy.

These two vignettes illustrate how multiple features of the hospital setting can offer opportunities for building rapport. Other components of inpatient treatment discussed elsewhere in this volume, including family involvement, group process, and psychiatric nursing, should also be considered. Therapeutic relationships with inpatients can be maximized if all of these diverse influences are recognized and used effectively.

The Treatment Team

Virtually all inpatient units utilize a multidisciplinary team to deliver treatment; however, the degree of cooperation and cohesion among the disciplines varies widely. Some programs devote a good deal of their resources to promoting teamwork, whereas others allow rather autonomous, or even competitive, functioning in the milieu. Comprehensive treatment models such as the therapeutic community, the reactive environment, and cognitive therapy generally encourage the formation of well-integrated treatment teams.

Table 2.1 lists steps that can be taken to build effective multidisciplinary teams. Role definition may appear to be fairly simple at first glance: physicians prescribe drugs, psychologists give tests and conduct group therapy, social workers interview families, and so forth. Yet, there is considerable overlap between the disciplines in most hospital settings, especially in the delivery of psychotherapy. Another area of potential role confusion is in leadership and decision making. Well-functioning teams develop a clear picture of each member's treatment philosophies and techniques. They recognize procedures that require unique training and competence while also identifying treatment areas where many staff members may pool their therapeutic efforts. A thorough understanding and respect for other disciplines helps to promote collaborative teamwork (Wright, 1987; Wright & Schrodt, 1989).

The team must develop an efficient system for making rational and timely decisions. Areas of treatment responsibility need to be carved out, mechanisms of decision making specified, and the leadership hierarchy established. The 6-West Adult Psychiatry Team at the Norton Psychiat-

TABLE 2.1. Steps in Building an Interdisciplinary Team

Define roles
Understand and respect other disciplines
Specify decision-making procedures
Communicate regularly
Utilize treatment plans
Develop clear treatment philosophy
Encourage support systems
Strive for consistent leadership and low staff turnover

ric Clinic can be used to illustrate this process. This general hospital psychiatry unit is affiliated with the University of Louisville School of Medicine.

Table 2.2 contains a listing of team members, their areas of clinical responsibility, and their major decision-making powers. An abbreviated list of team members is used because of space limitations. This team has developed its procedures during a number of years of working together. The senior psychiatrist is the team leader and may overrule or veto decisions of others. However, in practice, this rarely happens. Each member is aware of his or her area of clinical and decision-making responsibility so that they can work independently while still functioning as a unit. Decisions are usually made after consultation with fellow therapists.

Frequent and thorough communication is critical for effective teamwork (Wright, 1987; Thase & Wright, 1991). Opportunities for discussion of clinical situations can be built into the daily routine so that staff members know when and where they can meet each other and what decisions will be made at each meeting. A listing of team conferences for decision making on the 6-West unit at the Norton Psychiatric Clinic is provided in Table 2.3. Some decisions are routinely made at specific meetings. For example, assignment of admissions to teams is made at the Morning Staff Meeting. The patient's daily schedule is also determined at this meeting. The physician chooses from a list of therapeutic options after discussing these with the treatment team. The overall treatment plan is determined at the Therapeutics Conference. Other decisions, such as the nurse instituting emergency suicide precautions for a deteriorating patient, must be made rapidly without processing by the entire team. These decisions are reviewed in later meetings.

Treatment planning is a particularly effective method of coordinating staff efforts. The various disciplines meet together to set specific goals and to delineate responsibility for different components of the therapeutic program. Treatment planning in the cognitive milieu is discussed in Chapter 3.

A clear treatment philosophy also helps build team cohesion. Karasu (1986) has noted that psychotherapy is most effective if the practitioner ascribes to a definite theory and develops a high level of expertise in this approach. Conceptual and technological purity is much harder to attain in the multidisciplinary inpatient setting than in individual work with outpatients. Allowance needs to be made for the diversity of personality backgrounds and educational experiences of staff members. However, energetic leadership and a heavy investment in staff training can help the team develop a shared model for psychiatric treatment.

TABLE 2.2. Role Definition and Decision Making, 6-West, Norton Psychiatric Clinic

	Senior psychiatrist	Nurse	Psychologist	Social worker	Pastoral counselor
Unique clinical responsibilities	History and physical Coordinate medical care with other physicians Administer ECT Discharge summary Team leader	Initial nursing assessment Administer and monitor drugs Medical nursing procedures Discharge instructions	Psychological testing	Family system evaluation Family therapy Halfway house placements Nursing home placements	Contact patient's pastor or priest Pastoral evaluation Pastoral counseling
Shared clinical responsibilities	Treatment planning Cognitive therapy Communication with family Support hospital milieu Safety and quality control Communication with insurers	Treatment planning Cognitive therapy Communication with family Support hospital milieu Safety and quality control	Treatment planning Cognitive therapy Communication with family Support hospital milieu Safety and quality control	Treatment planning Cognitive therapy Communication with family Support hospital milieu Safety and quality control Communication with insurers	Treatment planning Cognitive therapy Communication with family Support hospital milieu
Decision-making responsibilities	Admission Activity level Suicide precautions Laboratory tests Medications Daily activity schedule Discharge	Safety precautions in emergency Prn drugs Special ward meetings Nursing care plan	Choose tests Frequency and content of addiction treatment program	Initiate family therapy Options for outpatient placement	Visitation by pastor or priest Extent of pastoral counseling

TABLE 2.3. Decision Making in Team Conferences, 6-West, Norton Psychiatric Clinic

Frequency	Meeting or activity	Decisions made
Daily	Morning staff meeting	Assign new admissions Determine patient's daily activity schedule Change privilege levels
Twice weekly	Therapeutics conference	Develop treatment plans Revise treatment plans Set discharge dates
Daily	Physician rounds (includes discussions with nurses, social workers, and other staff)	Order medications and lab tests Change suicide precautions and privilege levels
Weekly	Departmental meeting	Revise policies and procedures

It can also be beneficial to promote development of mutual support systems among staff members. Inpatient work is highly stressful. Patients are demanding and often dangerous to themselves or others. Those with mania or severe personality problems test limits and are prone to drive wedges between their caregivers. The pace of activity is often hectic, especially when a number of new admissions arrive or when there is a large cluster of patients with severe symptomatology on the unit. Facing these conditions without support from others is a daunting task. It is made even worse if the staff member anticipates being undercut or criticized at every turn. Although constructive criticism is sometimes needed, this may not be effective unless the staff member perceives a broad base of support for his or her actions.

An atmosphere of collegiality can contribute significantly to the development of a supportive environment. However, specific measures are also helpful. Team leaders can take responsibility for monitoring the unit's stress level so they can change case loads, temporarily hold admissions, or meet with individuals who appear to be having difficulty. Recognition and reward of staff contributions also can help create a supportive climate on the inpatient unit.

Changes in the composition of the team, especially those in leadership positions, is one of the most serious threats to the unit's functional capacity (Friis, 1986b). It takes a good deal of time and effort to form a tightly integrated and fully capable treatment team. In our experience, the loss of an important team member is almost always disruptive.

Therefore, we encourage consistent leadership and low staff turnover. When changes do occur, there are opportunities for exploring new ideas that may strengthen the team's capacity to serve.

SUMMARY

The introduction of cognitive therapy for inpatient use has opened a new stage in the evolution of hospital psychiatry. This chapter has reviewed previous treatment models in an effort to abstract information that can be useful in the construction of cognitively oriented inpatient programs. Methods such as long-term psychoanalytically oriented therapy, token economies, and therapeutic communities have given way to multifaceted programs that emphasize rapid, cost-effective treatments. However, elements of earlier approaches can be found in most current hospital settings. Examples of widely used procedures include analysis of transference issues and other therapeutic relationship problems, use of behavioral reinforcers, and recognition of social and ward-community influences.

Crisis intervention and psychopharmacology have played major roles in reducing the length of hospital stays, but these paradigms have not provided an organizing theory for inpatient psychiatry. Many units have adopted a multimodal approach, sometimes termed "rational eclecticism." This model incorporates findings from diverse areas of research and clinical practice.

Cognitively oriented treatment milieus utilize the specific theories and techniques of cognitive therapy to guide the treatment process. Cognitive therapy has been integrated on a theoretical and pragmatic basis with biological psychiatry, the other major treatment method used in cognitive milieus. Elements of older treatment models, such as the therapeutic community and the token economy, are incorporated to a lesser extent into cognitively oriented hospital programs.

Inpatient treatment units have universal goals of reducing symptoms, improving coping skills, and, if possible, returning the patient to the home environment. Building an effective treatment alliance is a central feature of most programs, although therapeutic relationships may vary depending on the model utilized. Formation of a coordinated treatment team is another common ingredient. Guidelines are offered in this chapter for establishing effective therapeutic relationships and cohesive treatment teams.

We conclude that inpatient units function most effectively when they have a clear philosophical orientation, consistent leadership and staffing, well-defined methods for making decisions, highly collaborative relationships with patients and families, strong mutual support systems, and treatment teams that can integrate their efforts in the service of quality care. Subsequent chapters in this volume demonstrate how the cognitive model promotes the development of these attributes.

REFERENCES

Abroms, G. N. (1969). Defining milieu therapy. *Archives of General Psychiatry, 21*, 553–560.

Allen, J. G., Deering, C. D., & Buskirk, J. R. (1988). Assessment of therapeutic alliances in the psychiatric hospital milieu. *Psychiatry, 51*, 291–299.

Almond, R. (1971). The therapeutic community. *Scientific American, 224*, 34–42.

Ayllon, T., & Azrin, N. H. (1965). The measurement and reinforcement of behavior of psychotics. *Journal of Experimental Analysis of Behavior, 8*, 357–383.

Beck, A. T., Rush, A. J., Shaw, B. F., & Emery, G. (1979). *Cognitive therapy of depression*. New York: Guilford Press.

Beers, C. (1908). *A mind that found itself*. New York: Longmans Green.

Bjork, D., Steinberg, M., Lindenmayer, J., & Pardes, H. (1977). Mania and milieu: Treatment of manics in a therapeutic community. *Hospital and Community Psychiatry, 28*, 431–436.

Blackburn, I. M., Eunson, K. M., & Bishop, S. (1987). A two-year naturalistic follow-up of depressed patients treated with cognitive therapy, pharmacotherapy, and a combination of both. *Journal of Affective Disorders, 10*, 67–75.

Bowers, W. A. (1989). Cognitive therapy with inpatients. In A. Freeman, K. M. Simon, L. E. Beutler, & H. Arkowitz (Eds.), *Comprehensive handbook of cognitive therapy* (pp. 583–596). New York: Plenum Press.

Bowers, W. A. (1990). Treatment of depressed inpatients. Cognitive therapy plus medication, relaxation plus medication, and medication alone. *British Journal of Psychiatry, 156*, 73–78.

Carlson, C. G., Hersen, M., & Eisler, R. M. (1972). Token economy programs in the treatment of hospitalized adult psychiatric patients. *Journal of Nervous and Mental Disorders, 155*, 192–204.

Cerletti, U. (1950). Old and new information about electroshock. *American Journal of Psychiatry, 107*, 87–94.

Clark, R. A. (1973). *Mental illness in perspective: History of schools of thought*. Pacific Grove, CA: Boxwood Press.

Cohen, S., & Khan, A. (1990). Antipsychotic effect of milieu in the acute treatment of schizophrenia. *General Hospital Psychiatry, 12*, 248–251.

Davis, M. H., & Casey, D. A. (1990). Utilizing cognitive therapy on the short-term psychiatric inpatient unit. *General Hospital Psychiatry, 12*, 170–176.

Denber, H. C. B., Turns, D., & Seeman, M. V. (1959). A therapeutic community: Analysis of its operation after two years. In H. C. B. Denber (Ed.),

Research conference on therapeutic community (pp. 57–76). Springfield, IL: Charles C. Thomas.

Denber, H. C. B., Turns, D., & Seeman, M. V. (1968). The therapeutic community: Nine years after. *The Psychiatric Quarterly, 42*, 531–537.

Deutsch, A. (1949). *The mentally ill in America*. New York: Columbia University Press.

Dobson, K. S., & Shaw, B. F. (1986). Cognitive assessment with major depressive disorders. *Cognitive Therapy and Research, 10*(1), 13–29.

Friis, S. (1986a). Measurements of the perceived ward milieu: A reevaluation of the Ward Atmosphere Scale. *Acta Psychiatrica Scandinavica, 73*, 589–599.

Friis, S. (1986b). Factors influencing the ward atmosphere. *Acta Psychiatrica Scandinavica, 73*, 600–606.

Friis, S. (1986c). Characteristics of a good ward atmosphere. *Acta Psychiatrica Scandinavica, 74*, 469–473.

Glick, I. D., Hargreaves, W. A., Raskin, M., & Kutner, S. J. (1975). Short versus long hospitalization: A prospective controlled study. II. Results for schizophrenic inpatients. *American Journal of Psychiatry, 132*, 385–390.

Glick, I. D., Hargreaves, W. A., Drues, J., & Showstack, J. A. (1976a). Short versus long hospitalization: A prospective controlled study. IV. One year follow-up results of schizophrenic patients. *American Journal of Psychiatry, 133*, 509–514.

Glick, I. D., Hargreaves, W. A., Drues, J., & Showstack, J. A. (1976b). Short versus long hospitalization: A prospective controlled study. V. One year follow-up results of non-schizophrenic patients. *American Journal of Psychiatry, 133*, 515–517.

Goshen, C. E. (1967). Progress and stagnation in psychiatry during the past fifty years. *Maryland State Medical Journal, 16*(2), 55–58.

Gralnick, A., & D'Elia, F. (1969). A psychoanalytic hospital becomes a therapeutic community. *Hospital and Community Psychiatry, 20*, 144–146.

Greenley, J. R. (1973). Power processes and patient behaviors. *Archives of General Psychiatry, 28*, 683–688.

Gunderson, J. G. (1978). Defining the therapeutic processes in psychiatric milieus. *Psychiatry, 41*, 327–335.

Hersen, M. (1976). Token economies in institutional settings. *Journal of Nervous and Mental Disease, 162*, 206–211.

Hersen, M., Eisler, R. M., Smith, B. S., & Agras, W. S. (1972). A token reinforcement ward for young psychiatric patients. *American Journal of Psychiatry, 129*, 228–233.

Herz, M. I., Endicott, J., & Spitzer, R. L. (1975). Brief hospitalization of patients with families: Initial results. *American Journal of Psychiatry, 132*, 413–418.

Herz, M. I., Endicott, J., & Spitzer, R. L. (1977). Brief hospitalization: A two year follow-up. *American Journal of Psychiatry, 134*, 502–507.

Hollon, S. D., & Najavitis, L. (1988). Review of empirical studies on cognitive therapy. In A. J. Frances & R. E. Hales (Eds.), *American Psychiatric Press review of psychiatry*, Vol. 7 (pp. 643–666). Washington, DC: American Psychiatric Press.

Jones, M. (1953). *The therapeutic community: A new treatment method in psychiatry.* New York: Basic Books.

Karasu, T. B. (1986). The specificity vs. non-specificity dilemma: Toward identifying therapeutic change agents. *American Journal of Psychiatry, 143*(6), 687–695.

Kazdin, A. E. (1972). Non-responsiveness of patients to token economies. *Journal of Behavior Research and Therapy, 10*, 417–418.

Kleespies, P. M. (1986). Hospital milieu treatment and optimal length of stay. *Hospital and Community Psychiatry, 37*, 509–510.

Leeman, C. P., & Autio, S. (1978). Milieu therapy: The need for individualization. *Psychotherapy and Psychosomatics, 29*, 84–92.

Lehman, A., & Ritzler, B. (1976). The therapeutic community inpatient ward: Does it really work? *Comprehensive Psychiatry, 17*, 755–761.

Liberman, R. P., McCann, M. G., & Wallace, C. J. (1976). Generalization of behavior therapy with psychotics. *British Journal of Psychiatry, 129*, 490–496.

Lieb, J., Libsitch, I., & Saby, A. E. (1973). *The crisis team*. Hagerstown, MD: Harper & Row.

Lindemann, E. (1944). Symptomatology and management of acute grief. *American Journal of Psychiatry, 101*, 141–148.

Lloyd, K. E., & Abel, L. (1970). Performance on a token economy psychiatry ward: A two year summary. *Journal of Behavior Research and Therapy, 8*, 1–9.

Lucero, R. J., Vail, D. J., & Scherbert, J. (1968). Regulating operant-conditioning programs. *Hospital and Community Psychiatry, 19*, 53–54.

Margolis, P. M., Daniels, R. S., Carson, R. C., & Meyer, G. C. (1963). The patient–staff meeting: A technique for encouraging communication in the psychiatric hospital. *Psychiatry, 26*, 19–25.

Maxmen, J. S., Tucker, G. J., & LeBow, M. (1974). *Rational hospital psychiatry.* New York: Brunner/Mazel.

Miller, I. W., Norman, W. H., & Keitner, G. I. (1989). Cognitive–behavioral treatment of depressed inpatients: Six- and twelve-month follow-ups. *American Journal of Psychiatry, 146,* 1274–1279.

Miller, I. W., Norman, W. H., Keitner, G. I., Bishop, S. T., & Dow, M. G. (1989). Cognitive-behavioral treatment of depressed inpatients. *Behavior Therapy, 20,* 25–47.

Miron, N. B. (1968). The primary ethical consideration. *Hospital and Community Psychiatry, 19*, 226–228.

Moline, R. A. (1976). Hospital psychiatry in transition: From the therapeutic community toward a rational eclecticism. *Archives of General Psychiatry, 33*, 1234–1238.

Myers, K., & Clark, D. H. (1972). Results in a therapeutic community. *British Journal of Psychiatry, 120*, 51–58.

Perris, C., Rodhe, K., Palm, A., Abelson, M., Hellgren, S., Livja, C., & Soderman, H. (1987). Fully integrated in- and outpatient services in a psychiatric sector: Implementation of a new mode for the care of psychiatric patients favoring continuity of care. In A. Freeman & V. Greenwood

(Eds.), *Cognitive therapy: Applications in psychiatric and medical settings* (pp. 117–131). New York: Human Sciences Press.

Schneck, J. M. (1975). United States of America. In J. G Howells (Ed.), *World history of psychiatry* (pp. 432–475). New York City: Brunner/Mazel.

Schrodt, G. R., Jr., & Wright, J. H. (1987). Inpatient treatment of adolescents. In A. Freeman & V. Greenwood (Eds.), *Cognitive therapy: Applications in psychiatric and medical settings* (pp. 69–82). New York: Human Sciences Press.

Scott, J. (1988). Cognitive therapy with depressed inpatients. In W. Dryden & P. Trower (Eds.), *Developments in cognitive psychotherapy* (pp. 177–189). London: Sage Publications.

Shaw, B. F. (1981). Cognitive therapy with an inpatient population. In G. Emery, S. D. Hollon, & R. C. Bedrosian (Eds.), *New directions in cognitive therapy* (pp. 29–49). New York: Guilford Press.

Shea, M. T., Elkin, I., Imber S. D., Sotsky, S. M., Watkins, J. T., Collins, J. F., Pilkonis, P. A., Leber, W. R., Krupnick, J., Dolan, R. T., & Parloff, M. B. (in press). Course of depressive symptoms over follow-up: Findings from the National Institute of Mental Health Treatment of Depression Collaborative Research Program. *Archives of General Psychiatry.*

Simons, A. D., Murphy, G. E., Levine, J. L., & Wetzel, R. D. (1986). Cognitive therapy and pharmacotherapy of depression: Sustained improvement over one year. *Archives of General Psychiatry, 43,* 43–48.

Swartzburg, M., & Schwartz, A. (1976). A five-year study of brief hospitalization. *American Journal of Psychiatry, 133*, 922–924.

Thase, M. E., Bowler, K., & Harden, T. (1991). Cognitive behavior therapy of endogenous depression: Part 2. Preliminary findings in 16 unmedicated patients. *Behavior Therapy, 22,* 469–477.

Thase, M. E., Simons, A. D., McGeary, J., Cahaline, J. F., Hughes, C., Harden, G., & Friedman, E. (1992). Relapse after cognitive behavioral treatment of depression: Potential implications for longer courses of treatment. *American Journal of Psychiatry, 149,* 1046–1052.

Thase, M. E., & Wright, J. H. (1991). Cognitive behavior therapy with depressed inpatients: An abridged treatment manual. *Behavior Therapy,* 22, 579–595.

Van Putten, T. (1973). Milieu therapy: Contraindications? *Archives of General Psychiatry*, *29*, 640–643.

Weisman, G., Feirstein, A., & Thomas, C. (1969). Three-day hospitalization—a model for intensive intervention. *Archives of General Psychiatry*, *21*, 620–629.

Whitely, J. S. (1970). The response of psychopaths to a therapeutic community. *British Journal of Psychiatry*, *116*, 517–529.

Wilmer, H. A. (1958). Toward a definition of the therapeutic community. *American Journal of Psychiatry*, *114*, 824–834.

Wright, J. H. (1987). Cognitive therapy and medication as combined treatment. In A. Freeman & V. Greenwood (Eds.), *Cognitive therapy: Applications in psychiatric and medical settings* (pp. 36–50). New York: Human Sciences Press.

Wright, J. H., & Beck, A. T. (1983). Cognitive therapy of depression: Theory and practice. *Hospital and Community Psychiatry, 34,* 1119–1127.

Wright, J. H., & Schrodt, G. R., Jr. (1989). Combined cognitive therapy and pharmacotherapy. In A. Freeman, M. K. Simon, H. Arkowitz, & L. Beutler (Eds.), *Comprehensive handbook of cognitive therapy* (pp. 267–282). New York: Plenum Press.

Wright, J. H., & Thase, M. E. (in press). Cognitive and biological therapies: A synthesis. *Psychiatric Annals.*

Wright, J. H., Thase, M. E., & Beck, A. T., (1992). *Inpatient cognitive therapy: Structures, processes, and procedures.* Paper presented at the World Congress of Cognitive Therapy, Toronto, Canada.

Zeldow, P. B. (1976). Some antitherapeutic effects of the token economy: A case in point. *Journal of Psychiatry, 39,* 318–324.

Chapter 3

The Cognitive Milieu: Structure and Process

Jesse H. Wright, M.D., Ph.D.,
Michael E. Thase, M.D.,
John W. Ludgate, Ph.D., and
Aaron T. Beck, M.D.

A variety of different treatment milieus have been designed for using cognitive therapy (CT) with hospitalized patients. The first inpatient cognitive therapy program was established in 1980 at the Norton Psychiatric Clinic of the University of Louisville. Subsequently, inpatient units with a cognitive orientation have been developed in a wide range of environments, including for-profit hospitals, public facilities, and university medical centers (Miller, Bishop, Norman, & Keitner, 1985; Schrodt & Wright, 1987; Perris et al., 1987; Bowers, 1989; Thase, Bowler, & Harden, 1991). Most of these units have been organized for the delivery of short-term care. However, several European treatment centers have offered extended therapy for chronically ill patients (see Chapter 14).

In this chapter, we describe and evaluate the four predominate types of milieus that are used for inpatient CT. These are termed the *primary therapist, staff, "add-on,"* and *comprehensive* models (Wright, Thase, & Beck, 1992). Guidelines for initiating a cognitive therapy unit (CTU) are also detailed. This is followed by suggestions for maximizing the cognitive focus of the inpatient experience.

INPATIENT COGNITIVE THERAPY UNITS

Primary Therapist Model

This model has been utilized in the early phases of development of the CTU in academic centers (e.g., University of Louisville, University of

Pittsburgh) where psychiatrists, joined by other nonphysician faculty members, introduce cognitive therapy as a research or teaching program to an eclectic milieu (Wright, 1989). Other forms of treatment—such as biological psychiatry, interpersonal therapy, or traditional behavior therapy—may also be used. The director of the unit, usually a psychiatrist, has received, or is receiving, extensive training in cognitive therapy. An ongoing educational program, including case supervision, is arranged for the primary therapists (those who provide individual, group, or family therapy) in the treatment setting. General staff training is also done, so that other members of the treatment team are conversant with CT principles and can support the work of the primary therapist. However, the major responsibility for provision of cognitive therapy rests with the primary therapist. There is a full representation of the multidisciplinary team at treatment planning meetings. These sessions serve as a forum for integrating cognitive therapy with other approaches (Thase & Wright, 1991).

Advantages and disadvantages of the primary therapist model are listed in Table 3.1. These units have developed in teaching centers that have a closed staff. A limited number of primary therapists (for example, two attending psychiatrists, two resident psychiatrists, one psychologist, two social workers, one pastoral counselor, and two nurse therapists at the 20-bed CTU of the Norton Psychiatric Clinic) make it possible to train most, if not all, primary therapists to be proficient in cognitive therapy. If the unit director and other unit leaders (e.g., major admitting psychiatrists, head nurse, chief psychologist, and others) en-

TABLE 3.1. Primary Therapist Model

Advantages	Disadvantages
Ward leaders endorse and utilize cognitive therapy	Possible conflicts with therapists who hold other treatment philosophies
Rapid introduction of cognitive therapy principles	Patient may be confused if there are competing treatment philosophies
Conducive to outcome research	Power of all staff not fully directed at delivery of cognitive therapy
Training and supervision encourage high level of competency	Training and supervision are time consuming, expensive
Fits with traditional expectation of patient for treatment from doctor or other primary therapist	Not well suited to other than closed-staff units

dorse cognitive therapy and devote themselves to learning this treatment method, then the rest of the primary therapists usually follow suit.

The programs at the University of Louisville and University of Pittsburgh experienced minimal dissension from staff members as cognitive therapy was introduced. However, there is a potential for conflict at facilities where therapists strongly hold an alternate treatment philosophy. Examples might include those who are heavily committed to psychodynamically oriented individual therapy or systems approaches to family treatment. Well-entrenched professionals who are unwilling to look at new approaches or who have a personal "ax to grind" with primary cognitive therapists could present serious obstacles to the development of a primary therapist model CTU. Biological psychiatry can be fully integrated with cognitive therapy in the primary therapist model if the unit psychiatrists use both methods of therapy and develop a theoretical approach that encompasses the two forms of treatment (see Chapters 2, 7, and 8).

One of the positive features of this model is that a few individuals who have been previously trained in cognitive therapy can rapidly introduce cognitive procedures to the inpatient setting. Full training of all staff members is not required. Typical start-up time for such units is 2 to 6 months.

The primary therapist model has also been conducive to research, especially when the emphasis has been on intensive individual CT (three to five times per week). Patients have been treated with, and without, concomitant pharmacotherapy in these treatment programs (see Chapter 1 for review of outcome research). Primary therapists who have had considerable previous experience and who enter a vigorous training program in cognitive therapy are likely to reach a high level of competence. Such programs often use rating procedures such as the Cognitive Therapy Scale (Young & Beck, 1980) or supervision by off-site experts to insure that a high standard of practice is used.

The positive aspects of intensive training are tempered somewhat by the expense of this process. Supervision time, workshops, and seminars do not directly generate income. Costs of program development must be considered, but cognitive therapy may lead to a marketing advantage that can offset the start-up expenses of the unit. One cognitive therapy inpatient director noted that his program was so successful that other area hospitals attempted to start CT "clones" to recapture "market share."

As compared to the staff or "add-on" models, the primary therapist approach fits with the patient's usual expectation that his or her psychiatrist or other primary therapist will administer the therapy. Yet, it can be argued that the rest of the staff (who are with the patient 24 hours of the day) have the potential to provide the bulk of treatment interventions, and, therefore, the emphasis should be placed on therapy by this group of professionals. We now turn to a treatment model that utilizes a large number of staff members in the delivery of cognitively oriented therapy.

Staff Model

The Mesa Vista Hospital in San Diego, California has been a pioneer in the use of the staff model for inpatient cognitive therapy. This specialty referral unit is part of a large, free-standing psychiatric hospital. Patients are admitted to the CTU by psychiatrists who may have little or no training in cognitive therapy. The physicians continue to treat the patient with pharmacotherapy while the cognitive therapy is provided by staff members. Most of the cognitive treatment is delivered by psychiatric nurses under the supervision of Raymond Fidelio, M.D., a psychiatrist who received advanced training at the Center for Cognitive Therapy, University of Pennsylvania. A psychologist provides group cognitive therapy.

In this program, the milieu is considered to be the most active ingredient of therapy. Very high staff morale and patient satisfaction are reported (Fidelio & Creech, 1989). In this regard, the experiences using the staff model of cognitive therapy are similar to those described by proponents of the therapeutic community (see Chapter 2). A unified model for treatment and an involvement of all staff in the therapy program apparently result in improved satisfaction for both patients and staff.

Advantages of the staff model are listed in Table 3.2. Perhaps most importantly, this form of treatment encourages consistent use of CT principles in multiple staff–patient encounters throughout the day. Therapy is broken out of the confines of the usual 50-minute session and is distributed to nurses, aides, social workers, occupational therapists, activities' therapists, and others who interact with the patient during as many of the working hours of the day as possible. For example, the daily schedule for a patient who is enrolled in the staff model program might include several CT opportunities, such as group therapy, occupational therapy, and psychoeducational sessions.

Of at least equal importance, the patient is engaged in impromptu, brief interchanges with staff members who can monitor progress with homework assignments, use guided discovery to elicit automatic thoughts following a family visit, or help the patient list options to manage a problem that has developed on the ward. These interactions are especially effective when they address an issue with some imme-

TABLE 3.2. Staff Model

Advantages	Disadvantages
High staff morale	Possible conflict with admitting psychiatrists
Persons who spend most time with patients have most responsibility for cognitive therapy	Not conducive to outcome research
Curriculum for therapy usually well developed	Training and supervision is time consuming, expensive
Daily activities designed to support and reinforce the principles of cognitive therapy	Staff training and experience generally lower than for primary therapists
Cohesive treatment philosophy	Staff turnover

diacy—one that is brought out by a family visit, a conflict with another patient, or some other important stimulus from the inpatient experience. The staff member can identify distorted cognitions almost as soon as they occur (i.e., while they are still tightly linked to dysphoric or "hot" affect). This provides an opportunity for rapid and effective intervention while the automatic thoughts and associated feelings are still fresh in the patient's mind.

The staff model is utilized on inpatient services that are dedicated largely, if not completely, to treating patients who can benefit from cognitive therapy. Patients are screened before admission. Those with organic mental disorders, mental retardation, or severe psychotic symptoms are usually sent to other units. This allows the staff to dedicate the majority of their efforts to provision of cognitive therapy without interference from the demands of caring for a diverse population of inpatients. Daily activities, group therapies, and psychoeducational programs are designed to heighten the chances of the patient's understanding and using basic cognitive theories and techniques. The curriculum for therapy, including informational packets, readings, and patient handbooks is also well developed.

Although this type of inpatient cognitive therapy has been reported to be quite successful, results have not been documented with outcome research. The nature of the staff model makes it unlikely that substantive research will be done on this treatment method. Since all staff provide CT, and all patients receive this approach, the unit becomes so heavily oriented to cognitive therapy that comparison with other treatment methods on the same unit becomes impossible. The only solution would be to assign similar patients randomly to two different units. This strategy would have scientific merit, but it is impractical and is unlikely to be accomplished.

Separation of the therapy program from the treatment offered by the attending psychiatrist is a clear disadvantage of the staff model. This division presents a source of potential conflict and patient confusion. Another concern centers on the use of personnel with relatively little training or experience in professional psychotherapy. There is a risk that such individuals will apply partially or superficially understood techniques without a careful consideration of the consequences of the intervention (see Chapter 15 for a discussion of staff training issues).

One of the challenges of the staff model is the development of an accurate case conceptualization that can be communicated and understood by a wide variety of staff members, who can then apply procedures that can be customized or "tuned" to the individual patient. Despite vigorous efforts of the clinical director or other ward leaders, and the dedication of staff members, there are a host of ways in which this process can break down. Considerable attention must be paid to treatment planning, staff communication sessions, and clinical supervision. Staff turnover can be another serious problem. A well-functioning cognitive milieu requires a staff that knows cognitive therapy well and has developed productive working relationships over a period of months or years. Rapid or substantive turnover can significantly diminish the overall effectiveness and cohesion of the milieu.

"Add-On" Model

Many cognitive therapy units use the "add-on" model in which cognitive therapy, in the form of a specialty track or module, supplements an existing milieu. One of the advantages (Table 3.3) of this type of inpatient cognitive therapy is that it is the least difficult to establish. It usually does not require a major investment in primary therapist or staff training or a retrofitting of the entire milieu. One or a few individuals who have had previous training in CT, or have been sent for training at another center, are brought into the milieu to administer the therapy. Some programs (e.g., Butler Hospital, University of Iowa) have been started in order to engage in outcome research. Results of standard treatment were compared with an inpatient program augmented with cognitive therapy. Several "add-on" CTUs have been started in private facilities where there is an interest in cognitive therapy but where there are competing treatment philosophies and open-staff admitting privileges (e.g., Santa Ana Hospital, CPC Laguna Hospital). Some programs have emphasized group therapy (e.g., University of Cincinnati, Santa

TABLE 3.3. "Add-on" Therapist Model

Advantages	Disadvantages
Shortest start-up time	Unit leaders may not utilize cognitive therapy
Least disruption of existing milieu	Potential for conflicts with unit leaders, admitting physicians, other therapists
Low cost	Patient confusion about treatment methods
Compatible with outcome research	Power of all staff not fully directed at delivery of cognitive therapy
Portability	Difficulty growing into more fully developed milieu

Ana Hospital), whereas others have developed strong individual therapy programs (e.g., University of Iowa, Butler Hospital). At the University of Pittsburgh's program, an "add-on" CT therapy group is available for all depressed inpatients, whereas the more intensive individual primary therapist program is available for selected patients.

Although the "add-on" model is relatively easy to implement and may be somewhat portable (for example, a group cognitive therapy module that works well on one unit could be used on other units in the same hospital), it has major disadvantages (Table 3.3). Several program directors have noted that if the ward leaders do not utilize cognitive therapy, or if there is intense competition between treatment philosophies, CT may be viewed as only an appendage or an adjunct to the core treatment program. Much of the effort of the cognitive therapy staff must be spent in defending the approach. Patients can become confused about the goals and procedures of treatment in milieus where therapists are struggling for power or control.

Probably the greatest disadvantage of the "add-on" model is that only a limited amount of the potential of cognitive therapy is utilized. In contrast to other models described here, only a small portion of the patient's day is devoted to cognitively oriented therapy. Growth into a fully developed comprehensive cognitive milieu is possible (see below), but there are several barriers to this process. These include ongoing struggles between competing treatment philosophies and lack of commitment from the ward or hospital leadership for a cognitive milieu. Programs that use the primary therapist and staff models have had more success in evolving into comprehensive cognitive therapy milieus.

Comprehensive Model

Well-established CTUs such as those at the University of Louisville and the Mesa Vista Hospital have moved in the direction of a comprehensive model as their treatment procedures have been refined. However, a truly comprehensive cognitive therapy program, in which all therapeutic activities are steeped in the cognitive approach and there is little or no "noise" in the system from other directions for therapy, has yet to appear.

The major features of this ideal model would be: (1) ward leaders, primary therapists, adjunctive therapists, and the entire staff are well-trained and experienced in cognitive therapy; (2) the milieu is designed to fully complement cognitive therapy; (3) individual, family, and group therapies are centered by cognitive theory and technique; (4) the psychoeducational program is designed to complement these therapies and reinforce learning of cognitive therapy principles; and (5) primary therapists and other staff members resolve disputes about theoretical issues and develop a common treatment philosophy (Table 3.4).

Practical issues have prevented most programs from reaching their full potential as comprehensive CTUs. For example, the University of Louisville CTU has been able to achieve a high level of training of all primary therapists, adjunctive therapists, and many of the staff members. There is a widespread and deep acceptance of the basic tenets of cognitive therapy. Much of the milieu is able to promote cognitive therapy principles. However, the unit is located in a general hospital, and patients of all diagnostic categories must be admitted. The demand on staff to care for psychotic and organically impaired patients dimin-

TABLE 3.4. Comprehensive Model

Advantages	Disadvantages
All primary therapists and staff use cognitive therapy	Training and supervision is time consuming, expensive
Milieu designed to fully support cognitive therapy	Full implementation may take several years
Curriculum for therapy well-developed	Not conducive to outcome research
Minimal conflict between therapists, disciplines	Much effort expended on maintaining milieu
Cohesive treatment philosophy	Other valuable approaches may not be utilized

ishes their capacity to perform cognitive therapy. Nursing staff turnover has also created problems in insuring continuity of the cognitive program.

The comprehensive model requires an extensive and enduring investment in training and supervision. Of the four models described here, this approach takes the most time to develop. In addition, considerable attention must be paid to the milieu in order to avoid regression to less clearly specified forms of treatment. Another problem with the comprehensive model is that the intense commitment to cognitive therapy may possibly lead to neglect of other valuable approaches to treatment. For example, the psychiatrists may not keep abreast of advances in psychopharmacology, or family therapists may not learn about alternate methods of resolving interpersonal conflicts.

We therefore think it unwise to advocate the organization of inpatient units solely for the delivery of cognitive therapy. Instead, it appears reasonable to strive for widespread application of cognitive techniques in an environment where the therapists have a broad base of knowledge in the general principles of hospital psychiatry and familiarity with other major forms of therapy. Within this framework, the multidisciplinary team can construct a comprehensive, cognitively oriented milieu that is firmly rooted in cognitive theory but does not ignore past contributions or worthwhile new developments in psychiatric treatment.

INITIATION AND GROWTH OF THE COGNITIVE MILIEU

"Breaking Away": Establishing a New Form of Inpatient Treatment

There are many forces that can undermine the efforts of those who wish to introduce cognitive therapy to the inpatient setting. Fear of change, biases against psychotherapy in general or cognitively oriented treatment in particular, staff inertia, lack of resources for training, and territorial conflicts can be formidable obstacles in developing a new cognitive therapy program. Careful design and gradual implementation of the treatment program are likely to improve the chances of success. A recommended sequence of steps to be taken in forming a new CTU is listed in Table 3.5.

Step One: Describe Rationale

Why should a standard inpatient program be converted to a cognitive therapy unit? Hospitals that have successfully managed this transition

TABLE 3.5. Steps to Develop a Cognitive Therapy Unit

1. Describe rationale
2. Establish goals for milieu
3. Identify program components and requirements
4. Develop timetable for implementation
5. Perform economic analysis
6. Obtain administrative approval for program
7. Begin training and recruitment
8. Develop cognitive therapy materials
9. Initiate treatment

have had solid reasons for supplanting an older model with a cognitively oriented approach to treatment. Early CTUs were established in academic centers as research and teaching programs. Favorable results of outcome studies with both outpatients and inpatients (see Chapter 1) and increased demand for training in cognitive therapy in psychiatry and psychology graduate programs helped solidify the justification for CTUs in academic institutions.

The majority of CTUs have originated in nonacademic settings where a different set of influences has promoted use of cognitive therapy procedures. Economic factors have been a driving force behind the creation of many of these CTUs. The short-term nature of cognitive therapy and the demonstrated utility of this form of treatment are very desirable features for hospitals that wish to distinguish themselves from others by providing high-quality, cost-effective care.

Table 3.6 includes a partial list of reasons for starting a CTU. After evaluating the program's unique situation, an individualized rationale should be developed that can easily be understood by administrators, staff members, referring professionals, insurance carriers, and others who have a significant impact on the hospital milieu.

Step Two: Establish Goals for Milieu

It is useful from the outset to have a clear idea of the goals for the cognitive milieu. A realistic appraisal of the resources and constraints of the local setting will help the organizers of the program to steer a course that will lead to a favorable outcome. This could include consideration of the four models of inpatient cognitive therapy described earlier in this chapter. Which model fits best with the goals for the treatment program? Is there an alternate model that might be developed?

A sample list of goals for a primary therapist model unit might

TABLE 3.6. Reasons for Starting a Cognitive Therapy Unit

Cognitive approach fits well with psychopharmacology
Collaborative relationships with patients
Educational materials available
Heightened staff morale
Improved specificity of treatment
Marketing advantage
Potential for relapse prevention
Pragmatic treatment model
Psychoeducational emphasis
Research
Short-term treatment approach
Treatment efficacy
Treatment manual available
Useful for treatment resistant patients

include: (1) develop a core group of therapists with high level of cognitive therapy expertise; (2) initiate CT research; (3) offer a training program in cognitive therapy; (4) educate staff in basic CT principles; and (5) enlist staff to assist with cognitive therapy. A hospital that wishes to establish a staff model might have different goals: (1) offer alternate treatment program that will increase patient referrals; (2) train nurses, aides, and other staff to provide "on the spot" cognitive therapy; (3) develop a cohesive milieu; (4) document improvements in patient and staff satisfaction with treatment; and (5) communicate advantages of cognitive therapy to admitting physicians.

Only a few goals are given as examples here. A full listing of specific objectives (including areas such as therapy formats, multidisciplinary team relationships, length of stay, and degree of cognitive orientation of the milieu) will facilitate the development of an effective plan for implementation of the inpatient program.

Step Three: Identify Program Components and Requirements

This stage involves specification of the cognitive therapy components of the milieu. A description of resources that will be required and methods that will be used to complete the transition is also needed. A detailed plan including the form and frequency of therapeutic modalities, training program, hierarchy of responsibility for therapy, psychoeducational methods, and treatment planning mechanisms is recommended. The design for use of principles from the therapeutic community, biological psychiatry, or other theoretical perspectives should also be articulated.

Step Four: Develop Timetable for Implementation

The next step is to plot out a time course for phasing cognitive therapy into the milieu. It is usually best to introduce new procedures gradually. Individuals who are resistant to change can learn about cognitive therapy in a relatively nonthreatening way if the therapists use pilot projects to demonstrate the usefulness of this approach before attempting to spread cognitive therapy to the entire milieu. However, it may be possible in some instances to convert a milieu rapidly to a cognitive model. This has been done at facilities such as the Mesa Vista Hospital, where a strong leader received considerable support from both administration and staff. On other units, where there have been substantial conflicts between treatment philosophies or power struggles between disciplines, changes in the milieu have proceeded at a slower pace.

A suggested timetable for implementation of a cognitive milieu is outlined in Table 3.7. This plan describes the start-up procedures for a

TABLE 3.7. Implementation Timetable for a Primary Therapist Model Unit

Time periods	Steps
Start	Begin training program for primary therapists Initiate weekly supervision group Form task force to develop psychoeducational program and materials
6 weeks	Workshops for primary therapists Begin orientation program for staff
8 weeks	Form task force to develop group therapy protocols Primary therapists start pilot cases Begin using psychoeducational materials
14 weeks	Workshops for primary therapists and staff Staff assists with individual and group therapy homework assignments
16 weeks	Primary therapists begin to submit videotapes of sessions for supervision and assessment with Cognitive Therapy Scale[a] Task forces on psychoeducational programs and group protocols submit reports
18 weeks	Individual cognitive therapy utilized whenever indicated Cognitive group therapy introduced to milieu
20 weeks	Psychoeducational program including group sessions, cognitive therapy materials, patient handbook fully implemented
24 weeks	Workshop for individual and group therapists All program components continue

[a]Young & Beck (1980).

hypothetical unit that has decided to begin with a primary therapist model that will subsequently be developed into a more comprehensive cognitive milieu. The timetable might vary considerably if there are different goals for the cognitive milieu. Also, the local environment plays a major role in dictating the pace of activity in developing a CTU. The sequence described in Table 3.7 is designed for a situation in which there is solid administrative backing for the project, the ward leadership fully accepts the value of cognitive therapy, and only a modest amount of resistance to cognitive therapy is anticipated among staff members.

Step Five: Perform Economic Analysis

Consideration of the costs and potential financial benefits to the institution is an important part of the process of initiating a CTU. Many facilities use the *proforma* approach to predict the economic impact of a new program. Unit leaders join with the department of finance to write a detailed 3 to 5-year budget for the CTU. Often, the first year's operations will be less profitable than that of later years because of expenditures for starting the program (e.g., training or recruitment, visiting faculty, materials, and marketing). Once the CTU is fully operational and is known in the community, revenue from increased referrals will be expected to override the costs of developing and maintaining a cognitive milieu. The CTU will need to achieve budgetary objectives in order to continue operation.

Step Six: Obtain Administrative Approval

Working through the first five steps prepares the CTU leaders to present a well-orchestrated plan to hospital administration or other agencies that must approve and fund the program. In our experience, hospital administrators are often quite interested in the clinical aspects of a proposed CTU and can understand rather quickly the advantages of a cognitive therapy program. The logical nature of the treatment often fits more closely with the administrator's operational style than other less specific therapies. Ideally, hospital administrators will not only give budgetary approval but will also develop a sense of ownership for the project that will lead to creative suggestions, an institutional affirmation of the value of the program, and support for future growth.

Step Seven: Begin Training and/or Recruitment

A training program is essential unless a well-experienced cognitive therapist is imported to the milieu to develop an "add-on" model for treatment. Even in this case, it is helpful to initiate an educational series for staff members. For most CTUs, the training of therapists should be well under way before initiating either group or individual cognitive therapy. Table 3.7 outlines a sample training sequence. A full description of training procedures is contained in Chapter 15.

Step Eight: Develop Cognitive Therapy Materials

The hospital setting is particularly well-suited for implementing the psychoeducational components of cognitive therapy. Patients have adequate time to complete readings, work on assignments, and attend teaching sessions. Furthermore, the principles of cognitive therapy can be reinforced through repeated opportunities for learning throughout the milieu. Many CTUs develop a course that includes a series of presentations to patients and families, use of workbooks, and other psychoeducational procedures. Patients often report that they refer to their cognitive therapy workbooks long after discharge. They find these materials very useful in managing new stresses and avoiding return of symptoms. Psychoeducational interventions are illustrated in later chapters of the book.

Step Nine: Initiate Treatment

The timetable developed in Step Four gives a general template for the introduction of various components of cognitive therapy to the milieu. Many CTUs begin with a few cases of individual therapy. As therapists gain experience, more patients are included in the cognitive therapy program. Other CTUs use the group format as the beginning form of therapy. It is important at this phase to evaluate thoughtfully the results of initial efforts and to make modifications in the treatment program where necessary.

Growth of the Cognitive Milieu

Attention can now be directed toward full development of the cognitive milieu. Although growth can be achieved in a number of areas, we focus here on three opportunities for enhancing the cognitive milieu: (1) enrichment of the daily schedule; (2) use of adjunctive therapies (i.e., multidisciplinary team); and (3) integration of the cognitive milieu through treatment planning. Other potential areas for development, including family therapy, psychiatric nursing, and specialty inpatient programs (e.g., geriatric, eating disorders, substance abuse) are discussed in detail elsewhere in this volume.

Enrichment of the Daily Schedule

As the cognitive milieu matures, a gradually increasing share of the patient's day should be devoted to the process of cognitive therapy. In the early phases of development of a primary therapist or "add-on" model, the patient may be engaged in cognitive therapy for only a small portion of the available time. But, as the milieu moves toward a comprehensive model, there will be a myriad of experiences in which the patient can be exposed to the cognitive approach to treatment.

An example of a unit that is evolving in the direction of the comprehensive approach to treatment (University of Louisville) can be used to illustrate how cognitive therapy can become a pervasive force in the milieu. On this unit, the daily schedule is arranged to complement and reinforce what is learned in individual or group cognitive therapy sessions. Homework assignments are carried out in therapeutic activities, where the responsible staff members are well versed in cognitive therapy principles (see next section). In addition, specialized group therapies are designed to fulfill focused objectives.

A sample daily schedule and a list of major therapeutic activities that take place each week are contained in Tables 3.8 and 3.9. In the early part of the day, patients engage in personal care, eat breakfast, and have time to work on cognitive therapy homework. Typically, they read materials such as *Coping with Depression* (Beck & Greenberg, 1974) or *Feeling Good* (Burns, 1980) and carry out individualized CT procedures such as recording thoughts or completing graded task assignments.

TABLE 3.8. Sample Daily Schedule: University of Louisville CTU

7:30 a.m.	Wake-up and personal care
8:00 a.m.	Breakfast
8:30 a.m.	Reading, homework, personal care
9:30 a.m.	Unit community meeting
10:00 a.m.	Occupational therapy
11:00 a.m.	Individual therapy
12:00 noon	Lunch, homework
1:00 p.m.	Group therapy
2:30 p.m.	Crafts, recreational, or horticultural therapy
3:30 p.m.	Reading, homework
4:00 p.m.	Exercise group
5:30 p.m.	Dinner
6:30 p.m.	Reading, homework
7:00 p.m.	Visit hour
8:30 p.m.	Stress management or medication group
9:30 p.m.	Reading, homework, individual consultation with nurse

TABLE 3.9. Therapeutic Activities: University of Louisville CTU

Cognitive group therapy	Medication group
Crafts	Men's group
Creative expressions group	Occupational therapy
Daily activity scheduling	Out-trip
Exercise	Pastoral counseling
Family night psychoeducational programs	Recreational therapy
Family therapy	Social skills group
Family visits	Stress management
Focus group	Therapy sessions with nurse
Homework	Unit community meeting
Horticultural therapy	Women's group
Individual therapy	

A unit-community meeting, which includes virtually all patients and most staff, is held Monday through Friday from 9:30 to 10:00 a.m. Procedures for this group are derived from both the therapeutic community and cognitive therapy. Patients are encouraged to share responsibility for their treatment and to help one another in the recovery process. A spirit of collaboration is reinforced by keeping an open forum for patient input. The successes and difficulties of treatment, and the problems that are encountered in living on an inpatient psychiatry service are discussed. Interpersonal issues that arise during the hospitalization serve as opportunities to apply principles of cognitive therapy. This meeting is also used to welcome new patients to the unit and to begin their orientation to CT. In their last unit-community meeting, patients who are ready for discharge discuss their plans for the future and say goodbye to their fellow patients.

Individual therapy, group sessions, recreational therapy, and consultations with a nurse take place on a daily basis; other therapeutic activities such as family therapy and pastoral counseling are arranged as needed. Daily schedules are individualized to match the patient's level of functioning and his or her progress through the treatment program. Most patients are able to benefit from the unit-community meeting, occupational therapy, crafts, recreational therapy, and exercise. However, those depressed persons with severe psychomotor retardation or psychotic features may be confused or overwhelmed if they are immediately entered into more demanding treatments such as cognitive group therapy or a "creative expressions" (i.e., literature and art therapy) session.

The treatment team uses a menu of various therapies from which they select a program that best fits the needs of each patient. For example, at both the University of Louisville and University of Pittsburgh CTUs, there is an option of attendance at regular group cognitive therapy or an alternative therapeutic experience held at the same time—a "focus" group. These CTUs are in academic settings in which the case mix is somewhat heterogeneous. Affective disorder is the predominate diagnosis; but some individuals may have schizophrenia, mania, or other psychotic illnesses. The focus group is designed for the latter group of patients. Highly structured exercises are used to build self-esteem or enhance mastery of activities of daily living.

The frequency and complexity of therapy sessions are increased as patients become accustomed to the unit, learn basic principles of cognitive therapy, and develop greater trust and rapport with the treatment team. Repeated evaluations by the primary therapists and other staff members are required in order to titrate the intensity of the cognitive therapy program to the patient's level of symptoms and personal resources. At times, the therapists need to consider additions to the standard repertoire of CT procedures. Examples might include preparation of cognitive therapy materials for the deaf or visually handicapped, adapting methods for use with an illiterate person, arranging a conjoint cognitive therapy session with a patient and employer, or use of computer-assisted CT for reinforcement of learning.

The University of Louisville CTU is an example of how cognitive therapy procedures can be expanded throughout the milieu. Other programs with a comprehensive orientation may have a somewhat different format, but all attempt to develop a cohesive treatment system in which CT can be applied with intensity, consistency, and thoroughness. The use of adjunctive therapies and the implementation of effective treatment planning strategies are integral to this approach.

Adjunctive Therapies

The availability of adjunctive therapies is an important feature of inpatient psychiatric treatment. The outpatient cognitive therapist rarely has the opportunity to involve an entire team of specialists (e.g., activities therapists, occupational therapists, expressive therapists, pastoral counselors, and others) in the treatment process. Adjunctive therapy has a long tradition in the psychiatric hospital. The general goals of adjunctive therapy are to (1) identify patient strengths and weaknesses, (2) promote adaptive behavior, (3) collaborate with the primary therapist by assisting the patient to carry out experiments or tasks in structured activities, and (4) provide alternate therapy experiences for patients who do not respond fully to more formal psychotherapy.

The role of the adjunctive therapist in a CTU is dependent on the prevailing treatment model. On comprehensive CTUs, the adjunctive therapists are well versed in cognitive theory and technique. In contrast, adjunctive therapists on an "add-on" model CTU may have received limited training in cognitive therapy. With the former model, the adjunctive therapist may be a major part of the cognitive therapy program. For example, activities therapists and occupational therapists at the University of Louisville CTU serve as group cotherapists and are involved in multiple one-to-one cognitive therapy encounters with patients throughout the day. With the "add-on" model, it is less likely that an adjunctive therapist will engage in standard cognitive therapy interventions. Nevertheless, it is important for the adjunctive therapist to have at least a rudimentary understanding of cognitive therapy principles so that treatment procedures can be coordinated.

In our experience, the cognitive therapy approach is readily accepted by activities therapists, occupational therapists, vocational rehabilitation counselors, and others who have been trained to promote skill development. The objectives and procedures of these types of adjunctive therapy are quite similar to those of cognitive therapy. However, expressive therapists may have more difficulty adapting to a cognitive orientation, because their discipline is rooted heavily in psychoanalytic theory. We will briefly discuss the use of the major types of adjunctive therapy in the CTU.

Activities Therapy

Recreational therapists and related disciplines (e.g., horticultural therapists, arts and crafts specialists) engage the patient in a wide range of therapeutic situations such as exercise, crafts, gardening, games, and trips outside the hospital. Usually, a significant portion of the patient's day is devoted to these pursuits. The activities therapists should be instructed in the use of the Daily Activity Schedule, a cognitive therapy procedure used in most CTUs. Ideally, the activities therapist will be able to assist the patient in completing mastery and pleasure ratings on the Daily Activity Schedule and will also involve the patient in discussing and planning changes in behavior.

Patients can be asked to predict how well they will perform or how much they will enjoy certain activities (e.g., bowling, woodwork, or a shopping trip). If the patient is feeling different after completing the task, the activities therapist can use guided discovery to help identify why a mood shift has occurred. If a negative prediction is confirmed, the activities therapist can work with the patient to identify what factors interfered with their accomplishment or performance. These data then can be used to problem solve and, if necessary, plan for additional assignments where skills can be built by coaching, feedback, modeling, cognitive rehearsal, and role playing.

The activities therapist can be resourceful and creative in trying to set up success experiences for the patient by breaking tasks down into small steps (i.e., graded task assignments). Group feedback is another useful tool in activities therapy. Discussions of therapeutic activities in a group setting may provide valuable information to challenge patients' erroneous conclusions that they performed poorly, accomplished little, or looked foolish.

Occupational Therapy

Occupational therapists who work in a psychiatric setting are primarily concerned with teaching skills to promote self-reliance and independence. These therapists have received extensive training on how to deal with actual physical, intellectual, or social deficits. In fact, they are probably better prepared than most psychiatrists, psychologists, or social workers to teach adaptive skills to persons with significant handicaps. Occupational therapists can augment the cognitive therapy program in a number of ways. First, they can provide a detailed assessment of functional capacity. This evaluation often gives more practical information than does extensive psychological testing. Can the patient manage daily activities of living, handle financial matters, or complete job-related tasks? Accurate data in this regard help the cognitive therapist to determine whether the patient's concept of self-efficacy is valid. With inpatients, there is a frequent admixture of true performance deficits and cognitive distortions about abilities.

During the treatment phase of occupational therapy, there is a natural partnership between the occupational and cognitive therapist. Both are interested in reducing symptoms and improving coping skills. The occupational therapist uses psychoeducational procedures, demonstrations, and *in vivo* rehearsal to build functional ability and self-esteem. Socratic questioning may also be used to uncover the patient's cognitive responses to the occupational therapy exercises. The cognitively-oriented occupational therapist will be able to point out maladaptive cognitions and help the patient to develop more balanced thinking. In addition, the occupational therapist can assist the patient in carrying out specific assignments from individual or group cognitive therapy.

Expressive Therapies

In art therapy and other expressive therapies (e.g., music, dance, drama), a strong emphasis is placed on providing an acceptable outlet for intense feelings. These therapies (especially art therapy) have also been interested in using art forms as a way of expressing hidden (or "unconscious") conflicts or themes. Freudian or Jungian theories have often been applied to understanding the art productions of psychiatric patients.

The potential conflicts with a cognitive model for therapy are readily apparent. In cognitive therapy, expression of feelings, by itself, is not considered to be a primary element of treatment, and psychoanalytic or symbolic interpretations are usually not given much credence. However, differences between expressive and cognitive therapists have been bridged in many CTUs. There are several reasons why the two seemingly disparate approaches can work together. First, art or other expressive media can be used to elicit cognitions in a visual mode when thoughts are not readily accessible through straightforward questioning. Second, the expressive therapist in a cognitively oriented inpatient program can begin to learn and use cognitive theories to interpret the significance of art productions, dance movements, or psychodrama experiences. Themes such as perfectionism, fear of failure, and the need to please others are seen repeatedly in responses to expressive therapy procedures. The expressive therapist may thus be able to help in the identification of significant underlying schemas.

Finally, the expressive therapist can use art or other media to stimulate intense affect by generating particularly meaningful cognitions. One of the common misconceptions about cognitive therapy is that this form of treatment is highly intellectualized and that affect is avoided whenever possible. To the contrary, experienced cognitive therapists know that emotion is often the "royal road to cognition" (Beck, 1991). Thus, the expressive therapist can assist the cognitive therapist by using techniques that elicit vivid affective responses.

Pastoral Counseling

A pastoral counselor or chaplain can be an important part of the treatment team for patients who have significant spiritual or religious problems. For example, patients may experience guilty ruminations relating to past sexual activities that were at variance with their moral or religious principles. Issues such as abortion, infidelity, and divorce often weigh heavily on individuals with strong religious beliefs. Other patients may be struggling with the recent death of a loved one or be facing their own mortality. Cognitive therapy can be combined with existential psychotherapy to approach these kinds of concerns. This type of blended therapy can be performed by a pastoral counselor who is aware of CT principles, a cognitive therapist who is experienced in dealing with existential or spiritual problems, or by a joint effort of the pastoral counselor and the cognitive therapist. Readers are referred to Frankl (1985) for a description of this form of cognitively oriented psychotherapy.

For some patients (especially those who are older and deeply religious) the pastoral counselor or chaplain may, at least at first, have a higher level of credibility than the secular therapist. Having such patients work with a pastoral counselor who is familiar with the cognitive model may be a critical step in developing an effective treatment program. The pastoral therapist can help a patient see the difference between pathological guilt and a genuine sense of responsibility. Also, when errors have been made (vis-à-vis the patient's value system), the pastoral counselor can engage the patient in a process of atonement and forgiveness.

Treatment Planning

The procedure of developing the patient's treatment plan serves to organize and integrate the contributions of all therapists working within the cognitive milieu. Written documentation of the treatment plan is required by the Joint Commission for Accreditation of Healthcare Organizations (JCAHO) and state agencies. However, even if such plans were not required, regular meeting of the treatment team is essential for providing a sustained, high-quality therapeutic program.

In our experience, treatment teams function optimally when they utilize a consistent, yet flexible, format and a well-specified agenda. A team caring for 10 patients might meet for 30 minutes each day, to review briefly the progress of all patients and address the formal treatment plans of perhaps two patients in detail; or they may meet for less frequent but longer sessions (e.g., two 60-minute meetings each week). In either case, it is important that all members of the multidisciplinary team be represented at each patient's detailed review.

The emphasis on the cognitive case formulation (Persons, 1989) varies depending on the type of CTU milieu and the nature of the patient's problems. When the "add-on" model is used, the cognitive therapist's input at team meetings is particularly important because the other team members may not be able to support the therapy properly without hearing about the formulation and plan for interventions. Moreover, anticipated roadblocks or points of "resistance" may be reviewed, and possible treatment strategies discussed among the full treatment team. It is, of course, easier to implement a cognitively oriented inpatient treatment plan when the primary therapist model is used, particularly when the attending psychiatrist or team leader is a cognitive therapist. In such settings, the treatment team meeting also can be a useful place for the primary therapist and/or team leader to teach other staff members about the cognitive model of psychopathology. An example of a written treatment plan for Mr. S., a 42-year-old shop owner admitted to a CTU for treatment of a disabling, antidepressant-resistant, depressive disorder is provided in Table 3.10.

In this case, the treatment team identified several different types of problems. Developing a problem list for the treatment plan is one of the most important functions of the interdisciplinary team. On some units, the preferred strategy is to "lump" problems into broad classifications; on others, the clinicians delineate circumscribed targets for treatment. Generally, our procedure is to strive for as much specificity as possible. We usually list problems in the following order:

1. *The primary presenting problem.* This is frequently a diagnostic category such as depression, schizophrenia, or anorexia nervosa. Alternately, the major symptoms can be described without indicating a firm diagnosis (e.g., suicide attempt, aggressive behavior, or psychosis). At times, there are two or more major presenting problems.

2. *Interpersonal problems.* There is almost always a marital, family, or occupational issue. A brief description of the problem helps the team to focus on possible solutions. Examples might include marital separation, suspected abuse, financial disputes, or conflict with a child.

3. *Behavioral or personality problems.* On many occasions, behavioral or social skills deficits, or sequelae of a personality disturbance, can be culled out for special attention. Although at times there may be some overlap with the primary diagnosis or presenting problem, significant interventions are more likely if the treatment plan highlights a defined concern. In the case of Mr. S., medication noncompliance and social withdrawal were targeted. Examples of other problems that could be selected are borderline personality traits, severe shyness, or excessive dependency.

4. *Medical problems.* Physical disorders are especially common in patients treated in psychiatric units of general hospitals (see Chapter 8). Including medical illnesses in the treatment plan helps the team to knit all the elements of the therapy program into a cohesive whole. Consultants and other medical specialists should be identified in the plan.

5. *Other.* Inpatients can present with a number of idiosyncratic therapeutic issues such as physical handicaps, educational deficiencies, or legal difficulties. These problems should be added to the treatment plan if they are causing significant distress or if they are having an impact on the patient's participation in the inpatient treatment program.

The next phase of the treatment planning process is to establish goals for therapy. The watchwords here are *clarity* and *reasonableness*. It is hard to measure whether a goal is met if it is stated in fuzzy or diffuse terms (e.g., better "communication," greater expressiveness, improved relationships). We think that goals are achieved more frequently if they are articulated in a manner that can be clearly understood by the patient and all of his or her therapists. It is also important to choose goals that have a reasonable chance of being accomplished during the hospitalization. The team should be asked to attempt to set target dates for reaching each of the objectives. Long-term goals may be designated for continued therapy as an outpatient.

Finally, treatment methods should be selected and matched to each of the goals. It is useful to indicate, by name, the therapists who will have responsibility for the major parts of the treatment plan. Usually, the treatment plan is written on a single sheet of paper that is filed in a patient's chart. It thus can be used by all staff members, including those who have not been able to attend the planning conference, as a quick reference to the design for therapy. The patient should be asked to review the plan, make suggestions, and agree to proceed with the scheduled treatment.

A well-orchestrated treatment plan is one of the fundamental elements of the cognitive milieu. Many of the basic features of cognitive therapy are incorporated in the plan. It provides the agenda for the entire hospital therapy program, and outlines the structure of treatment. The plan is a collaborative effort between the therapists and the patient. Therapy targets and treatment methods are evaluated empirically. Feedback is solicited from all parties, and the plan is reviewed at regular intervals. Changes are made as problems are resolved or new information is acquired. In an overall sense, the treatment plan serves as a schema for the hospitalization. Assumptions (or hypotheses) about the patient's problems and the therapists' preferred methods of treatment are set forth. These constructs guide the process to its conclusion. The team needs to continually reexamine these assumptions to determine whether they are accurate, adaptive, and effective.

SUMMARY

Four models (e.g., primary therapist, staff, "add-on," and comprehensive) for the cognitive milieu are described. These models represent broad categories of inpatient therapy programs and are presented here to guide the reader who may want to develop a cognitively oriented treatment unit. Advantages and disadvantages of the different types of

TABLE 3.10. Sample Inpatient Treatment Plan: Mr. S.

Date of plan	Problems	Goals[a]	Method	Nursing intervention	Target date
10/4/91	A. Refractory depression with suicidal ideation; has failed to respond to two TCAs, fluoxetine, lithium augmentation, and dynamic psychotherapy.	A_1 Reduce depressive symptoms by >50% (measured by BDI). A_2 Minimal suicidal risk. A_3 Rule out occult causes of refractory depression. A_4 Improve sufficiently to resume professional and personal relationships (long-term goal).	A_{1-2} Individual (5/wk, Dr. S.) and group (3/wk, Dr. B. and Ms. W.) cognitive therapy. A_{1-2} Consider MAOI (Dr. S.). A_{1-2} Activities therapy daily, Occupational therapy group (2/wk). A_3 Assess thyroid function, EEG, sleep studies, and MRI. A_4 Reevaluate following treatment with A_{1-2}.	A_{1-2} Review activity schedule, M and P ratings daily; assist with completion of DRDT forms. A_{1-2} Instruct on MAOI diet. A_3 Support patient and answer questions as they arise. A_4 N/A	A_1 10/18/91 A_2 10/09/91 A_3 10/07/91 A_4 11/10/91
	B. Marital discord; wife appears to be losing hope.	B_1 Determine level of marital dysfunction. B_2 Improve treatment-supporting role of spouse.	B_{1-2} Diagnostic couples session with MSW and conjoint therapy session (Dr. S. and MSW).	B_{1-2} Discuss reactions to sessions and clarify issues for therapy.	B_{1-2} 10/11/91
	C. Past noncompliance with prescribed medications.	C_1 Understated rationale for pharmacotherapy. C_2 Identify cognitions about medication.	C_1 Discuss with treatment team issues related to noncompliance.	C_1 Provide literature on antidepressants.	C_1 10/11/91 C_2 10/11/91

		C_{1-2} Attend medication education group. C_2 Individual cognitive therapy as in A_{1-2}.		
D. Withdrawn behavior; low self-esteem; unassertive.	D_1 Decrease time in bed during day by >80%. D_2 Engage in wide range of activities. D_3 Improve self-esteem by >25%. D_4 Learn assertiveness skills (measured by self-report)	D_{1-2} Daily Activity Schedule as in A_{1-2}. D_{1-2} Graded task assignments in milieu as in A_{1-2}. D_3 Social Skills group. D_4 Assertiveness group.	D_1 Monitor activities schedule as in A_{1-4}. D_1 Encourage patient to articulate needs.	D_{1-2} 10/11/91 D_3 10/18/91 D_3 10/18/91
E. Hypertension	E_1 Blood pressure to normal range.	E_1 Medical reevaluation (Dr. R.). E_1 Low-salt diet. E_1 Choose antihypertensive that doesn't aggravate depression or interact with antidepressants.	E_1 Monitor blood pressure daily.	E_1 10/07/91

[a]Goals listed here are short-term unless specifically labeled as long-term goal.

CTUs are detailed. We advise that all models for inpatient cognitive therapy develop an overarching treatment philosophy that can incorporate other useful therapeutic methods, such as biological psychiatry. A provincial attitude of "cognitive therapy only" is discouraged. Nevertheless, we think that cognitive therapy principles can serve as the major operational constructs for an inpatient unit.

Guidelines are offered for the initial development of a cognitive milieu. The process begins with careful planning. This includes description of the rationale, definition of goals, identification of program requirements, establishment of a timetable, and completion of a budgetary analysis. After obtaining administrative approval, a core group of cognitive therapists must be trained (or recruited) and educational materials prepared. Pilot cases are treated prior to full implementation of the CTU program.

Suggestions are also made for promoting growth of the milieu after the program is established. Many programs have been able to spread the influence of cognitive therapy within a unit by gradually introducing cognitive principles to an increasing share of the unit's scheduled therapeutic activities. Standard inpatient therapy groups, such as unit-community meetings and psychoeducational sessions, can be realigned to support the cognitive therapy perspective. Adjunctive therapies are especially important in this regard. Treatment planning offers another opportunity for encouraging development of the cognitive milieu. The problem-oriented, collaborative, and empirical nature of cognitive therapy is emphasized in the treatment-planning process.

The cognitive milieu is a new entry in a long series of treatment systems for inpatient psychiatry. Considerable additional clinical experience and outcome research will be required before the relative place of cognitive therapy in hospital psychiatry will be clear. However, a cognitive orientation to inpatient treatment appears to offer a pragmatic and cogent solution to the problem of providing an effective psychotherapy in a short period of time. The cognitive model also can serve as a clear and understandable organizing theory for the multiple disciplines, therapies, and activities of the inpatient milieu.

REFERENCES

Beck, A. T. (1991). Cognitive therapy: A 30-year retrospective. *American Psychologist, 46*(4), 368–375.

Beck, A. T., & Greenberg, R. L. (1974). *Coping with depression*. (Available from the Institute for Rational Emotive Therapy, 45 East 65th Street, New York, NY 10021.)

Bowers, W. A. (1989). Cognitive therapy with inpatients. In A. Freeman, M. K. Simon, L. E. Beutler, & H. Arkowitz (Eds.), *Comprehensive handbook of cognitive therapy* (pp. 583–596). New York: Plenum Press.

Burns, D. D. (1980). *Feeling good*. New York: William Morrow. Fidelio, R., & Creech, R. (1989). *Cognitive therapy on an affective disorders unit: First 15-month evaluation*. Paper presented at the World Congress of Cognitive Therapy, Oxford, England.

Frankl, V. E. (1985). Logos, paradox, and the search for meaning. In M. J. Mahoney & A. Freeman (Eds.), *Cognition and psychotherapy*, New York: Plenum Press.

Miller, I. V., Bishop, S. D., Norman, W. H., & Keitner, G. I. (1985). Cognitive-behavioral therapy and pharmacotherapy with chronic, drug-refractory depressed inpatients: A note of optimism. *Behavioral Psychotherapy, 13*, 320–327.

Perris, C., Rodhe, K., Palm, A., Abelson, M., Hellgren, S., Livja, C., & Soderman, H. (1987). Fully integrated in- and outpatient services in a psychiatric sector: Implementation of a new mode for the care of psychiatric patients favoring continuity of care. In A. Freeman & V. Greenwood (Eds.). *Cognitive therapy: Applications in psychiatric and medical settings* (pp. 117–131). New York: Human Sciences Press.

Persons, J. B. (1989). *Cognitive therapy in practice: A case formulation approach*. New York: W. W. Norton.

Schrodt, G. R., Jr., & Wright, J. H. (1987). Inpatient treatment of adolescents. In A. Freeman & V. Greenwood (Eds.), *Cognitive therapy: Applications in psychiatric and medical settings* (pp. 69–82). New York: Human Sciences Press.

Thase, M. E., Bowler, K., & Harden, T. (1991). Cognitive behavior therapy of endogenous depression: Part 2. Preliminary findings in 16 unmedicated patients. *Behavior Therapy, 22*, 469–477.

Thase, M. E., & Wright, J. H. (1991). Cognitive behavior therapy with depressed inpatients: An abridged treatment manual. *Behavior Therapy, 22*, 579–595.

Wright, J. H. (1989). *Cognitive therapy unit in a teaching hospital*. Paper presented at the World Congress of Cognitive Therapy, Oxford, England.

Wright, J. H., Thase, M. E., & Beck, A. T. (1992). *Inpatient cognitive therapy: Structures, processes, and procedures*. Paper presented at the World Congress of Cognitive Therapy, Toronto, Ontario.

Young, J., & Beck, A. T. (1980). *Cognitive therapy scale: Rating manual*. Unpublished manuscript, University of Pennsylvania, Philadelphia.

Part II

TREATMENT MODALITIES

Chapter 4

Individual Cognitive Therapy with Inpatients

John W. Ludgate, Ph.D.,
Jesse H. Wright, M.D., Ph.D.,
Wayne Bowers, Ph.D., and
Glenda F. Camp, Ph.D.

Individual therapy is one of the major components of most inpatient cognitive therapy programs. In this chapter, we describe cognitive therapy (CT) procedures for inpatients and illustrate how common target symptoms can be approached from a cognitive perspective. An emphasis is placed on treatment of anxiety and depression, the most common problems of hospitalized patients. Interventions for patients with personality disorders, substance abuse, chronic mental illness, and eating disorders are covered in other sections of this volume.

GENERAL PRINCIPLES OF INDIVIDUAL INPATIENT COGNITIVE THERAPY

The Inpatient Setting

Cognitive therapy with inpatients differs in several ways from the standard outpatient treatment of depression and anxiety (Beck, Rush, Shaw, & Emery, 1979; Wright & Beck, 1983; Beck & Emery, 1985; Bowers, 1989; Thase & Wright, 1991). Patients who are admitted to a psychiatric hospital pose a special challenge to the cognitive therapist. The presenting problems are usually quite severe, and there has often been a breakdown of coping mechanisms and support structures. Compared to individuals who receive outpatient CT, hospitalized patients are likely to have higher suicide risk, greater hopelessness, more disruption of physiological processes, and an increased level of social and occupational impairment. Cognitive therapy procedures must be geared to this high level of dysfunction.

The hospital milieu also influences the form of CT used with inpatients. The multidisciplinary team can either augment or impede the work of the individual cognitive therapist. Auxiliary therapists can reinforce principles learned in CT sessions. However, conflicts over competing treatment philosophies can confuse the patient and undermine efforts to use CT. The inpatient cognitive therapist needs to operate beyond the boundaries of the usual dyadic, patient–therapist relationship to be effective in the multilayered care delivery system of the psychiatric hospital.

Agendas for inpatient CT sessions include topics that are not encountered in work with outpatients. Issues such as the stigma of hospitalization, concerns regarding being away from family or spouse, or reactions to living in a hospital environment may require attention. The removal of the inpatient from his or her natural environment, although advantageous in many ways, also reduces the opportunities to deal directly with real-life situations. This feature of hospitalization is counterbalanced by the opportunity to use the inpatient milieu as a laboratory to learn and use cognitive therapy techniques.

Inpatient CT must also be tailored to the length of hospital stay. The duration of hospitalization is not under the direct control of the therapist but is often molded by the patient's life circumstances, the willingness of insurance carriers to underwrite continuing hospitalization, and the deliberations of hospital utilization review committees (Hersen,1985). A short length of stay (2–3 weeks in many current inpatient programs) places demands on the cognitive therapist to organize treatment in the most efficient manner possible.

Modifications of Cognitive Therapy for Inpatients

The following adaptations of standard outpatient CT (see Chapter 1 for a description of basic procedures) are offered as general guidelines for clinical practice with inpatients.

1. *Focus on symptom relief*. Goals for inpatient CT should take into account the short time period available for treatment and the patient's need to resume social and occupational functioning. The emphasis is on relieving symptoms and developing problem-solving skills that can be transferred to the outpatient setting. Long-term goals can be deferred until patients are well enough to leave the hospital and continue with outpatient therapy.
2. *Adjust length and frequency of sessions*. Because of the severity of

disorders, and the brief time for treatment during an inpatient stay, therapy sessions should be shorter (30 minutes or less) and more frequent (often daily) than the customary weekly or biweekly outpatient appointment. Longer sessions may be more productive after the patient starts to improve, but lengthy therapy encounters can overwhelm the severely ill hospitalized patient (Scott, 1989).

3. *Involve ancillary therapists*. Cognitive therapy in a hospital setting usually includes other treatment team members who serve as ancillary therapists. Interventions can be carried out throughout the day by various staff members (e.g., nurses, occupational therapists, social workers) who have opportunities to interact with the patient.

4. *Integrate therapeutic efforts*. The cognitive therapist may work in parallel with a pharmacotherapist, family therapist, consulting internist, group therapist, and others. The patient will be buffeted with ideas and suggestions from all of these sources. The individual therapist needs to take the major responsibility for developing a comprehensive case conceptualization and for insuring that the members of the multidisciplinary team work in concert.

5. *Assign homework in the milieu*. Homework assignments can be facilitated by staff members under the supervision of the primary therapist. The patient's efforts can be supported, and feedback on progress can be given promptly. Also, staff members can assist the patient in identifying and surmounting barriers to completion of the assignment.

6. *Use the hospital setting to identify "hot" cognitions*. The inpatient milieu provides a rich network of treatment activities, interpersonal events, and other stimuli that can induce automatic thoughts and intense emotion. For example, a 45-year-old man was terrified about a scheduled family visit. His therapist recognized that the surge in anxiety was related to dysfunctional thinking and was able to elicit a chain of negative automatic thoughts. Cognitive distortions were modified, and a role-playing exercise was used to prepare the patient for the visit. The inpatient setting allows the therapist to have much closer proximity to the actual events that generate cognitive distortion than is usually the case in treatment of outpatients.

7. *Take advantage of distance from environmental stressors*. Often patients will be admitted to the hospital because they are unable to cope with severe environmental stress and have developed disabling symptoms. Removal from the stressful situation allows time for reconceptualizing problem-solving strategies while in a "safe" environment. This point is illustrated in the case of a 36-year-old woman who was admitted after a suicide attempt. She described marked hopelessness about her home situation where she was faced with an abusive husband and two mentally retarded children. The hospital environment provided pro-

tection from her husband and respite from what appeared to be overwhelming child care responsibilities. She and her therapist were able to use this opportunity to build self-esteem, identify maladaptive behaviors, and practice new coping strategies.

SCREENING AND SELECTION OF PATIENTS

The Referral Process

The process by which inpatients are selected for cognitive therapy will vary depending on the organization of the hospital unit. In settings where the attending psychiatrist is not a cognitive therapist, or where CT is not the predominant treatment philosophy (e.g., "add-on" model—see Chapter 3), patients are usually referred by the physician to a cognitive therapy specialist for individual therapy. Although the referral source has deemed the patient suitable for this form of treatment, a more systematic evaluation process is often required to conclude that a trial of CT is indicated.

When the unit is more cognitively oriented (e.g. primary therapist and comprehensive models—see Chapter 3), patients who meet screening criteria for CT are routinely assigned to this type of treatment. If the staff model (see Chapter 3) is used, all patients receive cognitive therapy. Selection criteria for CT are applied before admission, and those who are not good candidates for cognitively oriented treatment are sent to other units.

Case Selection

Table 4.1 contains a list of diagnoses for which CT can be considered either a primary or an auxiliary treatment. We use the primary designation to indicate conditions for which CT may be employed without other adjunctive treatments such as pharmacotherapy. However, in practice most hospitalized patients receive combined psychotherapy and pharmacotherapy (see Chapter 7). For disorders in the primary category of Table 4.1, CT has either been previously established as an effective treatment or there is substantial literature that describes the clinical utility of the approach. In situations where cognitive therapy is considered to be an auxiliary treatment, there is little or no data to suggest that CT alone can be effective in treating the condition, but case studies or preliminary investigations indicate that it can help reduce symptoms associated with the disorder.

The most suitable candidates for the full CT treatment program

TABLE 4.1. Case Selection Criteria: Individual Cognitive Therapy

Cognitive therapy used as a primary treatment	Cognitive therapy used as an auxiliary treatment	Cognitive therapy not indicated
Major depression, nonpsychotic Anxiety disorders Most personality disorders Eating disorders Substance abuse	Major depression, psychotic Bipolar disorder Schizophrenia Schizoaffective disorder Mild dementia with depression anxiety	Severe dementia Acute delerium Moderate to severe mental retardation

are those with a diagnosis of major depression or anxiety disorders (Wright, 1988; Wright & Borden, 1991). Many forms of personality disorders also respond well to cognitive therapy (Beck, Freeman, & Associates, 1990; Young, 1990). However, in our experience, patients with antisocial personality structures are unlikely to have the capacity to form an effective, collaborative therapeutic relationship during a brief hospitalization. Individuals with borderline personality disorder are often admitted to the hospital when they become self-destructive. These patients can respond to CT if procedures are adjusted to account for potential distortions in the therapist–patient relationship. Personality disorders usually require long-term treatment (see Chapter 14). Thus, the inpatient stay is a relatively brief component of the total therapy experience for these individuals.

Cognitive therapy can also be regarded as a primary treatment for patients with eating disorders (Garner & Bemis, 1982, 1985; Fairburn, 1985; Agras, Schneider, Arnow, Raeburn, & Telch, 1989). Behavioral procedures are an important part of the therapy program for these individuals (see Chapter 13). There is a well-described methodology for use of CT for persons who are addicted to alcohol or drugs (Emery, Hollon, & Bedrosian, 1981; Marlatt & Gordon, 1985; Chapter 12 of this volume).

Factors that may favorably influence the course of CT with outpatients include good problem-solving ability, minimal impairment of learning and memory functioning, and a high desire for self-control (Wright & Salmon, 1990; Murphy, Simons, Wetzel, & Lustman, 1984; Sotsky et al., 1991). Inpatients rarely have a coalescence of all of these ideal features. Nevertheless, therapy procedures can be adjusted to work with the hospitalized patient "as is" (see coming sections in this chapter on Process of Inpatient Cognitive Therapy and Treating Target

Symptoms). The support of the family or a significant other and the patient's initial response to or identification with the cognitive model are also important (Teasdale, Fennell, Hibbert, & Amies, 1984). Outpatients who respond well to CT usually show significant improvement by the time they have had three or four sessions (Murphy et al., 1984). However, inpatients with more severe or complicated disorders may take longer to engage in therapy.

Limited research has been done regarding exclusion criteria for cognitive therapy. However, based on case studies and clinical experience, it appears that patients with organic brain syndromes, mental retardation, or severely impaired reality-testing (e.g., acute schizophrenia, florid mania, major depression with pronounced delusions or hallucinations) are unlikely to respond well to standard cognitive therapy. With some of these patients, modifications of techniques or addition of pharmacotherapy may allow CT to play a significant role in the overall treatment plan (Wright, 1987; Wright & Schrodt, 1989; Kingdon & Turkington, 1991a, 1991b). Later in this chapter, we describe cognitive and behavioral procedures for affective psychoses. Therapy of elderly patients with mild memory impairment is discussed in Chapter 11, and cognitive interventions for schizophrenics are detailed in Chapter 14. We recommend against attempting CT with patients who are admitted with severe dementia, acute delirium, or moderate to severe mental retardation.

DIAGNOSIS AND ASSESSMENT STRATEGIES

Assessment of inpatients who have depression and other psychiatric conditions is usually performed on several levels. The first step is to use the DSM-III-R categorization system developed by the American Psychiatric Association (1987). Questions regarding symptoms such as sleep, concentration, energy, loss of interest, or change in affect allow the therapist to establish an accurate diagnosis. The Beck Depression Inventory (Beck, Ward, Mendelson, Mock, & Erbaugh, 1961) and the Hamilton Rating Scale for Depression (Hamilton, 1960) can also give valuable information concerning the syndrome of depression, including the intensity of the disorder and range of symptoms. The Hopelessness Scale (Beck, Weissman, Lester, & Trexler, 1974) and the Scale for Suicide Ideation (Beck, Kovacs, & Weissman, 1979) provide data that are useful in estimating the risk of self-destructive behavior. Levels of anxiety can be measured with the Beck Anxiety Inventory (Beck, Brown, Epstein, & Steer, 1988) or the State–Trait Anxiety Inventory (Spielberger, 1983).

Other paper-and-pencil tests facilitate examination of cognitive structures and processes (Dobson & Shaw, 1986). The Automatic Thoughts Questionnaire (Hollon & Kendall, 1980) measures the frequency of certain negative thoughts characteristically reported by depressed patients. Maladaptive or dysfunctional beliefs can be quantified with the Dysfunctional Attitude Scale (DAS; Weissman, 1979). However, questions have been raised concerning the utility of the DAS in detecting changes associated with short-term hospitalization (Bowers, 1989; Miller, Norman, Keitner, Bishop, & Dow, 1989).

During therapy sessions, cognitions are assessed directly by involving patients in identifying and reporting negative thoughts. Assignments to monitor self-statements while in the session or to record thoughts and feelings in the interval between sessions are usually of considerable therapeutic value. The Daily Record of Dysfunctional Thoughts (Beck, Rush, et al., 1979) or modifications of this recording device (e.g., a sheet of paper used to record negative thoughts and feelings in two columns) provide clinically relevant methods of assessing the effect of dysfunctional cognitions on mood.

The involvement of hospital staff in assessment and monitoring is also important. One of the instruments most commonly used in cognitive therapy units is the Daily Activity Schedule (Beck, Rush, et al., 1979). Staff members assist patients in using this form to estimate the degree of mastery and pleasure associated with specific activities. Other information provided by the hospital staff during team meetings or informal conversations can be extremely helpful. For example, staff observations of the response to a therapeutic out-trip assisted with the treatment of Mr. D, a 45-year old man with an agitated depression. The patient's family reported that Mr. D had functioned very well prior to the onset of depression. He was a high school teacher who had experienced much success as a public speaker. Yet, on Mr. D's first therapeutic trip outside the hospital, staff members noted that he became highly anxious when he tried to communicate with others (e.g., order a meal at a restaurant, purchase sundries at a drug store). Further investigation by the individual therapist revealed a highly maladaptive chain of negative automatic thoughts in these situations (e.g., "They must be staring at me. . . . I'm pitiful. . . . How will I ever face my students again?").

STAGES OF THERAPY

The therapy phases for an inpatient are somewhat different from the general plan for CT outlined in Chapter 1. Fewer sessions are compressed into a shorter time period, and a number of additional ingredients are added to the usual treatment package. A template for the stages of inpatient treatment of depression is presented in Table 4.2. Considerable individual variability may be encountered in the patient's ability to grasp concepts or utilize CT techniques. The therapist needs to adjust the pace of therapy to account for these idiosyncrasies.

Most commonly, the early part of therapy is devoted to assessment, socialization to therapy, building a collaborative relationship, initiation

TABLE 4.2. Inpatient Cognitive Therapy of Depression: Treatment Stages

Early phase Sessions 1–3	Middle phase Sessions 4–10	Late phase Sessions 10–Discharge
Assessment Develop collaborative relationship Socialize to cognitive model Generate problem list Reduce hopelessness and suicide risk Initiate activity scheduling and recording Identify negative automatic thoughts Start therapy notebook Introduce homework Read unit cognitive therapy handbook Read *Coping with Depression* (Beck & Greenberg, 1974)	Continue activity scheduling and recording Identify and modify negative automatic thoughts Use daily record of dysfunctional thoughts Recognize recurrent themes in automatic thoughts Initiate graded task assignments Use milieu activities to identify cognitions, test hypotheses, practice changes in behavior Participate in group and family cognitive therapy (if available) Continue therapy notebook and homework assignments Read unit cognitive therapy handbook Read *Feeling Good* (Burns, 1980)	Reduce emphasis on activity scheduling and recording Continue graded task assignments Continue to identify and modify negative automatic thoughts Use daily record of dysfunctional thoughts Identify and modify schemas Continue use of milieu activities to facilitate cognitive therapy Continue to participate in group and family therapy (if available) Learn problem-solving skills Learn relapse prevention strategies Continue therapy notebook and homework assignments

of behavioral procedures, and demonstration of the cognitive model of depression or anxiety (Thase & Wright, 1991). Inpatients usually have disabling symptoms such as marked agitation, muscle tension, insomnia, or severe inertia that can be reduced through behavioral measures such as activity scheduling or relaxation training. Cognitive interventions may be more successfully implemented when physiological arousal is reduced and attention can be focused more easily on acquisition of new concepts (Thase & Wright, 1991). However, at times, inpatients are capable of doing intensive cognitive work, including the identification and modification of schemas, from the outset of treatment (Wright, in press).

During the first part of therapy, a problem list is developed, and the therapist begins to suggest procedures that can help to reduce symptoms. Eliciting automatic thoughts and emotions generated by a very recent life experience is a particularly helpful way of teaching the patient about cognitive therapy while starting to relieve his or her distress. The unit CT handbook and a brief pamphlet that explains cognitive therapy are frequently given to the patient as early homework assignments. Another important task in the beginning stage of therapy with an inpatient is reduction of hopelessness and risk for suicide. This topic is discussed in detail later in the chapter.

The middle portion of therapy with an inpatient is centered on maximizing the utility of cognitive and behavioral interventions throughout the milieu. The individual therapist introduces cognitive techniques such as thought recording, hypothesis generation and testing, and listing advantages and disadvantages of cognitions or behaviors. At the same time, learning is reinforced in multiple therapy settings in the milieu (e.g., group therapy, unit community meeting, family therapy). Additional readings and homework assignments are used to supplement these activities.

As the patient approaches discharge, there usually has been a substantial reduction in symptoms, plus gains in self-esteem, problem-solving capacity, and ability to function in social and occupational roles. Activity scheduling and recording become less important. At this point, the patient often is able to recognize recurrent patterns or themes of automatic thoughts and to identify underlying maladaptive schemas. Work can begin on schema modification, but full attention to change in this area may need to be reserved for outpatient follow-up treatment sessions. Perhaps the most significant goal for the last part of hospitalization is learning strategies that can help forestall relapse. Chapter 15 is devoted to this important component of inpatient treatment.

THE PROCESS OF INPATIENT COGNITIVE THERAPY

Cognitive and Behavioral Techniques

The full spectrum of techniques used in standard cognitive therapy (Beck, Rush, et al., 1979; Wright & Beck, 1983; Wright, 1988) may be considered for application in hospital settings. These procedures include guided discovery (Socratic questioning), recognition of cognitive errors, identification and modification of automatic thoughts, schema revision, activity scheduling, graded-task assignments, homework, and a variety of other interventions. Basic CT techniques have been explained in Chapter 1 and will not be recounted in detail here. Instead, we focus on cognitive therapy processes that require significant adaptation for inpatient use or that have a particular impact on the hospital milieu.

The Therapeutic Relationship

The principles of collaborative empiricism described by Beck and coworkers (Beck, Rush, et al., 1979; Wright & Beck, 1983; Schrodt & Wright, 1987) give inpatient CT a somewhat different tone from that of many other approaches to hospital psychiatry. Behavioral procedures such as activity scheduling or use of the level system (i.e., progressing through "privilege" levels) are done "with" instead of "to" patients. Also, the patient becomes an active partner in establishing the agenda and goals for therapy.

The therapist encourages the patient to give feedback about the treatment process. Are there problems on the unit? Is the therapist being understood? What suggestions does the patient have? Was the homework assignment on target? As the therapy progresses, the patient and therapist form a team that fosters personal growth, acquisition of problem-solving skills, and utilization of self-help techniques. The chances of problems such as excessive dependency or regression developing in the hospital environment are minimized by this approach.

Socialization to Therapy

Socializing patients to the cognitive model helps them understand the rationale for the treatment and assists with rapid entry into the most productive phases of therapy. Although a few patients may come to the unit with some prior knowledge of cognitive therapy, most will not have had any experience with this approach. Socialization to individual therapy takes place at the same time the patient is adapting to the rest of the milieu. Units that have a pervasive cognitive orientation make the job of the individual therapist easier by providing information in orientation groups, community meetings, and psychoeducational sessions (see Chapter 3). However, the individual therapist plays an important role in socialization to CT in all types of inpatient cognitive therapy units.

The most powerful way to introduce the patient to cognitive therapy is to illustrate the utility of the cognitive model with a situation or symptom that is deeply troubling the patient. "Learning by doing" usually has a pronounced effect if the patient can experience a significant change of painful affect. For example, a 45-year-old man was admitted to the unit after drinking a quart of Scotch and swallowing 25 sleeping tablets (flurazepam). He reported, "I've lost everything, I can't go on." During the course of the initial interview, the inpatient therapist identified a precipitating event (wife had left the patient) and a series of catastrophically negative cognitions (e.g., "I have no purpose left in life. . . . Without a woman, I'm nothing. . . . Who would want me?"). Marked depression and self-destructive behavior had followed this maladaptive cognitive response to his wife's departure. The therapist was able to use this highly charged therapy material to explain the links between life events, cognitions, emotions, and behavior. Cognitive errors such as selective abstraction and absolutistic thinking were identified; and Socratic questioning was directed at uncovering personal strengths, remaining interpersonal relationships, and opportunities for future growth.

In addition, it is usually helpful to give a brief explanation of the basic principles of cognitive therapy. The discussion should include a description of the different roles of patient and therapist and the need for effective collaboration. The importance of agenda setting and homework should also be emphasized. Socialization to the inpatient milieu is another necessary step in engaging the patient in therapy. This can be done, in part, with patient manuals, orientation groups, and sessions with nursing staff. The individual therapist's attention to this process can be advantageous in several ways: (1) the therapy bond is strengthened as the therapist shows concern for the patient's total treatment experience; (2) misunderstandings, confusion, and distortions about the milieu can be identified and corrected; and (3) a cohesive, multidisciplinary treatment approach is encouraged from the beginning of therapy. Bibliotherapy is also used as part of the socialization process. Pamphlets and books can help the patient learn the basic principles of cognitive therapy or understand disorders such as depression, anxiety, or bulimia. Commonly used materials include *Coping with Depression* (Beck & Greenberg, 1974), *Feeling Good* (Burns, 1980), *Cognitive Therapy and the Emotional Disorders* (Beck, 1976), and *Own Your Own Life* (Emery, 1982).

The Structure of Therapy

The use of structuring techniques is one of the hallmarks of cognitive therapy. There are several reasons why these procedures are especially important for inpatients. First, the hospitalized patient usually comes to treatment in a demoralized and confused state. Often marked disruptions of the regularity of the daily schedule have occurred. Work, sleep, meals, and use of leisure time are all in a state of disregulation. In addition, the inpatient is likely to have more pronounced forms of impaired concentration or learning and memory functioning than are seen with outpatients (Wright & Salmon, 1990).

The major structuring procedures used routinely in CT include agenda setting; feedback regulation; learning reinforcement; use of written diagrams, instructions, and assignments; and activity scheduling. Perhaps the most important structuring tool is the basic format of cognitive therapy itself. As opposed to nonspecific psychotherapies, CT offers pragmatic theories and well-defined treatment procedures that can be understood by both patient and therapist. Thus, the patient can follow a clearly marked path to recovery.

Structuring usually begins with setting an agenda. This helps guide the patient and therapist to an efficient use of therapy time. At the beginning of the session, the patient and therapist propose topics for the agenda. The items should be somewhat circumscribed so that the patient can attend to the therapeutic task without being overwhelmed by perceived difficulties. The therapist might say, "Let's make a list of the problems or issues that you want to discuss today." If the topics are very general (e.g., a troubled relationship, work conflicts, or low self-esteem), the therapist might then say, "It would help if we could focus on a specific concern that you have in this area." Reducing the field of discussion to manageable tasks can significantly diminish the patient's sense of hopelessness and helplessness (Wright, 1988).

The choice of agenda items depends on which issues are most troubling to the patient, the likelihood of solving a problem, the general severity of the patient's disorder, and the stage of therapy. Flexibility in setting and following the agenda is important, especially if an acute crisis arises. Initially, the therapist may take the lead in shaping the agenda. However, as therapy progresses, increasing responsibility for setting the agenda is given to the patient.

The therapist stops often during the session to both give and request feedback. These interchanges help to avoid confusion or misinterpretation. For example, after explaining a concept, a therapist posed the following question: "We have just talked about an example from your own experience of different types of cognitive errors; I want to make sure we are understanding one another; could you recap what you've learned?" Writing is another useful structuring device. The therapist can suggest that the patient keep a therapy notebook during the inpatient stay. This exercise reinforces the acquisition of CT concepts while the patient is in the hospital and helps tie together material from individual, group, and family therapy sessions. The therapy notebook also can be a valuable resource for review of CT procedures after discharge from the unit.

The Daily Activity Schedule provides another opportunity for structuring. Therapeutic use of the daily schedule is described in detail in Chapters 1 and 3. It is important for the individual therapist to interact with other team members and the patient in constructing a daily schedule that matches the patient's level of functioning and ability to utilize the various treatment opportunities in the milieu.

Cognitive Case Conceptualization

The conceptualization should include both a cross-sectional and a longitudinal or developmental analysis. A cross-sectional conceptualization involves breaking down each of the patient's problems into the following domains: situation, cognition, affect, and behavior. This method of formulating an inpatient case is shown in Table 4.3. Treatment inter-

TABLE 4.3. Cross-Sectional Cognitive Case Conceptualization

Problem	Cognitions	Affect	Behavior
Difficulty accepting hospitalization	"I'm weak because I had to come to the hospital." "I'm a burden on everyone."	Sadness Guilt	Social withdrawal in hospital
Relationship with husband	"He will leave me if I don't get better soon." "He is probably with someone else right now."	Anxiety Anger	Avoid discussing disorder with spouse Deliberate attempts to please spouse
Obesity	"I'm no good." "I'll never get control of this."	Depression Anxiety	Bingeing Self-induced vomiting

ventions should be systematically matched to the cognitive and behavioral pathology identified in the case conceptualization.

A longitudinal formulation of the patient's problems can be facilitated by asking the following key questions: (1) What are the patient's characteristic automatic thoughts? (2) What cognitive errors are involved in these thoughts? (3) What schemas or underlying assumptions are operating for this patient? (4) How were these acquired? These questions help the therapist to integrate the patient's history, negative automatic thoughts, distorted beliefs, and current life stressors in a logical and comprehensive manner. The goal is to understand how past learning experiences (and the resultant schemas) have contributed to the patient's current problems. A good case conceptualization not only provides a blueprint for intervention but also assists the therapist in predicting obstacles to treatment (Persons, 1989). The case conceptualization is only a set of theories about the nature and dimensions of the patient's psychological problems. This formulation needs to be validated or reconfigured after consideration of data uncovered by the therapy process. The inpatient setting allows excellent opportunities, including around-the-clock observation and the provision of many different challenges or tests to the patient, to refine the case conceptualization.

Mr. S, a depressed inpatient, listed poor self-esteem as one of his major problems. Staff members observed his reactions in a variety of hospital situations and reported that he became very self-critical whenever he thought his performance was being observed critically. This occurred in one instance when the patient group was trying to choose a movie to watch on the unit's VCR. Mr. S suggested in a tentative manner that the group select a classic movie, but he was quickly overruled by the majority who were interested in viewing a newly released thriller. He tried to maintain a facade of self-assurance. However, staff members noted increased body tension and a sad facial expression.

After the group discussion, one of the nurses sat down to talk with Mr. S. What had he been thinking when the others decided not to accept his suggestion? After several more questions, he revealed a series of automatic thoughts that suggested an underlying schema about perfectionism. Mr. S. had responded to the movie selection process by thinking: "I'm a real jerk for bringing up an idea that the others won't accept; if I decide to do something, I must succeed; there is no room for failure."

The information from this interchange was used to get a more detailed picture of the sources of Mr. S's low self-esteem. Mr. S and his therapist agreed that a modification of his maladaptive, perfectionistic schemas could lead to an improved self-concept and a reduction in depressive symptoms. They decided to generate a list of perfectionistic schemas, to write a table of advantages and disadvantages for each of the schemas, and to begin to explore the development of alternative views.

TREATING TARGET SYMPTOMS

Hopelessness

Suicidal ideation or attempts are among the most common presenting problems of inpatients. Because suicide risk is strongly associated with the level of hopelessness (Beck, Kovacs, & Weissman, 1975; Wetzel, 1976), the inpatient cognitive therapist frequently selects this symptom as the most important target for intervention during the first few days of hospitalization. One of the advantages of CT is that it can rapidly reduce hopelessness and thereby lessen the risk of suicide (Rush, Beck, Kovacs, Weissenburger, & Hollon, 1982). We regularly see patients who are admitted with abject hopelessness and intense suicidality but who, within a very brief time, develop a positive outlook for the future and a genuine desire to live.

Of course, precautions against suicide should be instituted until the suicidal crisis is past. During this period, the cognitive therapist begins to combat hopelessness in an active and direct way by: (1) establishing a strong collaborative relationship; (2) identifying environmental events that have triggered suicidal thinking; (3) eliciting negative cognitions associated with suicidality; (4) attempting to modify these negative cognitions; (5) generating a list of reasons to live; (6) developing alternate solutions to the patient's problems; and (7) obtaining a commitment from the patient to try the therapy process before taking any action to harm himself or herself.

These steps were followed with Mr. O, a 52-year-old man with a history of chronic schizophrenia, who was admitted to the hospital after becoming depressed, hopeless, and suicidal. He had taken an overdose of 40 lorazepam tablets and had been surprised to wake up alive. Mr. O told the admitting doctor: "There is no future. . . . My life is over. . . . Just let me die."

Mr. O's rapid slide into a suicidal state had been precipitated by two environmental events. His wife, who was also a schizophrenic, was admitted to the state hospital after a relapse, and a daughter had been arrested for drug abuse. Mr. O had been maintained on fluphenazine decanoate (Prolixin decanoate®) for several years. At the time of admission he had low-grade paranoia but no hallucinations. The predominant symptoms of schizophrenia were those of the "negative" variety: apathy, social isolation, and impaired interpersonal relationships.

Mr. O's hopelessness and suicidal ideation responded to cognitive therapy within the first 24 hours of treatment. No changes in the drug regimen were required. After taking a careful history and establishing a collaborative relationship, the cognitive therapist began to explore Mr. O's cognitions regarding the problems with his wife and daughter. Mr. O reported: "I've lost everything now. . . . I'll never see them again. . . . I don't know how I can survive without them." Mr. O continued with a string of self-negating statements: "I'm nothing. . . . I don't enjoy anything, and I can't even do one single thing right."

The therapist responded as follows:

DR. W: I can see from the way you are thinking now that things look pretty hopeless.

MR. O: That's right. I wish my overdose had worked.

DR. W: Part of the problem may be in the way you are viewing the situation. Let's take a look at some of your thoughts. First you told me that you had lost everything. What do you mean?

MR. O: My wife's gone. My daughter's gone. There's nothing left.

DR. W: Let's check to see if they're really "gone." You talk as if they're "gone" for good. Has your wife been in the hospital before?

MR. O: Yes, four or five times.

DR. W: How long does she stay?

MR. O: Oh, anywhere from just a couple of days to a month or so.

DR. W: And usually what is the effect of being admitted for treatment?

MR. O: She gets better for a while.

DR. W: Could you find out how long she will be in the hospital this time?

MR. O: I guess I could call—I didn't think to do that.

DR. W: If you have some information on your wife's condition, you could start to plan how to cope with her being away instead of jumping to the conclusion that she is gone for good.

MR. O: I guess you're right. Everything seemed to happen at once. I just got overwhelmed.

DR. W: That happens sometimes. If we take your problems one at a time, we can draw up ways to manage them. Now let's talk about your daughter.

They went on to discuss Mr. O's reactions to his daughter's drug abuse and to outline a plan for ways in which he could try to be supportive to her as she entered a drug rehabilitation program. The first session also involved the recognition of positive reasons for living. This is one of our routine interventions for hospitalized patients. Mr. O's list included the following items: (1) "My wife and daughter—I know they'll get out of treatment, and we'll be together again." (2) "My two grandchildren—I really love them and want to be around to see them grow up." (3) "I enjoy my ceramics—I want to try some new techniques and sell what I make at flea markets." (4) "My church is very important to me." By the end of the session, Mr. O was much less hopeless and was able to commit to further cognitive therapy. He was discharged after 1 week of hospitalization.

Anxiety and Panic

Severe anxiety, panic attacks, and phobias are seen frequently in hospitalized patients. Some patients are admitted after experiencing virtually constant severe anxiety that has not responded to outpatient interventions. Cognitive and behavioral methods (Beck & Emery, 1985; Clark, Salkovskis, & Chalkley, 1985; Wright & Borden, 1991) such as modification of distorted cognitions regarding "danger," relaxation, imagery, graded exposure, distraction, and rehearsal of coping skills are very helpful with these patients. An educational approach including explanations, illustrations, and bibliotherapy materials such as "Coping with Anxiety" (in Beck & Emery, 1985) or *Coping with Panic* (Clum, 1990) can be a very beneficial facet of the treatment of anxious patients. However, with inpatients, the level of anxiety is often so high that relaxation procedures, distraction, or pharmacotherapy may be required before proceeding in this direction.

The manner in which the cognitive model of anxiety might be introduced to help educate a patient about his or her disorder and its consequences can be seen in the following excerpt from a therapy session:

Ms. R: If I am very nervous, I get these terrible feelings . . . like everything seems unreal around me. Then I'm terrified that I am going to go really crazy.

Dr. L: And what happens then after you have those thoughts and feel scared?

Ms. R: I feel worse and worse. Then I get more strange feelings . . . like my sight seems different. After that, I worry even more.

DR. L: This is what we call the vicious cycle of anxiety. Your emotions, your bodily sensations, and your thoughts all build on one another. Let me make a diagram for you on paper of how the vicious cycle develops for you. Then we will look at a possible explanation of this "unreal" feeling that can help you cope with your fears of going crazy. If you could think differently about your anxiety, it might prevent the cycle from building up. How does this sound to you?

MS. R: Okay. I'd like to understand this thing better and start to control it, if I can.

The therapist then proceeded to diagram a cognitive model for anxiety (Wright & Borden, 1991) and to elicit examples from the patient's own experiences to illustrate the links between anxious thoughts, physiological arousal, and behavioral responses.

Relaxation therapy, training in respiratory control (Clark et al., 1985), and graded exposure can be carried out in individual therapy and also by other staff members who are trained to utilize these procedures. Many units have an expressive therapist, a biofeedback technician, or an occupational therapist who has special skills in anxiety management procedures. These individuals can augment the efforts of the individual therapist in bringing anxiety down to a manageable level. Removal from outside stress may lead to a reduction in panic attacks or episodes of anxiety while the patient is in the hospital. Thus, exposure to outside stimuli, either through imagery or on planned trips outside the hospital, is usually needed in order for the patient to confront the feared situations before discharge. If the patient's panic attacks or anxiety episodes are triggered in the inpatient setting, the therapist has the advantage of obtaining *in vivo* information about the situation–cognition–affect–behavior link. For example, when a patient experiences a panic attack during a hospital activity, a staff member can question the patient while the actual attack is in progress. What feelings (emotions) is he or she having? What sensations are being experienced? How are these sensations being interpreted? What is the feared outcome? When the cognitions and feelings are identified in this way, cognitive and behavioral interventions can be carried out "on the spot" to help reduce the level of anxiety.

Self-Esteem

Many of the adjunctive therapies and group activities available in the hospital milieu can complement individual CT by helping promote more realistic self-appraisal and an improved self-concept. The therapist can also instruct the patient in a variety of strategies for dealing with low self-esteem. These include keeping a daily journal of positive thoughts and events, recognizing assets on a checklist of positive traits, mastery and pleasure recording, carrying out behavioral tests of negative predictions of ability, and recognizing distortions in self-evaluative thinking (McKay & Fanning, 1987; Burns, 1980). For example, the patient who is very self-critical can be taught to recognize that he or she has frequent cognitive errors such as absolutistic thinking, personalization, and selective abstraction (Wright & Beck, 1983). The patient then can start to correct these distortions when they occur.

Mr. J was a 42-year-old man who was admitted to the hospital because of an agitated depression and suicidal ideation. His pronounced low self-esteem was captured in the repetitive self-statement: "I'm incapable of love." He was convinced of the validity of this cognition despite a solid marriage of over 20 years. Financial difficulties had stressed the marriage somewhat, but otherwise Mr. J's wife described the marriage in positive terms. She also noted that he had excellent relationships with his three children. Mr. J's therapist directly attacked the distorted self-concept by asking Mr. J to recount incidents in his life where he had been able to show or receive affection by family members. Together they also began to identify cognitive errors that reinforced his negative self-concept. Part of the therapy involved a reframing of his concepts about his role in significant relationships. Mr. J came to recognize that he had difficulties with openly expressing his feelings. Nevertheless, he had been able to establish long-standing loving relationships with his family members.

Interpersonal Problems and Social Skills Deficits

The group living arrangement of the hospital provides a microcosm for reenacting the interpersonal difficulties experienced by the patient. The inpatient setting can provide a structured, safe environment to work on these issues. For example, behavioral experiments to test out predictions regarding social situations can be carried out as homework assignments in the hospital milieu. Patients who make negative assumptions regarding how other people think about them can be encouraged to examine the validity of these cognitions by collecting data on how other people actually do react to them while in the hospital.

Cognitive–behavioral procedures can be used with benefit in the treatment of social anxiety, self-consciousness, and shyness. Particularly useful procedures include assertiveness training, decentering, role play, relaxation training, and cognitive behavioral rehearsal (Beck & Emery, 1985; Burns, 1985). Ms. M was a 27-year-old secretary who was admitted after she concluded that "No one would ever want me." She was reasonably attractive, had above-average intelligence, and had held a steady job for 8 years. Yet, she was painfully self-conscious and could not initiate any social activities. As a result, she had become increasingly lonely and isolated.

In addition to identifying and modifying distorted cognitions, Ms. M's therapist believed that social-skills training would be required to reverse actual behavioral deficits. They began with imagery procedures that reconstructed Ms. M's habitual maladaptive behavior in several key situations (e.g., expressing her opinion to others, starting a social conversation, meeting a potential friend). A list of alternate behaviors was generated, and role-play exercises were used to practice them. Auxiliary nurse therapists were used to help with the role plays. They "modeled" effective interpersonal behavior. Ms. M also attended an assertiveness training group. As a final step in the inpatient phase of therapy, she tried out some of her newly acquired skills *in vivo* as part of a graded task assignment.

SPECIAL ISSUES IN COGNITIVE THERAPY WITH INPATIENTS

Reactions to Hospitalization

Concerns about being a patient in a psychiatric hospital may emerge as topics for individual CT sessions. Guilt, shame, and self-deprecation related to the stigma of hospitalization are frequent agenda items early in therapy, whereas fears of leaving the hospital may become important as discharge nears. Other issues, such as problems in group living or conflicts with staff members, may become important during the hospital stay. Also, the patient may experience difficulties during family visitations or while on therapeutic passes outside the hospital. These issues should be included on the agenda for individual sessions and handled in a systematic manner employing usual CT procedures.

Multiple Therapies

Inpatients rarely receive CT "alone," without being influenced by other treatment approaches practiced in the milieu. When a number of different psychotherapies are conducted with the same patient, the multidisciplinary team needs to articulate a comprehensive treatment plan in order to ensure that a consistent message is given to the patient (see Chapter 3). Inpatients often receive combined cognitive therapy and pharmacotherapy. In such cases, the cognitive therapist should work with the pharmacotherapist to identify and manage conflicts arising out of combined treatment. Resolution can usually be achieved by developing an inclusive cognitive–biological treatment model that can be endorsed by the entire treatment team. Wright (1987) has described how a patient can be given a consistent treatment framework when CT and medication are used together. Combined treatment approaches are discussed further in Chapter 7.

Affective Psychoses

On most inpatient units, depressed patients with pronounced delusions are unlikely to be considered for a CT program, at least until some initial response to pharmacotherapy has occurred. However, cognitive interventions have been described for delusions and other psychotic symptoms (Wright, 1987; Perris, 1989; Wright & Schrodt, 1989; Fowler & Morley, 1989; Kingdon & Turkington, 1991a, 1991b). Bishop, Miller, Norman, Buda, & Foulke (1986) have observed that delusional thinking in a patient with psychotic depression can be treated with cognitive methods, particularly "examining the evidence" and generating alternative explanations.

Setting mutual goals is an important facet of the cognitive approach to affective psychoses. Finding some common ground regarding symptoms or other problems that the patient and the therapist want to change (e.g., sleep disturbance, lack of enjoyment, restlessness) is crucial. The use of structuring procedures, such as agenda setting, is also vital with such patients because they usually have disorganized thinking and behavior. Behavioral procedures that reduce tension or foster increased functioning are used heavily in the early part of treatment. Challenging the validity of delusions is usually reserved until a good collaborative relationship has been established and the patient has had experience in using guided discovery or other cognitive procedures to help with nondelusional issues.

Cognitive therapy was used as an adjunct to a combined antidepressant and antipsychotic medication regimen for Mrs. F, a 66-year old former dancing teacher who had somatic delusions. Despite an exhaustive medical evaluation and the frequent reassurances of her internist, she believed she had "cancer through my whole body." Physical symptoms were rather bizarre. Her complaints included: "My uterus is falling out; my stomach won't digest anything; and everything tastes like wool." She went on to say that "Nobody believes me, but I know I'm right."

The cognitive therapist began the treatment in a nonconfrontative way by collecting a complete history, without giving cues to Mrs. F that he disbelieved her complaints. This allowed him to identify several problems that he thought Mrs. F could accept as goals for therapy.

DR. W: You've told me about a number of different symptoms. You are concerned about cancer; but you've also mentioned not sleeping well, not being able to relax, not having energy, and losing interest in your usual activities.

MRS. F: That's right, I'm in pretty rough shape.

DR. W: Some of the symptoms that you mentioned can go along with depression, and you tell me you feel depressed.

MRS. F: Yes, it's all getting to me.

DR. W: Would you like to hear about ways that we can help relieve some of these symptoms.

MRS. F: I guess so, but nobody has been able to get to the bottom of this.

DR. W: I want to make sure you understand that we are not dealing now with the issue of whether or not you have cancer. We just want to get you feeling better so you can cope with this situation.

MRS. F: Well, I agree I need help. I'm so worked up I can hardly sit still.

They proceeded to practice relaxation and distraction procedures as a way of giving her short-term relief from her symptoms. An activity schedule was also introduced. After collecting base-line data, the therapist helped Mrs. F to arrange her day to include pleasurable and stress-reducing activities that were available on the unit. As Mrs. F began to feel somewhat better, rapport with the therapist improved, and they could begin to use guided discovery and other cognitive procedures. The somatic delusions were approached after Mrs. F had learned about the empirical basis of cognitive therapy.

MRS. F: I'm doing better, but I still can't get cancer off my mind.

DR. W: What kinds of thoughts go through your head when you worry about cancer?

MRS. F: I'm just obsessed with it, I guess. You know my mother died of colon cancer, and my sister had cancer of the pancreas. I'm all alone now, and it just seems like my time is up. My body doesn't feel right. It doesn't work like it should.

DR. W: Sometimes when people become depressed, they get all kinds of negative thoughts and fears, even about their health. What we can do is to look at your thoughts about your body in just the same way that we've checked out other areas—like guilty thoughts and low self-esteem. Would that be okay?

MRS. F: I don't see why not. Maybe I've let my fears run away from me.

This type of interchange would have been impossible at the beginning of therapy. The therapist had set the stage for this cognitive intervention by gradually building the therapeutic relationship and helping the patient to experience success in using cognitive and behavioral procedures.

DR. W: Let's start with your thoughts that your body doesn't work the way it should. I'd suggest we make a list of the sensations that bother you and then examine some of the alternate explanations for the problem.

MRS. F: Well, probably the worst thing is the constipation. Every time I have trouble with a bowel movement, I start to think I have cancer.

DR. W: Any other sensations that make you think you have cancer?

MRS. F: The pain in my stomach just won't go away, and I'm losing weight. That's about it. They've x-rayed me and used those scopes with the lights, but all they can find is a hiatal hernia. I just keep thinking they've missed something. I must have cancer; there's just too much wrong with me.

DR. W: I suppose there is a possibility that you have cancer even though all the tests were negative. I understand that you can never absolutely rule out cancer. However, there are some other possible explanations for your symptoms. Could we take a look at these?

MRS. F: All right.

Although CT has been used extensively with unipolar depressed patients, there have been only a few reports of treatment of bipolar disorder (Chorr, Mercier, & Halper, 1988; Wright & Schrodt, 1989). Bipolar patients are frequently encountered in an inpatient setting. When CT is used with this population, it is important that manic behavior or severe depression be controlled by medication so that the patient can concentrate sufficiently well to engage in the treatment process. Cognitive therapy can help bipolar patients acquire adaptive skills to cope with their mood cycles and plan activities congruent with these changes. It can also target some of the interpersonal problems that are seen in persons who have manic and depressed episodes (Wright & Schrodt, 1989).

Mrs. N was a 50-year-old woman with bipolar disorder who was admitted to the hospital after lapsing into a deep depression. She had been taking a combination of lithium carbonate and tranylcypromine, a monoamine oxidase inhibitor, but this regimen had not prevented the return of symptoms. Her psychiatrist reviewed different pharmacological options such as carbamazepine (Tegretol®) and valproic acid (Depakene®). At the same time, he attempted to modulate the depression with cognitive and behavioral procedures. During periods of depression, Mrs. N had a marked shift in her cognitive style. She became quite absolutistic, condemned herself for all her failings, and could remember little of her previous successes. The therapist approached this situation by explaining the effect of bipolar disorder on thinking processes and then engaging Mrs. N in exercises to interrupt her automatic, self-defeating cognitions.

One of their interchanges dealt with recognizing absolutistic thinking:

MRS. N: I've completely botched up my life.

DR. W: Here's another example of how extreme words just pop up into your mind and make you feel worse. Try to stand back from what you said and examine each of the words.

MRS. N: Okay, I'll try. I guess the "completely botched" is what you're concerned about.

DR. W: That's right. Those are pretty strong words. How accurate are they?

MRS. N: I've had my problems, but a lot of it wasn't my fault. I guess I've done some things right.

DR. W: That sounds more reasonable. People that get depressed often have very intense words, even inflammatory ones, that come into their heads on an automatic basis. It can help if we learn to spot them and try to reduce their influence—just like we did right now.

Physical or Sexual Abuse

It has been estimated that up to one-half of female inpatients have experienced sexual abuse (Beck, James, & VanderKolk, 1987; Jacobsen & Richardson, 1987). However, patients may not readily reveal histories of victimization unless a good relationship is established with their therapist, and the treatment team is sensitive to cues that abuse has occurred. Repetitive problems with low self-esteem, guilt and shame, self-abuse, chronic suicidal ideation, conflicted sexual relationships, and dissociative experiences may indicate that the patient has been a victim of sexual or physical trauma.

At some time during therapy with a patient who has experienced sexual trauma, a sensitively taken history about the abuse will probably be necessary. This allows the patient to unburden herself (or himself) of "secrets" that have rarely, if ever, been shared with others. This is often a critical step in beginning to cope effectively with being an abused person. The cognitive therapist can then turn attention toward post traumatic symptoms, such as intrusive thoughts, flashbacks, and avoidance of intimacy. Behavioral methods such as desensitization, relaxation therapy, and assertiveness training may be helpful in reducing these symptoms. In addition, victims of trauma, especially sexual abuse, usually need help in dealing with issues of self-worth, anger, and perceived lack of control over their lives. Standard cognitive interventions are applied to these types of problems. However, the successful resolution of sexual-abuse issues usually requires intensive work at the schema level.

Common schemas that we have observed in abused patients are: "I am defenseless. . . . I can't trust anybody. . . . I deserve what I get. . . . and I'm ruined for life." The inpatient phase of treatment is usually devoted to symptom reduction and identification of these underlying beliefs. Although some schema modification may be possible during the hospital stay, these concepts are usually so deeply embedded that extensive outpatient work will be required after discharge.

For patients who remain in physically abusive relationships, the focus of treatment should be on examining the assumptions and beliefs that prevent effective attempts to change the situation. For example, Ms. U, an inpatient who continued a physically abusive relationship, believed that "I can't make it alone" and "I have to be there for him because he is a sick man." Cognitive therapy with this patient was directed at modifying these beliefs. It also involved a cost–benefit analysis of her present coping strategies (e.g., drinking to "erase the pain") or possible alternative courses of action (e.g., going to live with her daughter or seeing a lawyer).

Transferring Gains to the Home Environment

Patients who are treated in a hospital setting may not be exposed to some of the real-life stressors that have contributed to their symptoms. Transfer of the gains of hospitalization to the outside environment is often an issue. A number of strategies can be employed to facilitate generalization of skills. These include (1) simulating real-life situations, as far as possible, within the institution; (2) employing role-playing, role-reversal, and imagery techniques; (3) instituting therapeutic leave or family visits as soon as they are feasible; (4) involving significant others in the treatment; (5) employing partial or day hospitalization as a steppingstone; (6) teaching skills with wide application; and (7) structuring therapy sessions in a manner that fosters a self-management approach.

Mild relapse following discharge from the inpatient unit is very common in depressed patients (Scott, 1989). It is important that the patient have realistic expectations in this regard so that he or she can plan for the possibility of symptom recurrence. Before discharge, problem lists should be rewritten to take into account the new situations and challenges that will occur after leaving the hospital. Transition and aftercare issues are discussed further in Chapter 15.

SUMMARY

This chapter describes individual cognitive therapy for patients who are hospitalized on an inpatient psychiatry service. Several of the important modifications of CT for inpatient applications include a focus on relief of the disabling symptoms that prompted hospitalization, shorter and more frequent sessions, use of the hospital milieu as a source of information and as an agent of change, and integration with other therapy approaches utilized on the inpatient service.

Cognitive therapy is indicated for a number of different diagnoses. This form of treatment is considered a primary therapy for depression, anxiety, personality disorders, addictions, and eating disorders. However, for patients with major psychoses, cognitive interventions are best utilized in an auxiliary role to pharmacotherapy. Adaptations of cognitive therapy for affective psychoses are described.

Cognitive therapy can help reduce target symptoms such as hopelessness, suicidal ideation, low self-esteem, severe anxiety, and interpersonal and behavioral deficits that are commonly experienced by inpatients. These symptoms are often the major reasons for hospitalization. The cognitive approach is also useful in building coping skills and preparing the patient to resume functioning in the home environment. Thus, cognitive therapy can offer the hospitalized patient a pragmatic avenue of recovery.

REFERENCES

Agras, W. S., Schneider, J. A., Arnow, B., Raeburn, S. D., & Telch, S. F. (1989). Cognitive–behavioral and response prevention treatments for bulimia nervosa. *Journal of Consulting and Clinical Psychology, 57*, 215–221.

American Psychiatric Association. (1987). *Diagnostic and statistical manual of mental disorders* (3rd ed., revised). Washington, DC: Author.

Beck, A. T. (1976). *Cognitive therapy and the emotional disorders*. New York: International Universities Press.

Beck, A. T., Brown, G., Epstein, N., & Steer, R. A. (1988). An Inventory for measuring Anxiety: Psychometric properties. *Journal of Consulting and Clinical Psychology, 56*(6), 893–897.

Beck, A. T., & Emery, G. (1985). *Anxiety disorders and phobias: A cognitive perspective*. New York: Basic Books.

Beck, A. T., Freeman, A., & Associates (1990). *Cognitive therapy of personality disorders*. New York: Guilford Press.

Beck, A. T., & Greenberg, R. L. (1974). *Coping with depression*. (Available from the Institute for Rational Emotive Therapy, 45 East 65th Street, New York, NY 10021.)

Beck, A. T., James, C., & VanderKolk, B. (1987). Reports of childhood incest and current behavior of chronically hospitalized psychotic women. *American Journal of Psychiatry, 144*(11), 1474–1476.

Beck, A. T., Kovacs, M., & Weissman, A. (1975). Hopelessness and suicidal behavior: An overview. *Journal of American Medical Association, 234*, 1146–1149.

Beck, A. T., Kovacs, M., & Weissman, A. (1979). Assessment of suicidal intention: The scale for suicide ideation. *Journal of Consulting and Clinical Psychology, 47*, 343–352.

Beck, A. T., Rush, A. J., Shaw, B. F., & Emery, G. (1979). *Cognitive therapy of depression*. New York: Guilford Press.

Beck, A. T., Ward, C. H., Mendelson, M., Mock, J., & Erbaugh, J. (1961). An inventory for measuring depression. *Archives of General Psychiatry, 4*, 561–571.

Beck, A. T., Weissman, A., Lester, D., & Trexler, L. (1974). The measurement of pessimism: The hopelessness scale. *Journal of Consulting and Clinical Psychology, 42*, 861–865.

Bishop, S., Miller, I. W., Norman, W., Buda, M., & Foulke, M. (1986). Cognitive therapy of psychotic depression: A case report. *Psychotherapy, 23*(1), 167–173.

Bowers, W. A. (1989). Cognitive therapy with inpatients. In A. Freeman, K. M. Simon, L. E. Beutler, & H. Arkowitz (Eds.), *Comprehensive handbook of cognitive therapy* (pp. 583–596). New York: Plenum Press.

Burns, D. D. (1980). *Feeling good*. New York: William Morrow.

Burns, D. D. (1985). *Intimate connections*. New York: New American Library.

Chorr, P. N., Mercier, M. A., & Halper, I. S. (1988). Use of cognitive therapy for a patient suffering from bipolar affective disorder. *Journal of Cognitive Psychotherapy, 2*(1), 51–58.

Clark, D. M., Salkovskis, P., & Chalkley, A. (1985). Respiratory control as a treatment for panic attacks. *Journal of Behavior Therapy and Experimental Psychiatry, 16*, 23–30.

Clum, G. (1990). *Coping with panic*. New York: Brooks-Cole.

Dobson, K. S., & Shaw, B. F. (1986). Cognitive assessment with major depressive disorders. *Cognitive Therapy and Research, 10*(1), 13–29.

Emery, G. (1982). *Own your own life*. New American Library: New York.

Emery, G., Hollon, S. D., & Bedrosian, R. C. (Eds.). (1981). *New directions in cognitive therapy*. New York: Guilford Press.

Fairburn, C. G. (1985). Cognitive–behavioral treatment for bulimia. In D. M. Garner & P. E. Garfinkel (Eds.), *Handbook of psychotherapy for anorexia nervosa and bulimia* (pp. 160–191). New York: Guilford Press.

Fowler, D., & Morley, S. (1989). The cognitive–behavioural treatment of hallucinations and delusions: A preliminary study. *Behavioural Psychotherapy, 17*, 267–282.

Garner, D. M., & Bemis, K. M. (1982). Cognitive behavioral approach to anorexia nervosa. *Cognitive Therapy and Research, 6*, 123–150.

Garner, D. M., & Bemis, K. M. (1985). Cognitive therapy for anorexia nervosa. In D. M. Garner & P. E. Garfinkel (Eds.). *Handbook of psychotherapy for anorexia nervosa and bulimia* (pp. 107–146). New York: Guilford Press.

Hamilton, M. (1960). A rating scale for depression. *Journal of Neurology, Neurosurgery and Psychiatry, 23*, 56–62.

Hersen, M. (1985). *The practice of inpatient behavior therapy: A clinical guide*. Orlando, FL: Grune & Stratton.

Hollon, S. D., & Kendall, P. (1980). Cognitive self-statements in depression: Development of an automatic thoughts questionnaire. *Cognitive Therapy and Research, 4*, 383–395.

Jacobsen, A., & Richardson, B. (1987). Assault experiences of one-hundred psychiatric inpatients: Evidence of the need for positive inquiry. *American Journal of Psychiatry, 144*(7), 908–913.

Kingdon, D. G., & Turkington, D. (1991a). The use of cognitive behavior therapy with a normalizing rationale in schizophrenia. *Journal of Nervous and Mental Disease, 179*(4), 207–211.

Kingdon, D. G., & Turkington, D. (1991b). A role for cognitive–behavioural strategies in schizophrenia? *Social Psychiatry and Psychiatric Epidemiology, 26*(3), 101–103.

McKay, M., & Fanning, P. (1987). *Self esteem*. Oakland, CA: New Harbinger Press.

Marlatt, G. A.,& Gordon, J. R. (Eds.). (1985). *Relapse prevention*. New York: Guilford Press.

Miller, I. W., Norman, W. H., Keitner, G. I., Bishop, S. D., & Dow, M. G. (1989). Cognitive–behavioral treatment of depressed inpatients. *Behavior Therapy, 20*, 25–47.

Murphy, G. E., Simons, A. D., Wetzel, R. D., & Lustman, P. J. (1984). Cognitive therapy and pharmacotherapy: Singly and together in the treatment of depression. *Archives of General Psychiatry, 41*, 33–41.

Perris, C. (1989). *Cognitive therapy with schizophrenic patients*. New York: Guilford Press.

Persons, J. (1989). *Cognitive therapy in practice: A case formulation approach*. New York: W. W. Norton.

Rush, J., Beck, A. T., Kovacs, M., Weissenburger, J., & Hollon, S. D. (1982). Comparison of the effects of cognitive therapy and pharmacotherapy on hopelessness and self-concept. *American Journal of Psychiatry, 139*(7), 862–866.

Schrodt, G. R. Jr. & Wright, J. H. (1987). Inpatient treatment of adolescents. In A. Freeman, & V. Greenwood (Eds.), *Cognitive therapy: Applications in psychiatry and medical settings*. New York: Human Sciences Press.

Scott, J. (1989). Cognitive therapy with depressed inpatients. In W. Dryden & P. Trower (Eds.), *Developments in cognitive psychotherapy* (pp. 177–189). London: Sage Publications.

Sotsky, S. M., Glass, D. R., Shea, T., Pilkonis, P. A., Collins, J. F., Elkin, I., Watkins, J. T., Imber, S. D., Leber, W. R., Moyer, J., & Oliveri, M. E. (1991). Patient predictors of response to psychotherapy and pharmacotherapy: Findings in the NIMH treatment of depression collaborative research program. *American Journal of Psychiatry, 148*(8), 997–1008.

Spielberger, C. D. (1983). *Manual for the state–trait anxiety inventory*. Palo Alto, CA: Consulting Psychologists Press.

Teasdale, J. D., Fennell, M. J. V., Hibbert, J. A., & Amies, P. L. (1984). Cognitive therapy for major depressive disorder in primary care. *British Journal of Psychiatry, 144*, 400–406.

Thase, M., & Wright, J. H. (1991). Cognitive therapy with inpatients: A treatment manual. *Behavior Therapy, 22*, 579–595.

Weissman, A. N. (1979). The dysfunctional attitude scale: A validation study. Doctoral Dissertation, University of Pennsylvania, Philadelphia.

Wetzel, R. D. (1976). Hopelessness, depression, and suicide intent. *Archives of General Psychiatry, 33*, 1069–1073.

Wright, J. H. (1987). Cognitive therapy and medication as a combined treatment. In A. Freeman & V. B. Greenwood (Eds.), *Cognitive therapy: Applications in medical and psychiatric settings* (pp. 36–51). New York: Human Services Press.

Wright, J. H. (1988). Cognitive therapy of depression. In A. J. Frances & R. E. Hales (Eds.), *American Psychiatric Press review of psychiatry*, Vol. 7 (pp. 554–90). Washington, DC: American Psychiatric Press.

Wright, J. H. (in press). Combined cognitive therapy and pharmacotherapy of depression. In A. Freeman & F. M. Dattilio (Eds.), *Casebook of cognitive behavioral therapy*. New York: Plenum Press.

Wright, J. H., & Beck, A. T. (1983). Cognitive therapy of depression: Theory and practice. *Hospital and Community Psychiatry, 34*(12), 1119–1127.

Wright, J. H., & Borden, J. (1991). Cognitive therapy of depression and anxiety. *Psychiatric Annals, 21*, 424–428.

Wright, J. H., & Salmon, P. G. (1990). Learning and memory in depression. In C. D. McCann & N. S. Endler (Eds.), *Depression: New directions in theory, research and practice* (pp. 211–236), Toronto: Wall & Emerson.

Wright, J. H., & Schrodt, G. R. (1989). Combined cognitive therapy and pharmacotherapy. In A. Freeman, K. M. Simon, L. E. Beutler, & H. Arkowitz (Eds.), *Comprehensive handbook of cognitive therapy* (pp. 267–283). New York: Plenum Press.

Young, J. E. (1990). *Cognitive therapy for personality disorders: A schema-focused approach*. Sarasota, FL: Professional Resources Exchange.

Chapter 5

Group Cognitive Therapy with Inpatients

Arthur Freeman, Ed.D.,
G. Randolph Schrodt, Jr., M.D.,
Mark Gilson, Ph.D., and
John W. Ludgate, Ph.D.

Group therapy is one of the cornerstones of the cognitive milieu. Inpatient cognitive therapy programs usually include a core group therapy experience, such as an open-ended group that meets several times a week, and a variety of other groups with a cognitive orientation. Some cognitive therapy units (CTUs) emphasize group therapy as the primary psychotherapeutic intervention during the inpatient stay. This chapter describes group cognitive therapy (GCT) procedures for hospitalized patients and illustrates treatment techniques in different types of inpatient groups. We begin with the presentation of a rationale for GCT. The middle portion of the chapter is devoted to a discussion of basic strategies and techniques for inpatient group therapy. A final section details several forms of GCT including core groups, unit-community meetings, and special-purpose groups. The reader will find that many of the group therapies explained here are applicable to both the inpatient and the aftercare phases of treatment.

RATIONALE FOR GROUP COGNITIVE THERAPY

Inpatient hospitalization automatically places patients into a treatment group, even if formal group therapy is not prescribed. When individuals live together for 24 hours a day in a relatively small area, it is hard to remain apart from spontaneous or planned group interactions. Inpatient therapists have recognized the importance of group processes for some time and have developed a variety of methods to capitalize on the group dynamics that are set in place by hospitalization.

Maxwell Jones, who originated the "therapeutic community," was one of the first to emphasize group therapy in hospital settings (Jones, 1953). He endorsed group therapy, in part, because it was an economical way to deliver treatment. There was a shortage of health professionals when the therapeutic community was first developed in England during and shortly after World War II. The spontaneous grouping of patients who are admitted to the hospital and the intense social relations of individuals who live together in a relatively small space were also offered as reasons for using group treatments (Jones, 1953). More recent models for inpatient psychiatry have continued to rely heavily on group interventions (Maxmen, Tucker, & LeBow, 1974; Moline, 1976; Yalom, 1983; Bowers, 1989).

The rationale for including GCT in current inpatient treatment programs rests partially on nonspecific operational principles such as universality, support, and peer feedback that are shared with other group therapies (Yalom, 1985). However, GCT has the advantage of being a short-term, problem-oriented approach that may be particularly useful in work with hospitalized patients. Several of the more important reasons for utilizing GCT for psychiatric inpatient programs are described below.

1. *Engagement in the therapeutic process.* When people are admitted to medical or surgical units, passivity is expected or even encouraged. Although diagnostic procedures, pre- and postoperative protocols and taking medication may require some effort on the part of the patient, the general implication is that treatment is "received." The same type of reaction can occur on a psychiatric inpatient service. Hospitalized psychiatric patients often feel overwhelmed, helpless, and hopeless. These individuals may develop the belief that something must be done "for" or "to" them. Group CT offers an opportunity to challenge this assumption. The group leaders (and, one hopes, group members) endorse the premise that self-control of thoughts, feelings, and behavior is possible. The problem-solving focus of GCT encourages patients to be active participants in their treatment. Effective collaboration between patient and therapist is one of the central features of cognitive therapy. The group setting promotes collaboration through a number of procedures, including agenda setting, role-playing, and self-help exercises.

2. *Diagnostic function.* The usual admission procedure for the inpatient unit involves one or more interviews with the doctors and nurses. The group experience adds a different dimension to the evaluation process. By directly observing the patient's behavioral interactions with

other patients, the clinicians gain a window into the patient's repertoire of interpersonal responses. The therapists do not have to depend on the patient's report of how others react to them or how they react to others. The scenario unfolds before the therapist's eyes. Patients who can appear quite intact in a one-to-one interview may have more trouble maintaining their stability when they are faced with the added stimuli of a group setting. Conversely, personal strengths, such as empathy skills, that are not readily apparent in individual therapy may be drawn out in the environment of group therapy.

3. *Universality.* Sharing perceptions and reactions in the group allows patients to see that they are not alone in their suffering and that other people have problems of a similar nature. Yalom (1985) has observed that patients regard the sense of universality as one of the most helpful features of group therapy. A form of resistance that can surface in individual therapy is illustrated by the statement: "You [the therapist] don't understand what I am going through." One patient continually used the phrase, "You don't know a person unless you have walked a mile in their shoes," as a way of disregarding the therapist's viewpoint. It is, however, far more difficult to ignore other patients who have had similar experiences (not the least of which is being in the hospital).

4. *Relatedness and support.* The group can help to foster a sense of relatedness for the chronically isolated patient and for the more social patient who is separated from family and friends while in the hospital. Also, even in the brief time generally allotted for inpatient treatment, the group can operate as a support for the patient who is faced with having to cope with significant life stress. A cognitive therapy group can be supportive in many ways, such as showing appropriate empathy or concern when a patient has experienced a loss, helping to counter hopelessness by spotting negatively distorted thinking, or suggesting alternative solutions to problems.

Beutler, Frank, Scheiber, Calvert, and Gaines (1984), in one of the best controlled studies of inpatient group therapy, found that some group experiences may be antitherapeutic. They observed that group tactics that attempted to increase affect and break down defenses were associated with a worsening of symptoms. However, groups that gave emotional support had the best clinical outcomes. Group CT offers the type of structure and support recommended by Beutler and colleagues.

5. *Peer feedback.* The group provides the first opportunity for many patients to obtain constructive peer responses to their behavior. Patients often assume that they are perceived in a certain way (usually negative) without ever checking this out in a reliable manner. It is important to see that the group gives accurate feedback. Unrealistic affirmations can

be as destructive as a continuance of negatively distorted self-concepts. Patients often comment that group feedback is a valued component of the therapy experience (Beutler et al., 1984). The positive aspects of the therapeutic interchange are not limited to the group member who receives feedback. Some patients come to realize that they have previously unrecognized abilities that they can use to help someone else. Group members frequently describe an enhanced sense of worth when they are able to assist another person.

6. *Psychoeducation.* The basic principles of the cognitive approach are taught and reinforced in a variety of experiments and group exercises. The group format is especially well-suited for presenting information on specific topics. Special psychoeducational programs can be designed for particular groups of patients that are served by the inpatient unit. For example, a unit that is dedicated to the treatment of chemical dependency can have didactic presentations on the biology of addiction, the twelve-step approach, and strategies of relapse prevention. An adolescent unit schedule might include a sex education class. Many group therapy programs develop written materials that help patients learn cognitive therapy skills in an orderly sequence. These learning aids are often combined in a folder or notebook that the patient receives on admission to the unit.

7. *Laboratory experience.* The group is a laboratory where patients can test out their automatic thoughts and experiment with different behaviors in a relatively safe environment. It is important to point out that although the group can provide opportunities for a broad range of cognitive and behavioral experiments, it also has the potential to be an arena for repeating dysfunctional behaviors or expressing primitive aggressive or narcissistic themes. A structured, problem-oriented approach, under the astute direction of a well-trained GCT leader, tends to forestall problems with "acting out."

8. *Modeling and social skills building.* Patients often model the behaviors of other group members or the therapists. In the process, the individual can learn effective coping strategies (e.g., assertiveness, empathic responses, goal setting, and problem solving). Basic social skills can be taught, discussed, and role played in the group. The opportunity for practice is important for all patients. However, those who have severe social skills deficits require the most assistance in building a higher level of social competence.

9. *Efficacy.* Controlled outcome research has established the efficacy of GCT for outpatients with unipolar depression (Shaw, 1977; Free, Oei, & Sanders, 1991). Several studies have compared GCT with other treatments. Rush and Watkins's pilot study (1981) suggests that

individual cognitive therapy leads to greater improvement than GCT, although later studies have found no difference between group and individual formats (Shaffer, Shapiro, Sank, & Coghlan, 1981; Brown & Lewinsohn, 1984).

Covi and Lipman (1987) found that both GCT and GCT plus imipramine were more effective than traditional, nondirective group therapy for depressed adults. In a study of depressed geriatric patients, GCT, antidepressant medication, and more traditional group therapy were all found to be superior to placebo (Jarvik, Mintz, Steuer, & Gerner, 1982). Group CT has also been shown to be as effective as pharmacotherapy (phenelzine and alprazolam) in the treatment of social phobia (Gelernter et al., 1991).

No controlled studies have been conducted as yet to establish the efficacy of GCT for inpatients. However, research with outpatients suggests that GCT is effective, cost-efficient, and generally associated with low drop-out rates. Although investigators have focused primarily on depression and social phobia, GCT protocols have been developed for a variety of other clinical conditions commonly encountered on inpatient units (Covi & Primakoff, 1988).

GROUP COGNITIVE THERAPY: BASIC PROCEDURES

Group Selection

Group selection is largely defined by the patient population of the particular milieu. In general, the optimum number of group members is 6 to 10 (although some psychoeducational family and community meetings have many more participants).

There are advantages and disadvantages to group homogeneity in terms of age, sex, diagnosis, and problem focus. For example, adolescents tend to work best in a group composed of peers, although they also may benefit from exposure to adults in groups such as AA meetings (see Chapter 12). Women's and men's groups often facilitate discussion of sensitive gender specific issues. Homogeneous groups that focus on problems such as depression or eating disorders can enhance identification and empathy among group members.

At the same time, homogeneous group selection can create certain problems. For instance, a group composed exclusively of depressed patients may lack the objectivity, energy, and hopeful encouragement provided by nondepressed members. Heterogeneity in group selection creates a more realistic social microcosm. Patients often benefit from the insights, strengths, and personal experience of patients who can provide feedback from a different perspective.

Patients with organic brain syndromes, acute psychosis, or mania are generally not suitable for GCT; however, they will often benefit from an activity group that focuses on reality testing and social interaction. Patients with severely disruptive personality disorders may need to be excluded from inpatient CBT groups. Linehan (1987) described a cognitive therapy group for borderline personality disorder patients that works well on an outpatient basis. However, the inpatient setting often does not allow the time for limit setting and redirection that these patients may require.

Length and Frequency of Sessions

The length and frequency of group meetings is dependent on a number of variables, including duration of hospital stay, therapeutic focus, hospital schedule, and space restrictions. Generally, we recommend that core groups meet for a minimum of 1½ hours. This allows the group to have time to set an agenda, do meaningful therapeutic work, and close the session with homework and review. Shorter groups of 45 minutes to 1 hour generally have difficulty in developing and gaining closure on therapy topics. However, groups with limited goals (e.g., orientation meetings for new patients, psychoeducational sessions for family members, assertiveness training) may be able to function effectively in 1 hour or less. These types of special groups may meet only once weekly. Groups that are designed to be a primary component of the inpatient stay are usually held two to three times weekly. Some inpatient programs that are devoted heavily to GCT have daily therapy sessions.

Location and Setting

The location and physical setting of the group are significant because they indicate to the patient the importance of this type of therapy. A group that meets in an unpleasant environment, such as a basement room where there are distracting noises or odors may get the impression that the hospital staff do not value group therapy highly. The group should be held in a room that has adequate and comfortable seating and is well lighted and ventilated. Sufficient room for the group members to get up and move around for role playing is another requirement. A chalkboard or easel, pads of paper, and pens and markers should also be available.

Therapist Staffing

Perris et al. (1987) and Yalom (1983) have noted that professional rivalry on the unit can have destructive and countertherapeutic effects. If the psychologists, psychiatrists, nurses, social workers, and other professionals cannot work together, why should the patient be expected to resolve conflicts in appropriate ways? The key issue in staffing the group is that the primary group therapist(s) be trained and experienced in cognitive therapy. Group therapists who are not familiar with cognitive therapy, or cognitive therapists who have not done group therapy, should first serve an apprenticeship as a cotherapist in GCT. The group can serve as an excellent educational opportunity for therapists in training. By working as a cotherapist, the novice can learn the therapy process *in vivo*. The cotherapist can also assist with role playing or modeling in the session.

The group leader can be a psychologist, physician, social worker, nurse, or other mental health professional who satisfies the criteria noted above. However, a therapist with a conflicting theoretical orientation can have very negative effects on the group. For example, during the vacation of a cognitively trained psychologist, a senior resident was asked to be a substitute group therapist. She quickly became frustrated with the cognitive group process and made it clear to patients that: "I'm not sure about this therapy. If you just take the medications, they'll do the job."

"Here-and-Now" Focus

The group adopts the same type of "here-and-now" focus that is used in other forms of cognitive therapy. When therapy is short-term treatment, it is extremely difficult for the group to obtain a historical perspective by reviewing childhood experiences. There isn't enough time for each member to reveal fully the details of his or her past. Historical issues are recapitulated, however, in the here-and-now through the influence of schemas. Some schemas are very obvious and will be recognized quickly by the therapist and the group members. Other schemas are not so clearly delineated and must be inferred from the patient's habitual cognitive style or behavior within the group. Although these dysfunctional patterns may have their roots in the past, the cognitive approach to therapy suggests that change is most likely if present functioning is the target of treatment interventions (Beck, Rush, Shaw, & Emery, 1979). There are some patients, especially abused individuals or those with severe personality disorders, who have such firmly held maladaptive beliefs that historical reconstructive work may be required (Beck, Freeman, & Associates, 1990). However, this is usually done in longer-term therapy after discharge from the hospital.

Pacing

Proper pacing of the sessions is one of the most difficult tasks for the inpatient group therapist. Invariably, the group will be composed of individuals with diverse diagnoses, assorted degrees of pathology, and different levels of motivation. The group therapist also must deal with a constant ebb and flow of patients. Some individuals will be in the group for the first time, and others will be nearing discharge. In many ways, the work of the inpatient group therapist can be likened to "hitting a moving target."

Procedures need to be developed both to welcome new patients and to go through a meaningful termination process for those who are about to be discharged. The therapist must take responsibility for structuring these activities so that the group does not take too much time with the entry and leave-taking procedures. The group begins with the therapist asking new patients to introduce themselves and to join other members in structuring an agenda for the session. Although new patients will have had some introduction to group therapy before coming to the first session (see Group Formats section of this chapter), a brief review of the ground rules and basic procedures is usually necessary. The welcoming activities can generally be accomplished in less than 5 minutes. Termination from group is usually not too difficult when the hospital stay has been brief. Although collaborative relationships (patient–therapist and patient–patient) form rather quickly in the inpatient setting, the patient is pointed toward discharge almost from the beginning of the hospital experience. Thus, prolonged discussions of termination issues can usually be avoided. A brief time, usually 5 minutes or less, can be set aside for saying goodbye to patients leaving the group. Individual group members will, of course, say their farewells at greater length outside of the group.

During the central part of the session, when agenda items are being discussed and cognitive and behavioral interventions are being implemented, the therapist tries to adjust the speed and complexity of procedures so that the majority of the patients will be able to benefit from the therapy. A balance must be struck between the needs (and capacities) of the more advanced or experienced members as compared to those who are profoundly ill, slow to grasp concepts, or new to the group experience. Unfortunately, it is not always possible to pace the group in a manner that is consistently helpful to all group members.

Several different procedures can be used when there are wide disparities in the composition of the group. First, the session can be divided into sections in which (1) basic principles are presented or reviewed, (2) generally relevant and understandable therapeutic work is done (e.g., listing automatic thoughts or cognitive distortions, considering advantages and disadvantages), and (3) more abstract or complex issues (e.g., schemas, implications of choosing alternate problem-solving strategies) are discussed. The therapist can clearly indicate to the group that some phases of the session will be most helpful for the new patient but will serve as a review for those with more experience, whereas other portions of the meeting may be somewhat confusing for those who are just starting GCT. Second, the therapist can arrange for either remedial or advanced work to be completed between sessions. Individualized assignments can be used to help beginning patients who are struggling with learning the cognitive model or other patients who desire a more challenging or diverse therapy experience. Group members can be recruited to help one another in accomplishing these exercises.

A third procedure that can help in keeping a productive pace for the session is to stop frequently to ask for feedback. Is the material being understood? Are there any members who are confused? Would reviews or additional explanations be of benefit? Does some of the discussion seem to be of limited interest or "off target?" Inpatient GCT is designed to be active and problem oriented in order to use the available time efficiently. However, the therapist must be on guard to avoid making excessive demands or moving at a speed that the patient cannot match. If the therapy is paced at a level beyond the patient's capacity, there is a risk that GCT will have a reverse effect of increasing hopelessness and helplessness. The goal is to pitch the content and the tempo of the session at levels that will promote a constructive learning experience for all members of the group.

Cognitive Techniques

One of the primary objectives of cognitive therapy is to teach the patient to identify negative automatic thoughts that occur in problem situations and to recognize the effects these thoughts have on his or her emotions and behavior. Understanding the nature of negative automatic thoughts is the first step in beginning to change dysfunctional cognitions. A large part of GCT is devoted to this process. The schemas that underlie the automatic thoughts may become apparent in some instances, but a full discovery of relevant schemas is unlikely in the short-term groups utilized in most inpatient cognitive therapy programs.

Material from the group setting may be used profitably by the individual therapist to clarify and modify schemas (see Chapter 4).

Ideally, each individual in the group assists with identifying and testing the thoughts of the other patients. The patient thus gains experience in thought monitoring while helping other group members. Many of the basic techniques of cognitive therapy described in Chapters 1 and 4 of this volume can be applied in the group setting. Several of these procedures are illustrated with vignettes from GCT.

1. *Understanding idiosyncratic meanings*. The therapist and other patients ask for clarification of what is meant by a word or idea that appears to be dysfunctional. Socratic questioning is used by the therapist, and the patients are encouraged to join in the process.

JOE: I get bummed out every time my family visits.

THERAPIST: Joe, what do you mean by being "bummed out"?

JOE: I don't know, I just don't feel very good.

THERAPIST: It might help Joe if he knew more details about his reaction. Could anyone help him understand what being "bummed out" means?

ALEX: Joe, maybe you could think back to the last time they visited.

MAUDE: That sounds like a good idea.

JOE: Well, it's just that they make me feel guilty . . . like I never measure up.

2. *Labeling of distortions*. The inpatient group provides many opportunities for recognizing, labeling, and changing cognitive distortions. The first step is to teach the group about the concept of cognitive distortions or errors (e.g., "all-or-none" thinking, overgeneralization, personalization, "mind reading," "jumping to conclusions"). This can be done *in vivo* during the session by Socratic questioning and by explanation of the nature of cognitive errors. Experienced group members can help perform this function, even without the therapist taking the lead. Reading assignments, thought records, and other homework may be used to reinforce learning about this form of cognitive pathology. Some inpatient groups list the most common distortions on a large chart in the group room; this emphasizes the importance of recognizing cognitive errors and also helps the patient group to use the same definitions and terms.

The following vignette illustrates methods of labeling distortions in an inpatient GCT session:

ALEX: I can never do anything right. I couldn't even figure out how to fill in the Daily Activity Schedule. Nothing ever works out the way I want it.

THERAPIST: We've been trying to learn how to recognize and label cognitive distortions. Can anybody describe the cognitive distortions that Alex just used?

SAM: Sure, it's funny how they're so obvious when someone else does it. Alex was using "all-or-nothing" thinking. I can't imagine that he *never* does anything right. In fact, he's helped me a lot by describing how he organizes himself at his job.

MARY: I think I heard Alex "overgeneralize." He talked about one minor problem with the activity schedule and then told us that "nothing ever works out the way I want it."

THERAPIST: Alex, what do you think?

ALEX: They're right. I do that kind of stuff all the time.

KEN: There you go again!

3. *Verbalization of internal dialogue (automatic thoughts).* This technique works extremely well in the group context. It involves having the group members put into words their internal negative dialogue. Other group members can set up "debates" with the negative voice. The patient can then reverse roles and have another group member be the negative voice and the patient be the rational responder. Other patients can serve as coaches for the adaptive responding. Once this technique is mastered, it makes an excellent homework assignment for the between-session time on the unit.

THERAPIST: Alice, you look like Maude's problem stirred up lots of thoughts. This might be a good opportunity to try to verbalize your private thinking and to get the group to help you with your reactions.

CARMEN: Give it a try. Getting thoughts out in the open really helped me yesterday after my parents visited.

ALICE: Okay. I'll try to just let it flow, like you did yesterday.

KEN: Go ahead.

ALICE: (*Describes negative automatic thoughts in detail as they occurred.*)

THERAPIST: Now that we know what Alice was thinking, how can we help her respond? (*Group develops ideas, and role-playing exercise commences.*)

4. *Questioning the evidence*. Each of the patients can be helped to identify and question the evidence that is being used to maintain ideas, actions, and feelings.

THERAPIST: Joe just brought out a negative self-statement—"I never measure up." Do any of the rest of you have similar ideas about yourselves?

MARY: I keep saying to myself, "I'm a loser, I'm a loser."

TIM: Yeah, I do it too. Anytime my dad sounds critical, I start thinking "I'm not good enough."

THERAPIST: We've had two other examples of negative self-statements. I'd like all of you to try to write down one or two of these types of thoughts. Then we'll put them on the chalkboard and try to look at the evidence for and against some of the ideas.

JOAN: I'll be the "secretary" and write on the chalkboard.

JOE: Thanks, I guess I can start off. I see lots of evidence that fits with the idea "I never measure up." My wife is always criticizing me: "You don't make enough money. . . . You're never home on time. . . . We never go anywhere." I used to hear the same kinds of things from my mother and father.

JOAN: We need something for the other side of the column.

JOE: Well, I almost always get good evaluations from my boss, and everybody seems to like the way I coach my son's soccer team.

THERAPIST: How about some input from the group?

KEN: Joe, you've been a great friend here in the hospital. You're always willing to help out others in the group.

MAUDE: From the way your son acts when he visits, you must be a good father.

THERAPIST: Any more evidence *for* Joe's statement?

ALICE: Joe keeps talking about how he can't do anything right—even when he tries to play golf or do something else to relax.

JOE: That's right, I'm always thinking about how others are judging me. I forget everything I've accomplished, and I can't ever enjoy myself.

THERAPIST: It looks like we're starting to get somewhere. We've seen that there's usually some evidence on both sides and that negative attitudes that go unquestioned can have very harmful effects. Let's go on now to some of the other group members' negative self-statements. We'll try to get started on the pro–con analysis here, and each of you can continue with the project for homework.

5. *Decatastrophizing*. This technique involves group members in the defusing of a catastrophic prediction or interpretation. One method of decatastrophizing is to pose the question, "What is the worst possible thing that would happen if . . . ? "This type of question should not be asked unless the therapist judges the patient and the group capable of (1) understanding the hypothetical and abstract nature of the question, (2) developing adaptive coping strategies for highly negative events, and (3) benefiting from the concept that "if I can handle the worst, I can manage anything else."

The "worst-case scenario" intervention is indicated when patients have the attributes listed above and when their fantasized consequences are largely a product of negatively distorted cognitions (e.g., "I'll be totally humiliated"; "I'll pass out"; "Everyone will laugh at me"). However, the procedure can be of considerable benefit even when an extremely deleterious outcome is possible.

THERAPIST: Joan, you've been trying to decide whether to confront your boyfriend about his drinking. It sounds like an important issue. You told us one of the reasons that you took the overdose was that you felt trapped in this relationship. What's the worst possible thing that could happen if you told him he needed to get help?

JOAN: He'd leave me, and I'd be all alone.

KEN: What if he did. What would be the big deal if that sleaze *did* leave?

CARMEN: What did he ever do for you?

JOAN: I don't know, but I still really care about him.

JOE: You could function just fine without him. You'd probably be in a lot better shape.

MAUDE: You deserve better than you're getting.

THERAPIST: Joan, the group seems to think that you could handle it well even if he did leave. How do you see the situation now?

JOAN: They're probably right. In fact, it's good to think that you can survive "without a man." But, what I really want to do is to tell him that I won't hang around if he doesn't stop drinking. I hope he'll change.

6. *Advantages and disadvantages*. Another useful problem-solving technique is to have patients list the advantages and the disadvantages

of maintaining a particular belief or manner of responding. This procedure can help to move them away from an all-or-nothing focus as they begin to recognize that thoughts or actions usually are neither entirely effective nor completely dysfunctional.

The search for advantages and disadvantages often leads to a deeper understanding of assumptions or habitual behaviors. With inpatients, this procedure is frequently directed at schemas or damaging actions that have played a significant role in precipitating admission to the hospital.

KEN: I'm starting to figure out why I feel like a failure.

THERAPIST: Can you tell the group what you've learned.

KEN: Yeah. It's hard to admit, but . . . I have to be *the best* at anything I do, or I think that I've failed.

MARY: I can identify with that. I always thought that I had to get all A's or be the first chair in the violin section. Otherwise, my parents or my friends wouldn't love me—or even like me.

THERAPIST: This kind of belief can set you up for lots of problems, but in a curious way it can also be of some benefit. That's one of the reasons these beliefs can hang around for a long time. Let's take a look at the advantages and disadvantages of Ken's assumption that he has to be *the best* at anything he does, or else he fails. (*Goes to blackboard and writes the group's ideas in two columns.*)

ALEX: Well, if you would believe that, you would probably try very hard.

JOAN: And you might have lots of successes.

CARMEN: But, what happens if you can't be the best? Then you're miserable, . . . and you might even give up and think about suicide like Ken did.

KEN: That's right. It makes me act like I'm a driven person. I don't have any fun, and I can't relax. I think I'm probably hard on others too. My wife says she can never please me.

SAM: Ken, you've got to admit that you might not have made all your money if you weren't always trying to come out on top.

KEN: I'm not sure it was worth it.

THERAPIST: I think you can probably see that listing the advantages and disadvantages is an important step in trying to change beliefs or assumptions that aren't working well for you. Let's spend a little more time working on the list, and then we can talk about helping Ken to modify this belief.

7. *Constructing adaptive self-statements*. Patients can be taught to give themselves specific instructions to control behavior or initiate new activities (Meichenbaum, 1977). This is especially useful for patients with impulse control difficulties. Self-instructions can be generated by the individual, the therapist, or the group.

THERAPIST: What do you need to tell yourself?

ALEX: I'm not sure.

THERAPIST: Does anybody have a suggestion?

MARIE: He just needs to stop the drinking.

THERAPIST: That's true. But what can Alex tell himself? What specific sentences should Alex learn?

JOE: He needs to tell himself about how it hurts him.

THERAPIST: Good. Do you think that it would be helpful if Alex would say over and over, "I want to take good care of my body."

ALEX: If I was able to say that it would probably help, but it's hard to remember to think in a different way.

THERAPIST: All the more reason for practice.

ALEX: Will it help?

THERAPIST: It's really an experiment. You can try it to see what happens.

8. *Reframing*. There are times that a seeming disaster can be turned to one's advantage. A prime example of this is admission to the hospital. When the patient sees being in the hospital as the final straw, the experience can be reframed as a beginning rather than an end.

MAUDE: My being here is just more than I can bear. I can't believe I've sunk so low that I need to be in a nuthouse.

KEN: Hey, that's enough of that stuff. We don't all think that way.

MAUDE: Yeah? How can being here be any good for me? I feel like it's the end of the road.

THERAPIST: Maude is bringing up an important point. What can you do when the hospital itself seems like the final blow?

KEN: Well I feel better about myself now than I ever have before. I've really learned to see things in a different way. You just need to give it a chance.

MARY: This is probably the best thing that has happened to me. If I wasn't here I would be going along in the same old way. Or, I might be dead.

9. *Examining options and alternatives*. Patients can be taught the problem-solving technique of developing lists of options and then examining the merits of making one choice over another.

MAUDE: When I think of trying to go back to work, I get overwhelmed. There's so much to do. I'll never catch up. The only answer is just to quit.

THERAPIST: Maude's facing a common problem: coping with return to work after you've been admitted to the hospital. Right now, she only can think of one solution—to quit. Does anybody have any other ideas about how she could manage the situation?

CARMEN: She could try to understand her thinking. Maybe she's sees going back to work in an "all-or-none" way. Maude says she could *never* catch up. That's pretty strong.

MARY: Carmen, that's a good suggestion.

SAM: Maude could also talk with her boss and be open with him about being depressed.

JOAN: I don't know about that idea. It might backfire.

THERAPIST: Joan's starting to consider how these plans might work out. Let's hold on analyzing the ideas for a short while until we identify a few more options.

JOE: Well, Maude, you could start back part-time so you don't have to handle everything at once. I think that's what I'd do.

MAUDE: No, they won't let me do that.

ALEX: Maybe you could break the job down into pieces, like we've done with other things that are hard to do. We could help you think about how to get started again.

THERAPIST: Maude, the group has come up with several ideas. How do they sound?

MAUDE: Well, I feel better just getting the sense that the rest of you wouldn't give up. I can try, but it's going to be hard.

THERAPIST: We've gotten a good start. Let's take a closer look at each of the options. We need to get more details on how Maude might be able to use the different ideas.

Behavioral Procedures

Behavioral techniques described for individual CT earlier in this volume (Chapters 1 and 4) are also used in the group setting. A detailed discussion of behavioral interventions is not repeated here. Instead, we briefly describe group applications of three major behavioral procedures: activity scheduling, graded-task assignments, and behavioral rehearsal.

Activity Scheduling

On most inpatient cognitive therapy units, the activity schedule is a basic part of the treatment program. It serves multiple purposes, including (1) structuring the patient's day, (2) organizing treatment in a logical manner, (3) stimulating increased levels of activity in depressed or withdrawn patients, (4) scheduling pleasurable activities, (5) teaching self-monitoring, and (6) providing cognitive material for individual, group, and family therapy. Usually the nurse and auxiliary therapists have primary responsibility for implementing the daily activity schedule. Nevertheless, group therapy may be used to review progress or to devise new activities for the schedule. Frequently the activity schedule will lead the patient to engage in behaviors that will stimulate automatic thoughts or schemas. These cognitions can then be brought to group therapy for examination and resolution.

Graded-Task Assignments

Graded-task assignments are derived from behavioral "shaping" and desensitization strategies. Each small, sequential step helps the patient to expand his or her activities in a gradual manner and to reach an eventual goal. It is important to avoid taking an overly ambitious initial step. The group can not only work to help to plan the graded tasks but help each other carry out the planned actions. For example, a patient who had difficulty in making interpersonal contact outlined a sequence of steps to improve his social skills. Step one was smiling at people on the unit as he passed by. The next step was to smile and nod. Step three involved saying hello while passing, and so forth. The patient was asked to assess the reactions of others to his actions and to record the cognitions that were evoked by the exercise. Another group member volunteered to walk along and to help evaluate the responses of the others. A successful completion of the assignment was reported at the next group session.

Behavioral Rehearsal

Group CT can be used to practice adaptive behaviors—for example, dealing directly with a significant other, a boss, or a friend. The group and the therapist can give feedback on the patient's performance and coach the patient on more effective response styles. With some patients, the other group members or the therapist may need to demonstrate or to model different behaviors. For example, patients can role play phone calls, family visits, or components of graded task hierarchies. The role play can be supervised by the therapist or performed as a homework assignment and reported back at the next therapy session.

Transference and Countertransference in GCT

The therapist should be prepared to manage extreme or charged interpersonal reactions within the group. Such responses are often manifestations of transference or countertransference. These terms, derived from psychoanalytic therapy, apply to GCT as generic descriptors of interpersonal responses that are derived from early experiences with significant others. Transference reactions can occur rather abruptly in the intense environment of the psychiatric hospital where the patient lives in close proximity to a wide variety of individuals and is exposed to a number of doctors, nurses, therapists, and other authority figures. These responses are important for diagnostic purposes and may also provide excellent opportunities for the identification of significant schemas. The therapist's role here is to (1) recognize transference reactions, (2) take actions to limit transference if this is likely to be destructive (procedures might include accurate feedback, explanations about the responsibilities of therapist and patient in cognitive therapy, and bringing the reaction "out into the open" for discussion), and (3) channel the group toward identification and modification of underlying schemas. Generally, the therapist must take the primary responsibility for working with transference reactions because short-term group members are unlikely to recognize these phenomena.

Countertransference can occur when the therapist has significant cognitive and emotional responses to the patient's transference.

Therapists should be aware of their own automatic thoughts and schemas and be able to maintain an empathic and rational demeanor even under the stress of the group interaction. If, for example, the therapist becomes angry at individuals in the group or starts to think that the next session will be onerous, a discussion with the cotherapist or another colleague is warranted. The same cognitive therapy techniques that are recommended to the patient are used by the therapist to explore and cope with thoughts and feelings evoked by the group experience.

Nonadherence to Treatment Recommendations

When patients fail or refuse to pursue the goals, expectations, and therapeutic prescriptions of the inpatient program, the therapist's responsibility is to ascertain the nature and source of the problem. Nonadherence may be a product of skill deficiencies (i.e., the patient is unable to perform an assignment because of a lack of ability). In this case, the therapist can suggest less complex or demanding treatment procedures and can also design interventions that will help the patient to develop necessary skills. Long-held behavioral patterns such as passive–aggressiveness can also lead to noncompliance. When this occurs, the therapist needs to identify the pattern and work with the patient to assess the advantages and disadvantages of maintaining the behavior.

It is rare to have an inpatient group in which all members are highly motivated for substantive growth. Most groups contain individuals who have been admitted involuntarily, are staying grudgingly in the hospital, or are ambivalent about a commitment to therapy. These types of patients present special challenges to the group therapist. A significant number (three or more in an 8- to 10-patient group) of poorly motivated patients can derail the group process. Thus, the therapist needs either to stimulate a more collaborative effort by using cognitive therapy procedures to modify the negative cognitions about treatment, or, when this is not possible, to alter the composition of the group by "selecting out" individuals who cannot apply themselves to the work of the group.

We have also seen situations where the patient's family or friends reinforce a negative view of treatment by directly disparaging the treatment program or by subtly undermining the patient's involvement in group therapy (I wouldn't want to hear about everyone else's problems. I hope you won't talk about me. You really don't want to tell all those people how you feel, do you?). When this occurs, the therapist may need to meet with family members or request that the family therapist help reverse the disruption of the group cognitive therapy process. The patient's response to the family communications can also be included on the agenda for GCT.

[1]We use the words adherence and compliance interchangeably to describe the degree to which the patient follows treatment recommendations. A proscriptive or controlling therapist stance for GCT is not recommended and should not be inferred from the use of these terms.

GROUP COGNITIVE THERAPY: FORMATS

Most cognitive therapy units have a core group that meets two or more times a week. We use the term core GCT to refer to groups that are considered to be a central component of the inpatient experience. Three forms of the core group are described: open-ended, rotating-theme, and programmed. On a short-term unit, all three types of core groups must, by necessity, be open-ended. However, the rotating theme and programmed groups add an additional structural element to the therapy. The unit-community meeting is another variation of inpatient group therapy. This format for GCT is an adaptation of treatment procedures developed for the "therapeutic community" (see Chapters 2 and 3). Many CTUs also utilize a variety of special purpose groups. Examples include family, outing (supervised excursions away from the hospital), homework, and assertiveness-training groups. These types of therapies may be used for psychoeducational purposes or to meet defined needs of a segment of patients on the unit (e.g., women, elderly patients, individuals with social skills deficits, those who are about to be discharged, etc.). Several illustrations of special purpose groups will be discussed. However, a full description of the entire range of inpatient groups is beyond the scope of the chapter. A list of the multiple groups in a well-developed CTU is contained in Chapter 3.

Core Groups

Open-Ended GCT

The traditional form of open-ended group therapy used with outpatients must be modified substantially to accommodate the fast-paced circumstances of psychiatric hospitalization. Whereas the outpatient group therapist might expect patients to stay in the group for 3 months or more, the inpatient therapist may only see patients for 1 to 3 weeks. In some cases, the hospitalized patient will be able to attend 10 or more sessions, but treatment courses of two to five sessions are not uncommon. The turnover in an open-ended outpatient group is usually kept to a minimum so that frequent comings and goings do not dominate the group process. In a hospital setting, the composition of the group is continually changing; it is a rarity to have an identical group composition for two sequential sessions. This flux in group membership presents significant challenges. Yet, inpatient group therapists have been able to develop procedures to socialize patients rapidly to the therapy, accomplish meaningful work in a limited amount of time, and manage the rapid interchange of patients in an effective manner.

The open-ended group is the most frequently used form of GCT in hospital settings. All of the basic procedures for GCT described earlier are utilized in the open-ended group. Patients are screened carefully in order to select group members who can enter rapidly into the therapy process. Advance preparation is also important. At a minimum, the patient is exposed to the cognitive model before attending GCT through one or more of the following: individual therapy, readings and other homework assignments, or instructional sessions with a nurse or auxiliary therapist.

At least two therapists are recommended for any of the core GCT groups. Reasons for having two, or even three, therapists include: (1) the intensity of the work is high; (2) therapists can help each avoid negative "countertransference"; (3) discussion among therapists promotes the development of accurate and effective cognitive case conceptualizations; and (4) cotherapists can assist patients with completion of homework assignments outside the group (especially if one of the cotherapists is a nurse or activities therapist). The cotherapy role is also useful in training programs for group cognitive therapists.

The therapist and cotherapist adopt a very active therapy style for an inpatient open-ended group. As the only permanent members of the group, they have the primary responsibility for transmission of the "group culture" (i.e., basic theories, rules, responsibilities, parameters of therapeutic relationships). The therapists must also structure the group process effectively and keep the pace of the session at a level that maximizes the chances for learning and minimizes the possibilities for confusion or overload.

Yalom (1983) recommends that each inpatient group session be viewed as a self-contained therapeutic experience, so that even if individuals can attend only one session, they are able to understand and respond to it. We agree with this viewpoint on group therapy with inpatients. Several suggestions for using GCT procedures to make each open-ended group session a "therapy within a therapy" are offered.

1. *Emphasize psychoeducational aspects of treatment.* One of the main purposes of the group is to teach cognitive therapy techniques that the patient can use for self-help in the hospital environment and after discharge. The therapist cannot hope to elucidate and work through all of the patient's distortions, interpersonal conflicts, or troubling behaviors during the brief hospital stay. Instead, the group therapist strives to help the patient understand the concepts of cognitive therapy that can be applied to solve these problems over the long term. The patient should leave each session armed with new information that will be of benefit, regardless of opportunities for further group therapy.

2. *Set a meaningful agenda.* Patients are instructed to come to the open-ended group with one or two agenda items in mind. After a brief introduction, including recognition of new members, the therapist moves immediately to setting the agenda for the session. Usually, the topics can be lumped into categories that can be rank-ordered according to their importance to the group.

Agenda setting usually consumes 5 to 15 minutes of the session. The therapist frames questions that help patients to state their topics clearly and succinctly and directs the group toward development of an agenda that is likely to be manageable for the individual session and productive in meeting the goals for GCT. Diffuse or amorphous topics are discouraged. If an event or interpersonal situation is described, the therapist can ask for the patient's predominant cognitive response in order to make the situation more understandable to the group. Table 5.1 includes illustrations of stated agenda items and highlights of the patient's cognitions about the issue or situation.

The agenda-setting process accomplishes much more than just the selection of topics for the session. Patients gain experience in identifying problems, verbalizing their concerns to others, and negotiating within a group. This activity also can help reverse attitudes of defeat or hopelessness if the patient is able to reduce an overwhelming or overgeneralized concern into an agenda item that is likely to respond to treatment.

3. *Focus on vignettes or concerns that have broad relevance.* Although an attempt is made to discuss at least briefly all chosen agenda items, a majority of the session is devoted to working with a few topics that are, of general interest, highly significant to group members, and illustrative of cognitive therapy principles. It is more important to select a limited number of items that can serve as teaching vehicles for the entire group than to attempt to cover all issues in an even-handed but superficial manner.

4. *Use homework to link GCT with the rest of the milieu.* An attempt is made to have each session lead to a homework assignment that can extend the work of the group into the larger milieu. Ideally, the patient will have the opportunity to return to the group to discuss the results of the assignment, but even if this isn't possible, there are other forums (individual or family therapy, sessions with a nurse, discharge conferences, etc.) to evaluate the impact of the homework. The self-help aspects of homework should be emphasized so that the patient will be encouraged to continue with these procedures after completing his or her brief course of GCT.

5. *Work on cognitive and behavioral changes that will prepare the patient for discharge.* Preparation for discharge is one of the major themes of the

TABLE 5.1. Open-Ended Group Agenda

Items suggested by patients	Groupings suggested by therapist	Hierarchy established by group
Maude: Reaction to call from boss ("Can I handle my job?")	Events that stimulate negative automatic thoughts	Events that stimulate negative automatic thoughts (Maude, Joe, and Ken)
Joe: Worry about a family session ("I'm afraid she'll leave me.")	Events that stimulate negative automatic thoughts	Low self-esteem (Mary and Ken)
Alex: The Activity Schedule doesn't make sense. ("How could it help to write down what I do all day?")	Homework	Homework (Alex, Joan, and all)
Sam: Concern about going home ("I want to go, but I'm afraid I'll get back into the same old routine.")	Preparing to go home	
Joan: Report on homework ("The graded task worked out well.")	Homework	Preparing to go home (Sam and Carmen)
Mary: Low self-esteem ("I always get down on myself.")	Low self-esteem	
Carmen: How do I handle a home visit ("I'll just get angry when I see all the mess he didn't clean up.")	Preparing to go home	
Ken: Going to occupational therapy ("They must think I'm a total basket case.")	Low self-esteem and events that stimulate negative automatic thoughts	

open-ended inpatient group. In a sense, rapid turnover is actually an *advantage*, because it continually keeps the group focused on the major goal of hospitalization: reduction in symptoms to allow discharge. New members can see that others make substantive progress before going home and that the inpatient stay will only be a short chapter in their lives. During their first session in GCT, patients will start to learn from more experienced group members how to make the transition back to the home setting. If the patient is able to attend only one or two group sessions, he or she will still be able to have the group help with preparation for discharge.

Rotating-Theme Groups

The rotating-theme group was developed specifically for use in hospital settings (Bowers, 1989). In this type of GCT, an external structure for the therapy agenda is used in an attempt to circumvent some of the problems that are encountered with rapid patient turnover. Several steps are involved in developing a rotating-theme group. The therapist's initial job is to ascertain the number of group sessions that can be held during a usual inpatient stay. For the sake of illustration, let us assume that group therapy is held three times a week, and most patients are able to attend eight group sessions during the course of an inpatient hospitalization. By focusing each of the eight sessions on a particular theme (e.g., the stigma of hospitalization, dealing with children, coping with parents, problems with school or work, or other common areas of difficulty), the therapist can structure a comprehensive group therapy experience. The topics for each session are posted on the unit bulletin board, and patients are asked to prepare in advance for each of the group meetings. Patients are instructed to write out two questions, problems, or thoughts relative to the selected theme and to bring what they have written to the next group session. Index cards are supplied for writing down ideas. Nurses and other staff members help prepare the patients by reviewing the material on the cards before the group meeting.

Although not every theme is fully relevant to every patient, the topic areas are of broad interest so as to capture the attention of most group members. Some patients, however, may have to wait for a future session before dealing with their primary problem. Writing down questions or ideas allows patients who have difficulty being spontaneous in the group to have a mechanism for expressing themselves. Patients who have been in other therapy groups may have difficulty making the transition to a theme-focused format because they have become accustomed to a less structured approach. In more traditional forms of group therapy, the outspoken individual may be able to force his or her issues to the forefront and dominate the group.

Initially, the topics for the sessions can be developed by the group therapists based on their experiences with the range of patients typically encountered in the hospital milieu. The topic list should be matched to the population mix. For example, themes for GCT on a unit that specializes in depression might include building self-esteem, choosing pleasurable activities, or coping with loss. On the other hand, themes for group therapy for an eating disorders program might include body image, meal planning, or thoughts about eating. The topic list evolves as the group therapists have the opportunity to experiment with various group themes. A shift in the composition of the patient group would suggest that the session themes be altered. Most inpatient units experience surges of admissions of certain types of patients. At one time the group may be made up of individuals with affective disorders; at another time, personality disorders, chemical dependency, or other conditions may predominate. A sample list of topics for a rotating-theme group for a unit where most patients have affective disorders is contained in Table 5.2.

The therapist prepares psychoeducational materials that are relevant to each theme and may outline the general content and procedure for the session in advance. However, it is also important to involve the group members in setting the agenda and providing input on the direction for therapy. The rotating-theme group is somewhat more structured than the open-ended group, but spontaneity and vigorous group interaction are still encouraged.

At the beginning of each group, the leader asks one of the group members to be the secretary for the day (a rotating assignment for group members or the cotherapist) and to record on a chalkboard the problems that the patients bring up for the agenda. Group members are then asked to read what they have written on their index cards. These are recorded by the secretary, and similar or redundant items are

TABLE 5.2. Rotating Theme Group: Sample Schedule

Session 1	Reactions to hospitalization
Session 2	Hopelessness versus optimism
Session 3	Building self-esteem
Session 4	Getting motivated again
Session 5	Fears and anxieties
Session 6	Setting and reaching goals
Session 7	Coping with family and friends
Session 8	Returning to work or school

grouped thematically by the leader. Usually, 10 members do not generate 20 distinct issues; a good deal of overlap almost always occurs. A hierarchy of agenda items is established, and the group begins to work. All of the guidelines and procedures for open-ended groups described earlier also apply to the rotating-theme group. The only major difference is that a general topic is used to speed the agenda-setting process and to provide a thematic structure for group sessions.

Programmed Groups

The third type of core inpatient cognitive therapy group provides a series of sessions that is designed to convey a defined body of knowledge about cognitive therapy. These groups are a hybrid between open-ended, rotating-theme, and more circumscribed, psychoeducational groups. Compared to other core groups, the programmed group relies the most on structure and didactic techniques and the least on spontaneous processes of group interaction. Covi, Roth, and Lipman (1982) have described the successful use of programmed content groups for depressed outpatients. In the outpatient setting, all of the patients go through the sequence of sessions in the same order and at the same time. This allows the leaders to develop a package of treatment sessions that is arranged like an educational course. Each session is a building block for the next. However, the situation is more complicated with inpatients. If there are eight programmed sessions, some patients may begin at session 1, whereas others may begin at session 7 or 8. The program must thus be designed so that patients can start anywhere in the sequence and not be significantly handicapped by missing earlier sessions.

A sample schedule for a programmed inpatient group is contained in Table 5.3. The basic cognitive model is described at the beginning of every meeting, so that new members will have at least an overview of the cognitive approach before launching into the session. After reviewing homework, the therapist briefly presents the topic for the day, such as identifying automatic thoughts or using graded-task assignments. This didactic material is designed to be understandable even if the patient has not had the benefit of earlier sessions in the sequence. Diagrams and handouts are used to accelerate the learning process.

The next step is to elicit agenda items from the patient group and to use this material to illustrate treatment procedures described in the session. The full degree of interactive agenda setting described for open-ended groups is usually not possible because of time limitations. Instead, the therapist is more directive and selects a limited number of vignettes or concerns that can be used to help meet the goals of the session. Specification of homework is the final phase of the programmed

TABLE 5.3. Programmed Group: Sample Schedule

Session 1: Introduction to the cognitive model
- Diagram of the cognitive model
- Illustrations of linkage between situation, thoughts, feelings, and behaviors
- Examples from patient's own experience
- Homework: Read *Coping with Depression*[a]

Session 2: Recognizing automatic thoughts
- Review cognitive model
- Review homework
- Definition of automatic thoughts
- Illustrations of automatic thoughts
- Elicit automatic thoughts associated with agenda items
- Homework: Three-column thought record (situation, thoughts, feelings)

Sessions 3–4: Modifying automatic thoughts
- Review cognitive model, definition of automatic thoughts
- Review homework
- Introduce Daily Record of Dysfunctional Thoughts (DRDT)
- Define and illustrate three methods of changing automatic thoughts (questioning the evidence, decatastrophizing, identifying positives)
- Work on automatic thoughts associated with agenda items
- Homework: DRDT, Chapter 3 of *Feeling Good*[b]

Session 5: Recognizing cognitive errors
- Review cognitive model, automatic thoughts
- Review homework
- List and define cognitive errors
- Identify cognitive errors associated with agenda items
- Homework: label cognitive errors on DRDT; identify behavioral goal for next session

Session 6: Reaching goals: The step-wise approach
- Review cognitive model; emphasize relationship between cognitive and behavior
- Review homework
- Introduce graded-task strategy
- Design graded-task assignments for agenda items
- Homework: follow through with graded-task assignments

Session 7: Cognitive–behavioral rehearsal
- Review cognitive model, emphasize relationship between cognitions and behavior
- Review homework
- Describe and illustrate rehearsal techniques
- Perform role plays and cognitive–behavioral rehearsal with agenda items
- Homework: rehearse strategies to meet a defined goal

Session 8: Recognizing schemas
- Review cognitive model, automatic thoughts
- Review homework
- Define and illustrate schemas
- Differentiate schemas from automatic thoughts
- Elicit schemas associated with agenda items
- Discuss methods of changing schemas
- Homework: list advantages and disadvantages for holding a schema; write out two alternatives for a schema

[a]Beck & Greenberg (1974).
[b]Burns (1980).

group. Usually, there is a standard assignment that is linked closely to the material presented in the group meeting. Individualized homework may also be arranged.

The programmed group is the most efficient of the three types of core groups in imparting basic information on cognitive therapy. However, this form of GCT also has several disadvantages. The most significant disadvantage is that it sacrifices time for process interactions between group members in order to accomplish educational objectives. There is a risk that some of the common operational principles of group therapy, such as universality, support, and peer feedback will be shortchanged. Also, patients may become frustrated if they do not have the opportunity to voice their primary concerns or to discuss what troubles them the most. In addition, the pace of the programmed group may be too fast for a significant portion of the group members; some individuals may become confused by the fairly rapid introduction of a number of new concepts. These problems can be circumvented to some extent if the therapist is adept at blending group process interactions with the psychoeducational effort and if the group is comprised of individuals who can both readily absorb didactic material and enter quickly into the interpersonal sphere of group activities.

Programmed groups are most suitable for CTUs that have relatively long lengths of stay and homogeneous patient populations. The ability to screen out patients with severe psychopathology, especially psychomotor retardation or impaired learning and memory functioning, is also advantageous. Under these conditions, patients are more likely to be able to proceed through the entire series of group meetings and therapists to have less difficulty presenting material that can be grasped by all members of the group. When programmed groups are used, it is advisable to have concurrent individual sessions to allow processing of each patient's own particular agenda for therapy.

Unit-Community Meetings

The community meeting is considered to be an integral feature of most inpatient psychiatric units (Oldham & Russakoff, 1987; Arons, 1982). It also can play a vital role in the cognitively oriented milieu (Davis & Schrodt, in press). This meeting is the largest formal group congregation in most CTUs; it includes all patients (except those who are severely psychotic, extremely agitated, or disruptive) and, preferably, most of the nurses, physicians, family therapists, and other professionals who work on the unit. The community meeting is task oriented and structured. In some units, the meeting may be presided over by elected patient leaders; in most cases, one or two permanent staff members call the meeting to order. Typically, introduction of new members is the first order of business. Patients are asked to state their name, and new members are encouraged to give a brief explanation of why they are in the hospital.

Not uncommonly, initial feelings of hopelessness and demoralization are alleviated by the supportive comments of fellow patients and staff.

After this brief introduction, the community meeting focuses on unit-wide issues rather than on direct resolution of personal difficulties. Individual concerns are channeled toward other therapeutic activities. The community meeting is used primarily to socialize patients to the unit and to provide a forum for dealing with interpersonal issues that arise during hospitalization. The orientation process includes discussions of ward rules and policies, explanations of the roles of the patients and staff, brief descriptions of principles of cognitive therapy, and clarifications of unit procedures. Experienced patients help the staff convey this information.

Problems that affect the community are also addressed. Concerns may range from the relatively mundane (e.g., meals arriving late, defective heating system) to the more serious (e.g., fear of a severely psychotic patient). Conflicts with other patients or with staff are commonly identified in the community meeting. These situations provide an *in vivo* experience in using cognitively oriented approaches to problem solving. The group leaders may select any of the GCT techniques described earlier; however, an emphasis is placed on helping the group to recognize cognitive distortions, identify options, and practice more adaptive behavior. Negotiation and compromise are encouraged whenever possible.

The patient's sense of helplessness can be aggravated by hospitalization if staff members are perceived as dictatorial or controlling. The unit community meeting can be a good place to dispel these perceptions, especially if actions are taken to share power and responsibility with the patients. A fully democratic decision-making process, as described by Jones (1953) for the therapeutic community, is impractical and probably unwise for short-term units (see Chapter 2). However, collaborative therapeutic relationships can be promoted by eliciting input, suggestions, and advice on the functioning of the milieu. The adult CTU at the University of Louisville uses a procedure of discussing and approving all privilege-level changes in the unit community meeting. Although the attending physician may veto the group's decision, in practice this rarely happens. This exercise in joint decision making increases the patient's investment in the therapeutic milieu and reinforces the collaborative nature of cognitive therapy.

Finally, the unit community meeting is used to help individuals manage issues related to discharge from the hospital. On the last day of hospitalization, patients are encouraged to review their treatment experiences and to share any "words of wisdom" they may have. Discharge often evokes ambivalent thoughts and feelings including hope, excitement, and apprehension—as well as a sense of loss of new friends made in the hospital. The camaraderie with fellow patients is often regarded as one of the significant experiences of a successful inpatient stay. An important goal of the unit community meeting is to help patients carry the positive aspects of their hospital experience with them after they return to their home environment.

Special Purpose Groups

Family Groups

The involvement of available family members in the hospital program can be quite advantageous. Family members meet as a group with a staff member to discuss their concerns about the patient, the hospitalization, the treatment program, and goals for the future. This group can be made available to family members for the patient's length of stay in the hospital, or, alternatively, an open-ended group can be offered that will continue even after discharge. Family groups are usually devoted primarily to such psychoeducational activities as imparting information on common psychiatric disorders, discussing the fundamentals of cognitive therapy, or giving details on psychotropic medication and possible side effects. These groups also provide support for families who are undergoing the stress of having one of their members in the hospital.

Outing or Travel Groups

The outing or travel group can take several forms. For patients who are agoraphobic or who have difficulty in social settings, these groups may involve going off the unit into real-life situations in which they can practice the coping skills they have learned on the unit. A scheduled trip to a local shopping mall can be an excellent source of data about how the patient is able to manage social stressors. The group is transported by hospital bus or car to the mall. Once there, skills such as assertiveness can be modeled by the therapist and then practiced by the patient (e.g., buying something and then returning it for a refund shortly thereafter, ordering food and then registering a complaint if it is not properly prepared). The travel group puts the patient directly into the real world while he or she can still experience the guidance and support of the hospital staff.

Homework Groups

We have found it helpful to have a homework group scheduled as the final therapeutic activity of the day, prior to the patients' going to sleep. This group, led by the night nursing staff, follows up on homework assigned in GCT or individual therapy. The work that the patients have done during the day is reviewed, and, when necessary, help is given in completing the assignments. This group provides reinforcement for doing homework. Additional benefits are gained by providing opportunities to examine the thoughts generated by the homework, discuss the problems encountered in doing particular assignments, and gain mutual support from other patients.

Other Groups

There are a number of other special purpose groups that utilize cognitive therapy principles. Examples include those that focus on (1) education about medication; (2) creative expression such as art, dance, music, or crafts; (3) occupational therapy; (4) women's or men's issues; and (5) transition to outpatient status. In a comprehensive cognitive therapy milieu, all of these groups are led by individuals with cognitive therapy training.

SUMMARY

Group cognitive therapy helps patients to engage rapidly in the overall treatment process, assists the treatment team in obtaining a multifaceted picture of the patient's disorder, and provides accurate peer feedback to group members. This form of inpatient cognitive therapy also promotes a sense of universality that helps to ease the patient's isolation and burden of shame and guilt. However, the main contribution of GCT is a resolution of symptoms through the identification and modification of cognitive–behavioral pathology.

This chapter describes basic procedures for GCT, including selecting and preparing patients for group therapy, structuring the length and frequency of sessions, and maintaining a "here-and-now" focus. Pacing group sessions is one of the most complex and difficult parts of GCT because of rapid patient turnover and wide variations in levels of symptomatic distress. Nevertheless, cognitive interventions such as identifying automatic thoughts, listing advantages and disadvantages, or examining alternatives can be used with benefit in most group sessions. Standard behavioral procedures such as graded-task assignments and rehearsal are also utilized widely in GCT.

Three major categories of inpatient GCT are detailed: core groups (open-ended, rotating-theme, and programmed), unit-community meetings, and special-purpose groups. Any of these types of groups is suitable for inclusion as part of a cognitive milieu. Factors such as length of stay, homogeneity of the patient group, and availability of other methods of delivering cognitive therapy should be considered in designing the group therapy components of a CTU. We conclude that group therapies should be developed as primary features of all inpatient cognitive therapy programs.

REFERENCES

Arons, B. S. (1982). Effective use of community meetings on psychiatric treatment units. *Hospital and Community Psychiatry*, *33*, 480–483.

Beck, A. T., Freeman, A., & Associates (1990). *Cognitive therapy of personality disorders*. New York: Guilford Press.

Beck, A. T., & Greenberg, R. L. (1974). *Coping with depression*. (Available from the Institute for Rational Emotive Therapy, 45 East 65th Street, New York, NY 10021.)

Beck, A. T., Rush, A. J., Shaw, B. F., & Emery, G. (1979). *Cognitive therapy of depression*. New York: Guilford Press.

Beutler, L., Frank, M., Scheiber, S., Calvert, S., & Gaines, J. (1984). Comparative effects of group therapies in a short-term inpatient setting: An experience with deteriation effects. *Psychiatry*, *47*(1), 66–76.

Bowers, W. A. (1989). Cognitive therapy with inpatients. In A. Freeman, K. M. Simon, L. E. Beutler, & H. Arkowitz (Eds.), *Comprehensive handbook of cognitive therapy* (pp. 583–596). New York: Plenum Press.

Brown, R. A., & Lewinsohn, P. M. (1984). A psychoeducational approach to the treatment of depression: Comparison of group, individual, and minimal contact procedures. *Journal of Consulting and Clinical Psychology*, *52*, 774–783.

Burns, D. D. (1980). *Feeling good*. New York: William Morrow.

Covi, L., & Lipman, R. (1987). Cognitive behavioral group psychotherapy combined with imipramine in major depression. *Psychopharmacology Bulletin*, *23*, 173–176.

Covi, L., & Primakoff, L. (1988). Cognitive group therapy. In A. J. Frances, & R. E. Hales (Eds.), *American Psychiatric Press review of psychiatry* (pp. 608–626). Washington, DC: American Psychiatric Press.

Covi, L., Roth, D., & Lipman, R. S. (1982). Cognitive group psychotherapy of depression: The close-ended group. *American Journal of Psychotherapy*, *36*(4), 459–469.

Davis, M. H., & Schrodt, G. R., Jr. (in press). Being where I can be safe. In A. Freeman & F. Dattilio, (Eds.), *Comprehensive casebook of cognitive therapy*. New York: Plenum Press.

Free, M. L., Oei, T. P. S., & Sanders, M. R. (1991). Treatment outcome of a group cognitive therapy program for depression. *International Journal of Group Psychotherapy, 41*, 533–547.

Gelernter, C. S., Uhde, T. W., Cimbolic, P., Arnkoff, D. B., Vittone, B. J., Tancer, M. E., & Bartko, J. J. (1991). Cognitive–behavioral and pharmacologic treatments of social phobia. *Archives of General Psychiatry, 48*, 938–945.

Jarvik, L. F., Mintz, J., Steuer, J., & Gerner, R. (1982). Treating geriatric depression. *Journal of the American Geriatrics Society, 30*, 713–717.

Jones, M. (1953). *The therapeutic community: A new treatment method in psychiatry*. New York: Basic Books.

Linehan, M. M. (1987). Dialectical behavior therapy in groups: Treating borderline personality disorders and suicidal behavior. In C. M. Brody (Ed.), *Women in groups* (pp. 145–162). New York: Springer.

Maxmen, J. S., Tucker, G. J., & LeBow, M. (1974). *Rational hospital psychiatry*. New York: Brunner/Mazel.

Meichenbaum, D. (1977). *Cognitive–behavioral modification: An integrative approach*. New York: Plenum Press.

Moline, R. A. (1976). Hospital psychiatry in transition. From the therapeutic community toward a rational eclectism. *Archives of General Psychiatry, 33*, 1234–1238.

Oldham, J. M., & Russakoff, L. M. (1987). *Dynamic therapy in brief hospitalization*. Northvale, NJ: Jason Aronson.

Perris, C., Rodhe, K., Palm, A., Abelson, M., Heelgren, S., Lilja, C., & Soderman, H. (1987). Fully integrated in- and outpatient services in a psychiatric sector: Implementation of a new model for the care of psychiatric patients favoring continuity of care. In A. Freeman & V. Greenwood (Eds.), *Cognitive therapy: Applications in psychiatric and medical settings* (pp. 117–131). New York: Human Sciences Press.

Rush, A. J., & Watkins, J. T. (1981). Group versus individual cognitive therapy: A pilot study. *Cognitive Therapy and Research, 5*, 95–103.

Shaffer, C. S., Shapiro, J., Sank, L. I., & Coghlan, D. J. (1981). Positive changes in depression, anxiety, and assertion following individual and group cognitive behavior therapy intervention. *Cognitive Therapy and Research, 5*, 149–157.

Shaw, B. F. (1977). A comparison of cognitive therapy and behavior therapy in the treatment of depression. *Journal of Consulting and Clinical Psychology, 45*, 543–551.

Yalom, I. D. (1983). *Inpatient group psychotherapy*. New York: Basic Books.

Yalom, I. D. (1985). *The theory and practice of group psychotherapy* (3rd ed.). New York: Basic Books.

Chapter 6

Inpatient Family Therapy

Part A. Inpatient Family Treatment: General Principles

Ivan W. Miller, Ph.D.,
Gabor I. Keitner, M.D.,
Nathan B. Epstein, M.D.,
Duane S. Bishop, M.D.,
and Christine E. Ryan, Ph.D.

"Joan," a 46-year-old married nursing aide, was admitted to the hospital for increased depression and suicidal ideation. On admission, she reported a history of chronic depression lasting for the last 10 years. An acute exacerbation had occurred during the last 3 months. She had a severe level of depression (Beck Depression Inventory = 31) as well as high levels of hopelessness and suicidal ideation. Identified problem areas included low self-esteem and interpersonal conflicts with her husband and co-workers. Joan was treated with a combination of antidepressant medication and individual cognitive therapy beginning when she was in the hospital and continuing on an outpatient basis. Cognitive therapy focused on reducing hopelessness and teaching her to monitor and evaluate her negative thoughts about herself and her future. She was quite responsive to the treatment and made excellent progress, so that by discharge her depression was much improved (BDI = 16), and by the third week after discharge, it was almost nonexistent (BDI = 5). At this point, the patient returned to work and reported feeling better than she had "in years." This low level of depression continued for the next 3 weeks, and the patient seemed well on her way to an impressive recovery. However, the following week, her level of depression increased substantially (BDI = 21). In a therapy session, the patient reported that her husband of 21 years had told her to stop coming to treatment because he didn't like how she was changing. He threatened to harm her physically if she continued. Despite the efforts of the therapist, the patient terminated treatment and never returned.

Although perhaps more extreme than usual, this case illustrates that psychiatric disorders and their treatment always occur within a social setting. Most often the primary social network consists of the patient's family. As in the case presented above, failure to adequately incorporate the patient's family into therapy can undermine the treatment plan. This chapter discusses how family system interventions can be included in the treatment of severe psychiatric illnesses. We begin with a brief review of the literature concerning families and psychiatric disorders and then present a series of guidelines for family treatment in an inpatient setting.

Because the most common illnesses treated on CTUs are affective disorders, this chapter refers primarily to "depression" and "depressed patients." However, our clinical experience with inpatient family therapy includes a broad range of psychiatric conditions. We consider virtually all of the content of this chapter to be applicable to other diagnostic categories of inpatients as well.

ROLE OF THE FAMILY IN PSYCHIATRIC DISORDERS

Theories about the role of the family in psychiatric illness have changed over time. Freud thought that the basis of most disorders lay in early child–parent experiences (Freud, 1917). This tradition continued through the 1970s. Concepts such as the "schizophrenogenic mother" and the "double bind" placed the emphasis on the family as *the* major cause of psychiatric disturbance. However, in the late 1970s and the 1980s the pendulum began to swing back because of both increased recognition of the biological aspects of psychiatric disorders and protests by the families of patients. The role of families in mental conditions was thus minimized by the "biological revolution."

Current models of the family and psychopathology reject the previous extreme positions (e.g., Keitner & Miller, 1990). Instead, psychiatric disturbances are thought to be biopsychosocial disorders. Although the relative etiological significance of the three components of the system is not always clear and may, in fact, vary for different patients, the presence of a severe psychiatric disorder always has a significant impact on the patient's biological, psychological, and social functioning (Keitner & Miller, 1990). Conversely, all three elements of the system will also have an influence on the patient's illness. Thus, for optimal treatment of a psychiatric condition, the entire biopsychosocial system must be considered.

ROLE OF THE FAMILY IN DEPRESSION

The role of the family in the development, maintenance, and treatment of depressive disorders has been the subject of increased interest in recent years (Keitner & Miller, 1990). Briefly, this research has revealed a number of important relationships between family systems and depressive disorders.

1. *During an acute episode, families of depressed patients have significantly impaired family functioning.* These effects have been described both in hospitalized patients (Keitner, Miller, Epstein, & Bishop, 1986; Keitner, Miller, Epstein, & Bishop, 1987) and in outpatients (Biglan et al., 1985; Birtchnell, 1988; Hinchliffe, Hooper, Roberts, & Vaughan, 1975; Hinchliffe, Vaughan, Hooper, & Roberts, 1977; Weissman, 1974). The level of family impairment is generally quite severe. Some studies suggest that families of depressed and substance-abuse patients exhibit a greater level of family dysfunction than do families of patients with other disorders (Crowther, 1985; Miller, Kabacoff, Keitner, Epstein, & Bishop, 1986). There does not appear to be a particular type of family dysfunction associated with having a family member who is depressed. There can be numerous difficulties in many aspects of family life, including problems with communication, problem-solving, self-disclosure, and levels of conflict (Keitner & Miller, 1990).

2. *After remission of the patient's acute symptoms, family functioning usually improves.* Again, these effects have been found both in samples of inpatients (Hinchliffe et al., 1977; Keitner, Miller, Epstein, et al., 1987; Merikangas, Prusoff, Kupfer, & Frank, 1985) and outpatients (Dobson, 1987; Rounsaville, Prusoff, & Weissman, 1980). But, for a substantial number of patients and families, family functioning does not return to baseline levels (Hinchliffe et al., 1977; Keitner, Miller, Epstein, et al., 1987; Merikangas et al., 1985). These families continue to experience more problems than normal families.

3. *The level of family functioning is a predictor of recovery from the acute episode.* High levels of family dysfunction during an acute episode have

been found to be associated with lower rates of full response to treatment (Keitner, Miller, Epstein, et al., 1987; Rounsaville, Weissman, Prusoff, Herceg-Baron, 1979; Swindle, Cronkite, & Moos, 1989). Even among those patients who do recover, poor family functioning is associated with a longer duration of treatment (Keitner, Miller, Epstein, et al., 1987).

4. *Family functioning is related to relapse vulnerability.* High levels of family dysfunction, particularly excessive criticism among family members, have been consistently associated with elevated rates of symptom recurrence (Hooley, Orley, & Teasdale, 1986; Hooley & Teasdale, 1989; Vaughan & Leff, 1976).

5. *Family variables may be an important factor in predicting suicidal behavior among depressed patients.* Depressed inpatients with a suicide attempt or current suicidal ideation prior to admission reported worse family functioning than those patients without current suicidality (Keitner, Miller, Fruzzetti, Epstein, & Bishop, 1987). In addition, depressed inpatients with poor family functioning were more likely to have recurrent suicidality during a 2-year follow-up period (Keitner, Ryan, Miller, Bishop, & Epstein, 1990).

We have recently presented a conceptual model for the role of family functioning in major depression that is applicable to most psychiatric disorders (Keitner & Miller, 1990). In this model, patient vulnerability and family competence are seen as independent, yet interacting factors. Certain individuals are vulnerable to the development of depression for a number of reasons (e.g., cognitive, genetic, early life experiences). Similarly, there is a range of premorbid family competency that may be influenced by a variety of factors. A patient's vulnerability to illness may be affected by family issues. Concurrently, a family's competence may be compromised by the disorder of one of its members.

According to this model, when a vulnerable patient develops an acute episode, the family has to respond to the patient's disorder. If the family is able to react effectively, then the episode may last a relatively short time. Conversely, if the family is unable to cope adequately with the patient's illness because of its own difficulties, then it is likely that the episode will be more prolonged, and the patient will be more likely to relapse. Subsequent episodes or lack of full recovery may further impair the family's competence, thereby setting up a vicious cycle. To summarize, patient vulnerability and family competence are seen as mutually reinforcing influences; they may act together to further the depression or provide a way of lessening its impact.

RESEARCH ON FAMILY TREATMENT FOR DEPRESSION

Despite research suggesting that the family is an important influence on depressed patients, there have been relatively few controlled studies that have investigated the efficacy of marital or family treatment for depressed patients. Three studies have reported that marital or family treatment "alone" (e.g., without psychotropic drugs or other adjunctive therapies) for depressed outpatients produced response rates equivalent to pharmacotherapy or individual treatment (Beach & O'Leary, 1986; Friedman, 1975; McLean, Ogstron, & Grauer, 1973). In the single study of inpatient family treatment reported to date, a research group at the Payne Whitney Clinic (Glick et al., 1985; Haas et al., 1988; Spencer et al., 1988) randomly assigned patients to family treatment, composed of six psychoeducational family meetings over a 5-week hospital stay, or to a control group. All other treatments were held constant. At discharge from the hospital, the *female* patients who had received the family treatment had better symptomatic and family functioning. This result was maintained at the 6- and 18-month follow-up evaluations. However, there was no benefit and even a worsening among *male* patients who had received the family intervention.

The results of a study by Jacobson, Dobson, Fruzzetti, Schmaling, and Salusky (1991) are particularly relevant to the selection of marital or family treatment with a cognitive therapy (CT) approach. They reported that among a sample of depressed outpatients with high levels of marital distress, individual CT alone produced clinically significant improvement in only 43% of patients, and *deterioration* in 29%. In contrast, a behavioral marital therapy intervention with this sample produced significant improvement in 75% of the patients; no patients manifested deterioration. This finding suggests that among a subsample of depressed patients who have high levels of marital or family distress, individual CT alone may not be sufficient in all cases. In some it may actually produce distress.

The results of the study by Jacobson et al. are congruent with our clinical experience in a study of cognitive and behavioral treatments for depressed inpatients (Miller, Norman, & Keitner, 1989). Although we did not include measures of marital or family functioning in this study, our clinical judgment was that virtually all of the patients who did not respond to a combination of medication and individual cognitive or behavioral treatment had significant family problems not addressed by our treatment protocol.

In summary, the available research indicates that marital or family therapies can be effective treatments for depression. More specifically, there are suggestions that a subset of patients with high levels of marital or family dysfunction may not respond to individual CT alone. Thus, for maximum treatment effectiveness, the therapy program for depressed inpatients should include a family assessment and intervention component.

GUIDELINES FOR CONDUCTING FAMILY TREATMENT ON INPATIENT UNITS

Which Family Therapy Model Should Be Selected for a Cognitive Therapy Inpatient Unit?

There are probably hundreds of types of family therapies. Our first recommendation concerning the choice of a family therapy model is to choose one method. Many family therapists use an "eclectic" approach that includes bits and pieces of a number of different types of therapies. Highly experienced and competent therapists can sometimes effectively use strategies from several different types of therapies. But more often than not, use of multiple models leads to an unfocused and disorganized approach that is confusing to the families and the therapist. We suggest that choosing one model and becoming an "expert" in its application is a far more efficient and effective strategy.

Given the many types of family therapy, how can one be chosen for use on a CTU? We recommend that unit leaders choose a therapy model with which the available family therapists are the most experienced and comfortable. In line with our comments above, it is probably more important to utilize one method well than to force therapists to fit into a model for which they have little training, competence, or desire to learn.

Family treatment on a CTU should either be cognitively oriented or similar in structure, style, and focus to cognitive therapy. If the latter course is chosen, the similarities between therapies should include several of the common characteristics of contemporary cognitive and behavioral treatments:

1. Focus on current problems.
2. Active, directive stance by the therapist.
3. Structured therapy approach.
4. Collaborative therapeutic relationship.
5. Focus on behavioral and cognitive change.
6. Therapist addresses problems in an open, straightforward manner.

7. Use of homework.
8. Time-limited treatment.

We believe there are four models of marital and family therapy that have been described in detail that meet these criteria: behavioral marital therapy (Beach, Sandeen, & O'Leary, 1990; Jacobson & Margolin, 1979); cognitive–behavioral therapy for couples (Baucom & Epstein, 1990; Beck, 1988; Dattilio & Padesky, 1990); interpersonal therapy (Gotlib & Colby, 1987); and problem-centered systems therapy of the family (Epstein & Bishop, 1981; Miller, Bishop, Keitner, & Epstein, in press). Each of these models presents a theoretical rationale and method of treatment that includes the common characteristics listed above and has a content and treatment approach that is congruent with cognitive therapy.

Although all of these treatment approaches appear suitable for use on a CTU, there are some important differences between them. One difference concerns the degree of CT rationale that is included in the treatment regimen. Whereas, in our view, none of these treatments is antithetical to a CT orientation, the cognitive–behavioral therapy for couples (Baucom & Epstein, 1990; Beck, 1988; Dattilio & Padesky, 1990) utilizes the most CT content in treatment interventions. Behavioral marital therapy takes a more behavioral/problem-solving approach but includes some cognitive procedures. Interpersonal therapy (IPT) and problem-centered systems therapy of the family (PCSTF) employ a somewhat broader formulation for treatment. They include a number of cognitive and behavioral procedures but use a systems orientation to conceptualize the family.

Another difference between these types of treatments can be found in their degree of emphasis on treating the complete family system. As their names suggest, behavioral marital therapy and cognitive–behavioral marital therapy have been described primarily as marital interventions, although similar procedures have also been used with entire families (Alexander, 1988). Cognitive–behavioral therapy is used with the whole family in many CTUs. This type of therapy is illustrated in Part B of this chapter. Both IPT and PCSTF have been designed explicitly as family therapies that usually include all family members in treatment.

In our experience, it is easier to integrate the family model with the other treatment interventions if the family treatment model is consistent with the orientation of the rest of the CTU. Thus, the choice between these models for a specific CTU will depend to some extent on the type of CTU. Cognitive therapy programs that employ a comprehensive or staff model (see Chapter 3) may have family therapists who are highly experienced in cognitive therapy or related approaches. For these types of CTUs, choice of one of the more cognitively oriented family treatment models is probably the optimal solution. On the other hand, units that are based on an "add-on" or primary therapist model are less likely to have access to cognitively oriented family therapists and to have a wider range of theoretical orientations among staff. In these situations, a choice of one of the more broadly based family therapies may be indicated.

None of these marital/family therapies was developed initially for inpatient family treatment. Although most of the therapeutic principles of these treatments are applicable to an inpatient setting, family therapy of hospitalized patients has a number of unique aspects. In the subsequent sections, we describe a series of basic guidelines for inpatient family treatment. These guidelines are based on our own experience using the PCSTF approach within an "add-on" inpatient program. However, we believe that these guidelines are applicable to inpatient cognitive therapy regardless of the particular family treatment model or type of CTU utilized.

How Should Family Therapists Be Selected?

There are several guidelines associated with the selection of family therapists. First, the family therapist should be a mental health professional with specific training and experience in conducting family therapy. Although this point seems obvious, it is important to emphasize that family treatment is a distinct type of treatment that requires specialty training and experience. Learning to conduct effective family therapy requires conceptual and executive skills that are specifically related to treatment of families.

Therapists must be able to perceive and organize data that are collected when multiple family members are present. They also need to be able to maintain objectivity and neutrality while empathizing with the family's situation. Another requirement is learning the concepts associated with a particular family treatment approach. Finally, the family therapist must be able to select and implement appropriate family intervention procedures. These skills are typically not obtained solely through reading or workshops; mastery is dependent on supervised, intensive clinical training. Without such training, family therapists can do more harm than good!

The next guideline concerns the relationship between the family therapist and other hospital staff. In our judgment, the family therapist should be involved as much as possible with the other aspects of the patient's treatment. This recommendation is based on the biopsychosocial orientation to depression presented at the beginning of this chapter. The ideal way to achieve an integration of the biological, psychological, and social aspects of treatment is for one individual to conduct all the therapeutic interventions for a patient. However, this option is not usually practical. Few practitioners are trained and experienced in pharmacotherapy, cognitive therapy, group therapy, and family therapy. It is more usual to find individuals who are experts in one (or sometimes two) treatment modalities. Those few individuals who are skilled in these multiple areas of expertise are usually involved in administration or have other commitments that interfere with an ability to conduct all aspects of the treatment program personally. For these reasons, most inpatient treatment is delivered using a treatment team model in which therapy is parceled out to a number of individuals who have a variety of therapeutic skills. Commonly, there will be a psychiatrist who is responsible for the pharmacotherapy, a psychologist who performs individual or group CT, and a social worker who serves as the family therapist, as well as nurses and mental health workers who are also involved with the patient.

There are several options for integrating family therapy with the other elements of inpatient cognitive therapy. On some CTUs, the family therapist also serves as a group therapist, or even a pharmacotherapist. However, in most situations the different components of treatment are linked through the treatment planning process (see Chapter 3). It therefore is important to select family therapists who can be cooperative and flexible as they participate in treatment planning and other multidisciplinary team processes (Thase & Wright, 1991). If the family therapist becomes fully involved in the overall treatment plan: (1) there are fewer chances for miscommunication between treatment team members; (2) family issues are more likely to be considered in other treatments; and (3) family therapy is more valued and supported by the other team members *and* the family.

When Should Family Treatment Be Started?

Family treatment should begin as soon as possible after admission. Whereas some clinicians argue that family treatment should be delayed until the patient is "less disturbed," we think it is best to begin family treatment shortly after admission. There are several reasons for this decision. First, we find that seeing the family early in the hospital stay often gives us important information that we can use in a comprehensive formulation of the patient's disorder. Family members are excellent sources of information, especially early in treatment when they may be more accurate historians than an extremely disturbed or disorganized patient. Furthermore, since family conflicts are often major issues for inpatients, assessment of the role of the family in the patient's disorder is critical. Another reason for involving the family as soon as possible is that this participation conveys an important message: the family hears that the treatment team is interested and open to learning what the family knows about the patient. This stance encourages cooperation and collaboration between the treatment team and the family and helps to minimize any intentional or unintentional "sabotaging" of treatment by family members. Early involvement of the family also indicates that the clinicians recognize that the patient's problems have an impact on all family members; this sets the stage for comprehensive family assessment and treatment.

Who Should Be Included in Family Treatment?

All members of the family should be included in family treatment. When seeing a family for the first time, we prefer to have present all the family members living at home. We also include other individuals living in the home, and we may subsequently add significant extended family and outsiders who are actively involved with the family. This allows us to obtain (1) a full range of views, (2) an indication of potential allies and supports, (3) direct observation of parent–child and sibling interactions, and (4) ideas for the general future course of action for all members of the system.

However, it is not always possible to include all members of the family in the therapy. Reasons for not seeing the entire family include illness and necessary "excused" absences of some members (e.g., employment or residence out of town, genuine inability to get off from work to attend a session). Also, there are some situations where it is clinically advisable to see only some of the members and to exclude others. The most common reason for limiting participation in family therapy is the need to work on the sexual relationship of the parents. In these situations, a separate session is scheduled for the parents, or the children are asked to wait outside for part of the meeting. Acutely psychotic patients also may be excluded during the first part of therapy.

There are many reasons for including all members in the therapy. Since the disorder of one family member affects the entire family, all the members are involved whether they like it or not. Some family members may be extremely helpful to the therapy process in the informal roles of cotherapists or auxiliary therapists. Indeed, this is one of the basic strengths of family therapy; members can be trained to intervene positively and to be more effective problem solvers within their own family rather than be rendered impotent or inadvertently add to the problems.

Also, we find that in many families there is one member who has the role of the "healer"—someone who carries a disproportionate load of the family burden. This person is often relieved to receive help in dealing with problems that he or she thought were overwhelming. It is impossible to know in advance which family member has taken on this role, so seeing all family members increases the likelihood of finding this source of information and support within the family.

How Are Family Sessions Structured?

The structure of family sessions is very similar to the structure of individual cognitive therapy. We begin each family meeting by setting an agenda for the session. The agenda setting involves solicitation of input from both the therapist and family members about their expectations and goals for the session. During the session, we systematically elicit feedback from the family regarding the members' thoughts and feelings. In family meetings, it is especially important to elicit feedback from *all* family members present. Because it is not unusual to find that some family members are more vocal than others, we make special efforts to encourage feedback from the quieter members of the family. Capsule summaries are used throughout the session to provide the family with an overview of the major points. Finally, most sessions end with the development and assignment of a homework task.

What Should Be the Focus of Inpatient Family Treatment?

Since most inpatient settings today have a relatively short length of stay, the goals of family interventions must be adapted to the brief time available. We have found that with a short hospitalization, inpatient family therapy should focus on six major goals: (1) establish a collaborative relationship with the family; (2) give support to the family for the burden that they experience; (3) address the family's presenting problem; (4) conduct a comprehensive assessment of the family system and its relationship to the patient's disorder; (5) provide the family with psychoeducational information about the patient's disorder; and (6) plan discharge.

Establish a Collaborative Alliance with the Family

As in individual CT, a major task in inpatient family treatment is establishing a good working relationship. Because of the severe and often chronic nature of the disorders treated on inpatient units, most families of inpatients have had previous experiences with mental health professionals. Some of these experiences may have been quite unpleasant because of mental health professionals who have ignored the family completely, uncritically accepted the patient's complaints against other family members, or blamed the families themselves as a result of ignorance about the likely causes of affective episodes and other psychiatric illnesses. Thus, it is not unusual for families to come to the first meeting with quite negative thoughts and feelings. Family members often have exaggerated fears regarding demands for self-disclosure (e.g., "I thought you wanted to know everything about my private life") or apportionment of blame (e.g., "I was afraid you would blame me for Joe's problems"). Other families can unrealistically disavow all responsibility (e.g., "Martha's depression is her own fault. I don't have anything to do with it. Why do you want to see me?").

It is critical that the family therapist elicit and identify these cognitions early in the first session. In our experience, these types of cognitions are so prevalent in families of inpatients that we begin the first family session by reassuring the families of the routine nature of the assessment. We start the session by thanking the family for coming and telling them that we see the families of *all* patients who are admitted to the unit. This statement serves to "normalize" the family meeting. Second, we explicitly tell families that we are not here to blame them for the patient's problems but to try to understand better what combination of factors may be contributing to the patient's *and the family's* current problems and distress. We then ask for each family member's thoughts and expectations about the family meeting. If family members have additional dysfunctional cognitions about family sessions, specific cognitive interventions may be required. Finally, during the family session, we take much care to recognize, listen, and address each family member so as to convey that we value his or her contribution and perspective.

One potential danger for inpatient family therapists is the tendency to ally themselves too readily with the patient. In contrast to outpatient treatment, where the patient and the family are usually seen the same number of times, in hospital settings the patient is more often the focus of attention and feels disproportionate alliance to the treatment team, including the family therapist. The patient may be perceived by the rest of the family as having a closer relationship to the treatment team, even if that is not the case. The family therapist needs to elicit the family's cognitions about the treatment alliance and to correct distortions if they are present. However, the reality of differences in levels of attention should also be acknowledged and discussed.

Recognition and Support of Family Burden

Living with a psychiatric patient is not easy. Often the presence of a family member with a psychiatric disorder creates extraordinary difficulties and burdens for other family members (Coyne et al., 1987; Fadden, Bebbington, & Kuipers, 1987; Jacob, Frank, Kupfer, & Carpenter, 1987). Social isolation, financial worries, fears about unpredictable behavior, and chronic tension characterize families of depressed patients (Jacob et al., 1987). The stress is especially severe for families of patients disturbed enough to require hospitalization. Explicit recognition and empathy for the burden that family members experience help increase the collaboration between the family and treatment team and can provide a sense of support for family members.

Address Presenting Problem(s)

Because most patients enter the psychiatric hospital in a crisis situation, often involving family issues or conflicts, it is very important to address the family's major presenting problems. The notion of a "presenting problem" simply refers to the family's primary concerns at the time of assessment. Often we directly ask each family member "What problems do you see in your family?" The psychosocial factors that have contributed to the patient's being hospitalized at this time are also identified. Depending on the nature, severity, and importance of family issues, problems can be (1) addressed immediately with cognitive–behavioral procedures (2) postponed pending a comprehensive assessment of the family (see below) or (3) reframed or articulated in a different manner.

Comprehensive Assessment

Possibly the most important goal of inpatient family treatment is to conduct a comprehensive assessment of the family, including both its strengths and weaknesses. As we have discussed elsewhere (Epstein & Bishop, 1981; Miller et al., in press), a thorough assessment of the family is an essential guide for the course of therapy. It is critical that the hypotheses about the relationship between the family and the patient's disorder be based on clear evidence gathered from multiple sources. One common difficulty is establishing the validity of a patient's negative comments about family members. Whereas these perceptions are sometimes true, they also can be a result of cognitive distortion related to an affective disturbance or other psychiatric condition. Clinicians should be wary of falling into the trap of assuming disturbed family relationships in the absence of verifiable data.

This issue is especially relevant in the inpatient setting where other treatment team members may draw erroneous conclusions about family dysfunction and its relationship to the patient's disorder. For example, a woman with a very chronic and treatment-resistant depression was hospitalized for several weeks. Many treatments were tried with limited success. When the patient's depression lifted somewhat, she was granted permission to go home on passes with her husband. These visits were associated with a worsening of her depression the next day. This pattern led some unit staff to believe that the husband was mistreating his wife and that the marital relationship was severely disturbed. Further assessment with both husband and wife failed to yield any evidence for these beliefs. Both partners denied conflict at home and reported that nothing much actually had happened. When the patient's depression finally improved substantially, she was able to go home and return feeling energized and well. The relationship between home visits and increased depression had not been a product of family dysfunction but was the result of the patient's level of depression and low stress tolerance.

Psychoeducation

One of the most important functions of family therapy is to provide members with information concerning the patient's disorder. The psychoeducational process imparts information concerning (1) symptoms and etiology of the patient's illness, (2) available treatment approaches, and (3) common problems experienced by families who have a member with a psychiatric disorder. This information improves the family's understanding of the patient's condition and leads to better collaboration and compliance with the treatment team.

Discharge Planning

In most cases, families of patients can be a major source of support after hospitalization, even if the patient does not live at home. Thus, we find it very useful to include families in discussions of discharge plans. Families are readily able to identify potential problems and resources. At the very least, involvement of the family in discharge planning maximizes the likelihood that the family will support the discharge program.

Family treatment is often continued on an outpatient basis. This is especially important in the case of severely dysfunctional families. Failure to provide adequate follow-up family treatment can undo whatever has been accomplished during the inpatient stay. One particularly tragic case reported previously by our group (Epstein, Keitner, Bishop, & Miller, 1988) illustrates this point all too well. A 17-year-old male was admitted to the hospital after a 6-month course of increasing depression, drinking, and drug abuse. More recently, he had had a series of car accidents, increasing conflict with his family, and a suicide attempt. Individual and family assessment indicated a relatively healthy family until about a year previously when the patient had become depressed following a series of significant losses.

The family, which had previously functioned well, could not cope with these changes in the patient's behavior and became increasingly angry and critical toward the patient. Their actions worsened the patient's depression and created a vicious cycle effect. After the patient was hospitalized, several family sessions identified this pattern and helped to restore positive behavior among family members. The patient's depression then lifted dramatically. On discharge, further follow-up family treatment was recommended in order to maintain and consolidate these changes. However, the family had logistic difficulties returning to the hospital for treatment, so a referral was made to a local mental health center. Apparently, a sound treatment relationship was never established, and the family discontinued treatment without notifying us. About 6 months following discharge, the patient shot himself. In retrospect, it appeared that in the absence of continued, satisfactory family treatment, the family returned to its previous dysfunctional patterns.

Do All Families Need Family Therapy?

No. Although there are common stressors associated with having a severely impaired psychiatric patient in the family, our clinical experience and research data suggest that families of psychiatric patients vary tremendously in their level of competence and in the type of family dysfunction associated with having a family member with a psychiatric disorder. Some families cope very well with the strains of having a psychiatrically ill member. With this type of family, we will schedule one or two sessions to complete a basic assessment, provide psychoeducational information, and answer any questions they may have. Subsequent contacts are usually by phone, the focus being on pragmatic details concerning treatment and discharge planning.

Other families cannot tolerate the increased burden of living with a psychiatric patient and show many signs of dysfunction. Still other families have significant problems even without the added stress of a member with a psychiatric disorder and manifest severe deterioration when faced with this stress. These types of families require more intensive family therapy interventions. Families with more severe dysfunction may need to be seen several times a week for the length of the patient's stay in the hospital *and* have continued outpatient family treatment.

No empirical evidence exists for any type of specific family dysfunction in specific diagnostic groups. In our studies of families of depressed and other psychiatric patients, we have found a wide range and severity of family dysfunction (Miller et al., 1986; Keitner et al., 1986; Keitner, Miller, Epstein, et al., 1987). Other investigators have reported similar findings (Biglan et al., 1985; Birtchnell, 1988; Hinchliffe et al., 1975, 1977; Hops et al., 1987; Weissman, 1974). Also, numerous types of family dysfunction have been related to poor treatment outcome, including expressed emotion (Hooley et al., 1986), perceived criticism (Hooley & Teasdale, 1989), and overall family functioning (Keitner, Miller, Epstein, et al., 1987). Thus, there is no compelling evidence to suggest that there is a unique form of family dysfunction that is (1) present in all families of psychiatric patients, (2) consistently matched to any particular disorder, or (3) predictive of course of illness.

What Types of Family Problems Are Common During Inpatient Treatment?

There are several clinical issues that occur relatively frequently among families of inpatients. These problems include attributions for the patient's behavior, disruptions in role functioning, treatment compliance, and coping with suicidal behavior.

1. *Attributions for the patient's behavior.* Families of psychiatric inpatients often have difficulty making attributions for the patient's behavior (i.e., for what problems or behaviors should they hold the patient accountable versus what problems or behaviors are really part of the disorder?). Negative symptoms (e.g., worrying, social withdrawal, irritability, oversensitivity, and unresponsiveness) are the most difficult for family members to comprehend. These types of symptoms are likely to be seen as under the patient's voluntary control and not as part of the disorder. Consequently, family members may draw erroneous conclusions about the meaning of the patient's behavior. For example, the loss of libido often found during the onset of a depressive episode is frequently viewed by the spouse as an indication of marital dissatisfaction (Holder & Anderson, 1990). Even though the interactions between psychiatric conditions, personality factors, and family dysfunction are complex, the issue of which behaviors should be attributed to the disorder and which behaviors are under the patient's control needs to be

explored carefully with the families in order to arrive at some common understanding.

2. *Disruption in role functioning*. When the patient is hospitalized (and often for a substantial period prior to admission), he or she is no longer able to fulfill his or her responsibilities in the family. These duties may include financial, household, or emotional support roles. Without the patient, usual family functioning is likely to be disturbed. Other family members have to assume additional responsibilities to maintain the family. The disruption in role functioning associated with hospitalization can have both negative and positive aspects. For most families, the patient's decreased functioning and absence create increased stress for other members. For these families, issues in family therapy revolve around instrumental problem solving (i.e., reorganizing family tasks to take the patient's absence or reduced functioning into account). Of even more importance are the family's concerns about the chronicity of the patient's disability and their fears that the patient will never be able to regain his or her previous level of functioning. The therapist should elicit the family members' expectations about the patient's future functioning and explore the validity of these predictions. In some cases, the patient's absence is viewed by the family as a positive event because the patient's behavior has been extremely stressful to the family. When this occurs, the family therapist needs to help the family and patient identify the causes of the conflicts and help the family prepare to reintegrate the patient back into the family unit.

3. *Treatment compliance*. Nonadherence to treatment recommendations is a frequent contributing factor to the need for hospitalization. In these situations, the patient's lack of compliance often becomes a family issue as well. There are two common patterns of family involvement in noncompliance. First, the family may have attitudes and beliefs about treatment that reinforce or even cause the patient's noncompliance. Inaccurate beliefs about the usefulness or effects of medication are frequent (e.g., "I don't think he's sick enough to need drugs," or "If Leo starts taking drugs, he'll end up like those junkies"). When there are maladaptive cognitions about pharmacotherapy, the family therapist needs to explore these beliefs and help the family develop more adaptive attitudes about the utility of the treatment plan. Frank, Prien, Kupfer, and Alberts (1985) have demonstrated that a family intervention can dramatically increase the chances of adherence to antidepressant pharmacotherapy.

Second, the family may recognize the need for treatment, but the patient does not. In this scenario, the patient's failure to comply may be seen as willful; therefore, family members become frustrated and angry. They may then engage in escalating attempts to control the behavior.

The goals of the family therapist are to help the family distinguish between the effects of the disorder and "volitional" causes of behavior; avoid destructive blaming or retribution; and problem solve to find more effective strategies for increasing the patient's compliance.

4. *Coping with suicidal behavior*. There are usually feelings of shock, grief, and anger among families with a member who has made a recent suicide attempt. Accompanying cognitions range from disbelief and puzzlement ("Why would she try to kill herself?") to self-blame ("What did I do wrong?" "Why couldn't I have prevented this?") to outrage ("How could he do this to me?"). Several types of interventions by the family therapist are useful in these situations. In cases where the patient has made a recent suicide attempt, it is important for the family therapist to ask about the patient's and family's thoughts about the attempt and whether they have questions about suicidal behaviors. Within the context of this discussion, it is often helpful to utilize psychoeducational techniques. Particular topics should include (1) how to respond to suicidal ideas and attempts, (2) the difficulty predicting suicide, and (3) potential warning indicators. The goals of the intervention are to modify maladaptive cognitions the family may have concerning the suicide attempt as well as to provide the family with accurate information about suicidal behavior. Discussion of suicide in family therapy sessions also encourages open, direct communication regarding this difficult topic. This could increase the likelihood of dialogue between the family and patient if suicidal thoughts return.

Who Is Responsible for Family Therapy in a CTU?

One of the major differences between outpatient and inpatient family treatment is that the responsibility for therapeutic interventions in the hospital setting is spread across multiple individuals and disciplines. Careful treatment planning should be used to designate which members of the interdisciplinary team are assigned to various components of the family treatment. Of course, a trained family therapist, usually a social worker, has primary responsibility for a thorough family assessment. In most cases, this individual also provides intensive family therapy, if indicated. However, the physician, nurse, and ancillary therapists also have important roles in family treatment.

For example, the psychiatrist may meet with family members early in the hospitalization to perform a variety of functions including collecting further history, communicating information about the treatment plan, and promoting a strong collaboration among the patient, family members, and therapists. In some cases, the psychiatrist may act as an auxiliary family therapist by focusing on specific issues such as treatment compliance or coping with medical illness. When the psychiatrist has had advanced training in family therapy, he or she may act as the primary therapist or cotherapist for intensive family treatment. At the very least, the psychiatrist should be aware of the plan for family therapy and support this work in communications with the patient and family members.

The psychiatric nurse frequently meets with family members throughout the hospital stay. The admission process, family visits, and discharge procedures provide opportunities to assess family functioning and intervene with supportive measures, psychoeducational efforts, or cognitively oriented treatment. Skilled psychiatric nurses who are experienced in cognitive therapy can interact with family members during acute crises while emotions and cognitions are "hot." A brief intervention on the unit can be followed by more thorough work on the issue in formal family therapy. Ancillary therapists such as occupational therapists, pastoral counselors, and activities therapists may also support the family treatment effort with inpatients. Part B of this chapter illustrates a comprehensive cognitively oriented approach to family therapy in a CTU.

SUMMARY AND CONCLUSIONS

Families can exert a major influence on the expression and course of psychiatric disorders. Virtually all families of psychiatric inpatients experience some level of family dysfunction. Patients from severely dysfunctional families have lower recovery and higher relapse rates. Because family therapies can produce a significant improvement in family functioning and reduce the risk for relapse, a family treatment component should be included in all cognitive therapy units.

We recommend the following guidelines for application of family therapy on a CTU:

1. A family therapy model should be selected that is cognitively oriented or is similar in structure, style, and focus to cognitive therapy.
2. The family therapists should be involved as much as possible in the other aspects of the patient's treatment.
3. Family treatment should begin as soon as possible after admission.
4. If possible, all members of the family should be included in family treatment.

5. The structure of family sessions should be similar to the organization of individual cognitive therapy sessions.
6. Inpatient family therapy should focus on six major goals:
   a. Establish a collaborative relationship with the family.
   b. Recognize and support the family's burden.
   c. Address the family's presenting problem.
   d. Conduct a comprehensive assessment of the family system.
   e. Provide the family with psychoeducational information about the patient's disorder.
   f. Plan discharge.
7. A comprehensive family assessment is indicated for each hospital admission, but all families do not require family therapy.
8. Common concerns for inpatient family treatment include:
   a. Attributions about the patient's behavior.
   b. Disruption in role functioning.
   c. Treatment compliance.
   d. Coping with suicidal behavior.
9. For the most effective outcomes, family therapy must be well integrated with other treatment components.

REFERENCES

Alexander, P. C. (1988). The therapeutic implications of family cognitions and constructs. *Journal of Cognitive Psychotherapy: An International Quarterly, 2,* 219–236.

Baucom, D., & Epstein, N. (1990). *Cognitive behavioral marital therapy*. New York: Brunner-Mazel.

Beach, S., & O'Leary, K. (1986). The treatment of depression occurring in the context of marital discord. *Behavior Therapy*, *17*, 43–49.

Beach, S., Sandeen, E., & O'Leary, K. (1990). *Depression in marriage*. New York: Guilford Press.

Beck, A. (1988). *Love is never enough*. New York: Harper & Row.

Biglan, A., Hops, H. L. S., Sherman, L., Friedman, L., Arthur, J., & Osteen, V. (1985). Problem solving interactions of depressed women and their husbands. *Behavior Therapy*, *16*, 431–451.

Birtchnell, J. (1988). Depression and family relationships: A study of young, married women on a London housing estate. *British Journal of Psychiatry*, *153*, 758–769.

Coyne, J., Kessler, R., Tal, M., Turnbull, J., Wortman, C., & Greden, J. (1987). Living with a depressed person. *Journal of Consulting and Clinical Psychology*, *55*, 347–352.

Crowther, J.H. (1985). The relationship between depression and marital maladjustment. *Journal of Nervous and Mental Disease*, *173*, 227–231.

Dattilio, F., & Padesky, C. (1990). *Cognitive therapy with couples*. Sarasota: Professional Resource Exchange.

Dobson, K.S. (1987). Marital and social adjustment in depressed and remarried women. *Journal of Clinical Psychology, 43*, 261–265.

Epstein, N. B., & Bishop, D. S. (1981). Problem centered systems therapy of the family. In A. Gurman & D. Kniskern (Eds.), *Handbook of family therapy* (pp. 444–482). New York: Brunner/Mazel.

Epstein, N., Keitner, G., Bishop, D., & Miller, I. (1988). Combined use of pharmacological and family therapy. In J. F. Clarkin, G. L. Haas, & I. D. Glick (Eds.), *Affective disorders and the family: Assessment and treatment* (pp. 153–172). New York: Guilford Press.

Fadden, G., Bebbington, P., & Kuipers, L. (1987). Caring and its burdens: A study of the spouses of depressed patients. *British Journal of Psychiatry, 151*, 660–667.

Frank, E., Prien, R. F., Kupfer, D. J., & Alberts, L. (1985). Implications of noncompliance on research in affective disorders. *Psychopharmacology Bulletin, 21*(1), 37–42.

Freud, S. (1917). *Mourning and melancholia* (1957 ed.). London: Hogarth Press.

Friedman, A. (1975). Interaction of drug therapy with marital therapy in depressive patients. *Archives of General Psychiatry, 32*, 619–637.

Glick, I., Clarkin, J., Spencer, J., & Haas, G., Lewis, A., Peyser, J., DeMane, N., Good-Ellis, M., Harris, E., & Lestelle, V. (1985). A controlled evaluation of inpatient family intervention, I: Preliminary results of the six-month follow-up. *Archives of General Psychiatry, 42*, 882–886.

Gotlib, I., & Colby, C. (1987). *Treatment of depression: An interpersonal systems approach*. New York: Pergamon Press.

Haas, G., Glick, I., Clarkin, J., & Spencer, J., Lewis, A., Peyser, J., DeMane, N., Good-Ellis, M., Harris, E., & Lestelle, V. (1988). Inpatient family intervention: A randomized clinical trial, II: Results at hospital discharge. *Archives of General Psychiatry, 45*, 217–224.

Hinchliffe, M., Hooper, D., Roberts, F., & Vaughan, P. (1975). A study of the interaction between depressed patients and their spouses. *British Journal of Psychiatry, 126*, 164–172.

Hinchliffe, M., Vaughan, P., Hooper, D., & Roberts, F. (1977). The melancholy marriage: An inquiry into the interaction of depression, II: Expressiveness. *British Journal of Medical Psychology, 50*, 125–142.

Holder, D., & Anderson, C. (1990). Psychoeducational intervention for depressed patients and their families. In G. I. Keitner (Ed.) *Depression and families: Impact and treatment*(pp. 157–184). Washington, DC: American Psychiatric Association Press.

Hooley, J., Orley, J., & Teasdale, J. D. (1986). Levels of expressed emotion and relapse in depressed patients. *British Journal of Psychiatry, 148*, 642–647.

Hooley, J., & Teasdale, J. (1989). Predictors of relapse in unipolar depressives: Expressed emotion, marital distress, and perceived criticism. *Journal of Abnormal Psychology, 98*, 229–235.

Hops, H., Biglan, A., Sherman, L., Arthur, J., Friedman, L., & Osteen, V.

(1987). Home observations of family interactions of depressed women. *Journal of Consulting and Clinical Psychology, 55*, 341–346.

Jacob, M., Frank, E., Kupfer, D., & Carpenter, L. (1987). Recurrent depression: An assessment of family burden and family attitudes. *Journal of Clinical Psychiatry, 48*, 395–400.

Jacobson, N., Dobson, K., Fruzzetti, A., Schmaling, K., & Salusky, S. (1991). Marital therapy as a treatment for depression. *Journal of Consulting and Clinical Psychology, 59*, 547–557.

Jacobson, N., & Margolin, G. (1979). *Marital therapy*. New York: Brunner/Mazel.

Keitner, G., & Miller, I. (1990). Family functioning and major depression: An overview. *American Journal of Psychiatry, 147*, 1128–1137.

Keitner, G., Miller, I., Epstein, N., & Bishop, D. (1986). The functioning of families in patients with major depression. *International Journal of Family Psychiatry, 7*, 11–16.

Keitner, G., Miller, I., Epstein, N., & Bishop, D. (1987). Family functioning and the course of major depression. *Comprehensive Psychiatry, 28*, 54–64.

Keitner, G., Miller, I., Fruzzetti, A., Epstein, N., & Bishop, D. (1987). Family functioning and suicidal behavior in psychiatric inpatients with major depression. *Psychiatry, 50*, 242–255.

Keitner, G., Ryan, C., Miller, I., Bishop, D., & Epstein, N. (1990). Family functioning social adjustment and recurrence of suicidality. *Psychiatry, 53*, 17–30.

McLean, P., Ogstron, K., & Grauer, L. (1973). A behavioral approach to the treatment of depression. *Journal of Behavioral Therapy and Experimental Psychiatry, 4*, 323–300.

Merikangas, K., Prusoff, B., Kupfer, D., & Frank, E. (1985). Marital adjustment in major depression. *Journal of Affective Disorders, 9*, 5–11.

Miller, I., Bishop, D., Keitner, G., & Epstein, N. (in press). *The McMaster approach to families: Theory, treatment, and research*. New York: Pergamon Press.

Miller, I., Kabacoff, R., Keitner, G., Epstein, N., & Bishop, D. (1986). Family functioning in the families of psychiatric patients. *Comprehensive Psychiatry, 27*, 302–312.

Miller, I., Norman, W., & Keitner, G. (1989). Cognitive-behavioral treatment of depressed inpatients: 6 and 12 month follow-up. *American Journal of Psychiatry, 146*, 1274–1279.

Rounsaville, B., Prusoff, B., & Weissman, M. (1980). The course of marital disputes in depressed women: A 48 month follow-up. *Comprehensive Psychiatry, 21*, 111–118.

Rounsaville, B., Weissman, M., Prusoff, B., & Herceg-Baron, R. (1979). Marital disputes and treatment outcome in depressed women. *Comprehensive Psychiatry, 20*, 483–490.

Spencer, J. J., Glick, I., Haas, G., Clarkin, J., Lewis, A., Peyser, J., DeMane, N., Good-Ellis, M., Harris, E., & Lestelle, V. (1988). A randomized clinical trial of inpatient family intervention, III: Effects at 6-month and 18-month follow-ups. *American Journal of Psychiatry, 145*, 1115–1121.

Swindle, R., Cronkite, R., & Moos, R. (1989). Life stressors, social resources, coping, and the 4-year course of unipolar depression. *Journal of Abnormal Psychology, 98*, 468–477.

Thase, M. E., & Wright, J. H. (1991). Cognitive behavioral therapy with depressed inpatients: An abridged treatment manual. *Behavior Therapy, 22*, 579–595.

Vaughan, C. E., & Leff, J. P. (1976). The influence of family and social factors on the course of psychiatric illness. *British Journal of Psychiatry, 129*, 125–137.

Weissman, M. (1974). *The depressed woman: A study of her relationships*. Chicago: University of Chicago Press.

Part B. Family Cognitive Therapy with Inpatients

Jesse H. Wright, M.D., Ph.D., and Aaron T. Beck, M.D.

The basic principles of family treatment on a Cognitive Therapy Unit (CTU) have been set forth by Miller, Keitner, Epstein, Bishop, and Ryan in Part A of this chapter. They note that some CTUs may not have family therapists who have been trained specifically in cognitive therapy (CT). Therefore, they recommend that a family therapy model that is compatible with CT, such as behavioral marital therapy (Jacobsen & Margolin, 1979), interpersonal therapy (Gotlib & Colby, 1987), or problem-centered systems therapy of the family (Epstein & Bishop, 1981), be employed.

In this section of the chapter, we give a more detailed explanation of how inpatient family therapy is conducted by experienced cognitive therapists. After briefly describing family cognitive therapy (FCT), we illustrate the team approach to cognitively oriented family treatment on a CTU.

OVERVIEW OF FAMILY COGNITIVE THERAPY

Family Cognitive Therapy (FCT) is a derivative of individual CT (Beck, Rush, Shaw, & Emery, 1979), cognitive therapy for couples (Epstein & Eidelson, 1981; Epstein, 1982; Schmaling, Fruzzetti, & Jacobsen, 1989; Baucom & Epstein, 1990), and behavioral approaches to marital therapy (Weiss, 1975; Epstein & Williams, 1981; Beach, Sandeen, & O'Leary, 1990). The primary emphasis in FCT is on cognitive and behavioral change at *both* the individual and family system levels (Teichman, 1984; Beck, 1988). The cognitive mediation model, described in earlier chapters, is expanded to the entire family network.

Epstein, Schlesinger, and Dryden (1988) have described four types of cognitions that family members may have when they appraise the significance of family events: (1) cognitions about oneself; (2) cognitions about oneself in relation to another family member; (3) cognitions that each member has about relationships among family subgroups; and (4) cognitions about oneself in relation to family subgroups. Although it could be argued that there are other possibilities, such as cognitions about the complete family system, the points made by Epstein, Schlesinger, and Dryden are that information processing within a family system is quite complex, and many possibilities for misunderstandings or miscommunication exist.

Therapeutic interventions in FCT are based on the assumptions that family members interpret and evaluate one another and that emotions and behavior are influenced by these cognitions (Epstein et al., 1988). It is not suggested that cognitive processes cause all family behavior but simply that cognitive appraisal is part of the interactive relationship among events, cognitions, emotions, and behavior. In the following section, we describe five major components of family cognitive therapy.

FAMILY COGNITIVE THERAPY PROCEDURES

Collaborative Empiricism

The principle of collaborative empiricism is utilized to engage the family members in understanding themselves and each other. With understanding comes a greater tolerance—even empathy—for each other's abrasive or dysfunctional behavior. At the same time, by directing family members into a problem-solving mode, the therapist is relieved of total responsibility for affecting change. By accepting shared responsibility, family members are less likely to regress to immature patterns of behavior and thinking.

Collaborative empiricism is modeled by the therapist in interactions with individual family members and work with the family as a whole. Also, behavioral assignments are given that can engage family members in collaborative work between sessions. The goal is to help the family become a cooperative team for the investigation and change of maladaptive beliefs.

Structure

Family cognitive therapy, like other forms of CT, utilizes structuring techniques to improve the efficiency of sessions, enhance learning, and maintain the focus on "here-and-now" problem solving. Structuring procedures are particularly important for inpatients and their families, because the degree of pathology is often quite high, hopelessness and helplessness may be intense, and there may be significant impairment of learning and memory functioning (see Chapters 1 and 4).

Agenda setting is one of the most important structuring operations. Usually in the beginning phase of FCT, the therapist assists the family to develop a problem list that is used as a guide for the entire therapy. Of course, the problem list is subject to revision as new information is uncovered. However, an initial problem list can serve as an overall structuring device for the therapy process. In addition, agendas are set at the beginning of each family session to help target the family's efforts toward manageable issues and tasks. Observations of family interactions during the problem list and agenda-formation stage help the therapist assess family roles, communication patterns, automatic thoughts, schemas, and adaptive and maladaptive behaviors. This information is used to direct the cognitive and behavioral interventions described later.

The therapist plays an active role in structuring sessions. The basic procedures of CT, such as psychoeducation, feedback, behavioral interventions, and homework assignments, provide a "built-in" structure. In addition, directive comments may be needed from time to time in order to keep the family focused on productive therapeutic work. However, a balance must be struck between the need to help the family organize their efforts to use CT and allowing family processes to unfold more naturalistically. We believe that family therapy should not be structured as tightly as individual therapy. Opportunities should be provided for the family to reveal their habitual patterns of interactions and to express thoughts and feelings openly.

Psychoeducation

Psychoeducational procedures are used in FCT (1) to communicate the basic concepts of cognitive therapy, (2) to teach new problem-solving strategies, and (3) promote behavioral change. Epstein et al. (1988) recommend that the family cognitive therapist present didactic material such as "minilectures" or handouts early in therapy. Reading assignments can include materials such as *Coping with Depression* (Beck & Greenberg, 1974), *Feeling Good* (Burns, 1980), *Intimate Connections* (Burns, 1985), and *Love Is Never Enough* (Beck, 1988). As the treatment proceeds, the therapist also uses modeling, role play, and behavioral interventions (described later) to teach the family new ways of communicating and solving problems.

Families of hospitalized patients should be provided with detailed information on the inpatient program, including unit "rules and regulations," visiting procedures, treatment methods, and, most importantly, the role of the family in the treatment milieu. A unit handbook and audio or videotaped orientations can be used to help with this educational effort. In some CTUs, a special weekly group is arranged to explain therapy procedures to families.

Cognitive Restructuring

The first level of cognitive restructuring involves eliciting and testing automatic thoughts. Socratic questioning is the main procedure used in this process. However, other standard cognitive therapy techniques, such as imagery, thought recording, or *in vivo* assignments may also be employed. Families are taught to recognize automatic thoughts, identify cognitive errors (e.g., selective abstraction, absolutistic thinking, personalization, magnification and minimization, arbitrary inference), "examine the evidence" for the validity of cognitions, and develop realistic assessments of family events. The treatment is directed at all four dimensions of family information processing identified by Epstein et al. (1988). Thus, family members may examine dysfunctional cognitions they have about themselves, their relationships to other family members, interactions among family subgroups, and so forth.

Family cognitive therapy is directed primarily at elucidating the meanings given to behavior. The meaning can often be discerned through obtaining automatic thoughts in the family therapy sessions or by questioning family members specifically about meanings of their interactions, as illustrated in the following example.

A middle-aged depressed woman reacted negatively when her

family (as well as the hospital staff) kept pressuring her to be more active as a way of combating her depression. The patient would react to the verbal entreaties with the statement, "You just don't understand." Her husband and adult daughter would become frustrated and then irritated at the patient's apparent resistance. In the family session, the discussion proceeded as follows:

DAUGHTER: Mom, you just don't want to get well. You resist every suggestion we make.

THERAPIST: What thoughts do you have about your mother getting well?

DAUGHTER: It's my responsibility. I try my hardest, but she just blocks me. She makes me feel guilty.

THERAPIST: *(to the patient)* What do you think when people urge you to get active?

PATIENT: All my life I have been everybody's slave. I would do what everybody wanted. Now that I'm sick, it's the same thing all over again. Everybody is telling me what to do—and I can't take it anymore. I want to be my own person.

By ascertaining the meaning behind the participants' behavior, the therapist was able to formulate the family problem more clearly. The patient's depression was in part a reflection of her despair over ever having a life of her own. Her unwillingness to "take orders" was derived from her belief that she had always been subservient to everybody else. She had been unable to verbalize her despair and her desire to express her individuality until she was encouraged to verbalize her thoughts by the therapist.

Once the meanings of the members' behavior were clarified, the family members developed a more adaptive concept of the problem and what to do about it. Husband and daughter began to work together to help the patient regain some sense of independence and, at the same time, engage in activities that would expedite her recovery. The daughter questioned her mother about what she would like to do, and the mother opted for spending more time taking walks and exercising as physical therapy rather than attending occupational therapy.

This example demonstrates that negative automatic thoughts often spill out after simple questioning by the therapist. We find that the intense emotions that are often expressed in family meetings *increase* the chances of uncovering salient cognitions. Thus, the interpersonal element enhances the effort of the therapist to discover maladaptive patterns of information processing.

The second level of cognitive restructuring concerns modification of basic beliefs (schemas). At times, beliefs can be inferred from repetitive patterns of automatic thoughts. In other instances, family members will directly articulate an assumption such as "I'm not appreciated," "John and Susanne are the favorites," "Our family can't communicate," or "You have to look out for yourself in this family to survive." There may be a certain degree of validity in such assumptions. However, usually the belief has an exaggerated or distorted quality to it that aggravates the problem and contributes to a "self-fulfilling prophecy" effect.

The techniques for modifying basic assumptions are similar to those used to change automatic thoughts. The family is encouraged to view the beliefs as hypotheses and to gather data that will either support or refute the assumption. Procedures may include collecting information through direct questioning in sessions, listing advantages and disadvantages, exploring options, and trying out new conceptualizations via behavioral experiments.

Behavioral Procedures

Behavioral interventions used in FCT are derived from both individual CT and behavioral marital therapy. Standard CT techniques such as activity scheduling, graded-task assignments, and cognitive–behavioral rehearsal can be very helpful in facilitating behavioral change. These procedures can be used with individual family members, subgroups, or the entire family. Behavioral contracts may be used in some cases if exchanges can be arranged in a "win–win" manner (Epstein et al., 1988).

Special behavioral interventions may be required when there are specific skills deficits (e.g., communication, assertiveness, problem solving). For example, the therapist may utilize communications-training methodology to help family members express messages (both positive and negative) clearly and to learn to listen effectively (Epstein & Jackson, 1978). Assertiveness training involves educational work on the differences between assertion, aggression, and submission (Epstein, 1980). The therapist also models assertive communication and uses role play and behavioral rehearsal to encourage skill acquisition (Epstein, 1981). Training in problem solving helps families to be able to define problems, generate alternate solutions, evaluate options, develop plans, and evaluate the results of their efforts (Epstein et al., 1988).

FAMILY COGNITIVE THERAPY WITH INPATIENTS: CASE ILLUSTRATION

Mrs. G. was a 68-year-old widow who was admitted to a CTU after outpatient treatment had failed to stem the tide of an escalating depression. Her two adult children were the primary movers in arranging the hospital admission. The children explained that their mother had become increasingly dysfunctional; they believed that she was no longer able to manage activities of daily living or to take her medication reliably. But the major problem that appeared to prompt admission was Mrs. G.'s incessant telephone calls to her children. She complained relentlessly, cried, talked about being lonely, and made "manipulative" statements that seemed to be designed to cause guilt (e.g., "I'm all alone now, nobody cares. . . . I've been a failure as a mother. . . . my children don't love me. . . . you never want to stay when you visit").

The patient reported most of the classic symptoms of depression including depressed mood, insomnia, decreased appetite and weight loss, low self-esteem and guilt, poor concentration, hopelessness, and helplessness. She had thoughts of wishing that she were dead but did not have suicidal plans or intent. Mrs. G. had been hospitalized three times previously for treatment of depression and had received electroconvulsive therapy once with moderate benefit. Over the last 5 years, she had been chronically depressed. The pattern of symptoms suggested a "double depression"—a chronic dysthymic disorder with superimposed periods of severe major depression. The most recent episode of major depression had lasted over 6 months despite trials of nortriptyline, fluoxetine, and supportive psychotherapy.

During the admission process, it became readily apparent that family issues were part of the problem. Mrs. G. was accompanied to the unit by her daughter Phyllis and son Michael. During the admission interview, the psychiatric nurse observed a high level of tension in all family members. They were superficially congenial but seemed to be struggling to control frustration and anger. The nurse decided to intervene.

NURSE: You've been very helpful in answering my questions, but everybody looks tense. You all look angry. What are you thinking about?

SON: *(Exasperated)* It's just been very hard for us the past few weeks.

MRS. G.: You can say that again.

DAUGHTER: Mother's illness has been a strain on *all* of us.

NURSE: You'll have a chance to talk with the social worker soon about these things, but it might be a good idea to at least identify a few of the problems now. That way the treatment team can start to help you as soon as possible.

DAUGHTER: Well . . . it's hard to say with everyone here, but Michael and I have been dealing with this for a long time—*too* long a time, and we've just about had it. We've tried our best, but no matter what we do, it's never good enough.

MRS. G.: *(Tearful and angry)* That's just what I thought. You two just put up with me; you don't really want me around. You might as well dump me in here and throw away the key.

SON: Mother, you know we love you. We just don't know what to do anymore. Phyllis is right, there's no way we can seem to satisfy you. I'm about at my wit's end.

NURSE: I can see your family's been under a lot of stress. Most families of our patients have the same types of problems. You feel helpless to change things and even a bit guilty about not being able to do it on your own. Does that describe your situation?

DAUGHTER: Yes, It does.

SON: You're right about feeling helpless. The things mother says to us really hurt sometimes. I feel like I've tried everything, and nothing's worked.

MRS. G.: *(Sarcastically)* Well, *I'm sorry*! *(pause, appears guilty)* I don't mean to upset you. I just feel miserable all the time.

NURSE: I'm getting the impression that everyone would like things to improve, but nobody seems to know how to do it.

DAUGHTER: That's right.

NURSE: You've decided to come to the hospital, so that's a start. But, let me try to give you a few pointers that might help you get going with your sessions with the doctor and the social worker. Would that be okay?

MRS. G.: All right.

SON: We need all the help we can get.

NURSE: The first thing to understand is that depression often makes people act in ways that nobody likes—being dependent, or irritable, or angry. If we can treat the depression, these problems should get better. In the meantime, we have to be careful not to blame ourselves or others for the effects of the depression.

DAUGHTER: You've hit the nail on the head. There's been lots of blaming going on.

NURSE: The second thing is that all three of you are using very strong, absolute statements like "No matter what we do it's not good enough" or "You don't really want me around." We've found that families of depressed patients often get into this exaggerated style of thinking. You can try to stand back from the situation and check to see if your thoughts are really accurate.

SON: Lots of times we've done things to help mother that she really seems to appreciate, but lately we haven't been able to get through to her.

MRS. G.: I know you're trying. I should be grateful, but I just panic and say the first thing that comes to mind.

NURSE: You'll be able to pick up on these issues in your therapy sessions. But for now, I'd suggest that you all read the unit handbook that explains the treatment approach and also take time to read the pamphlet *Coping with Depression*. The readings will help you learn how to get started with therapy.

SON: Okay. We appreciate the suggestions.

The nurse explained her interactions with the family to the admitting psychiatrist before he examined the patient and discussed the treatment plan with the family. Thus, the physician was able to support a family perspective for therapy from the beginning of the hospitalization. The family therapist heard about the initial efforts of the nurse and the doctor at a planning conference the morning after admission. They were able to identify two major family issues: (1) regressive, dependent behavior associated with depression had stimulated maladaptive and destructive family system responses; and (2) lack of compliance with pharmacotherapy had become a problem for the entire family. It was decided to complete a full family assessment and then reconvene the treatment team to organize a comprehensive approach to family treatment.

The family assessment was used to obtain an in-depth analysis of the presenting problem and a detailed history of family functioning—including strengths and weaknesses, communication patterns, and important family events. It was found that Mrs. G. had always tried to control her children to some extent and that there had been an undercurrent of anger about this for many years. Even when she was not depressed, Mrs. G. had been somewhat demanding of attention. She also had high expectations for her children's success. After she had become depressed, these activities had escalated sharply.

Her son, Michael, had married, but Mrs. G. had never approved entirely of his choice. There was only one grandson who was now away at college in another region of the country. Phyllis, Mrs. G.'s daughter, had never married. Both children were college graduates who had achieved modest success in business careers. Mrs. G.'s husband had been a powerful attorney who doted on his wife. He died suddenly of a heart attack when Mrs. G. was 55. Her depression started soon thereafter.

The family assessment also revealed a long-standing pattern of dysfunctional assumptions that had been magnified during Mrs. G.'s depression and appeared to be aggravating her symptoms. For example, Michael believed that his mother would never change. He had essentially stopped trying. He visited her but did the bare minimum. Mrs. G.'s daughter, Phyllis, who had very low self-esteem, had thoughts such as "I can never measure up." She kept trying to meet her mother's needs; however, she always saw herself as a failure. Michael's wife, Sarah, thought Mrs. G. was a mean, spiteful woman concerned about "nobody but herself." On the other hand, Mrs. G. had complex, ambivalent thoughts about her children. She loved them deeply and even cared a great deal for Sarah. She was also proud of their accomplishments. But, rigidly held expectations were, in her opinion, not being met (e.g., "My children should always respect me; their love is everything; I need them to be happy; if they loved me, they would give me their full attention"). Her critical comments were either driving her family away (Michael, Sarah, and their son) or causing low self-esteem and guilt (Phyllis).

The family therapist identified six primary goals for family treatment: (1) educate family about depression in order to reattribute at least part of the blame to the disorder; (2) identify and modify key maladaptive assumptions in the family system; (3) reduce number and intensity of critical comments; (4) reduce Mrs. G.'s dependent behavior and children's frustration, anger, and retribution (especially from son, Michael); (5) reduce family burden; and (6) improve treatment compliance. A comprehensive, milieu approach to family treatment was developed to accomplish these objectives (Table 6.1). It was thought that outpatient follow-up would be needed to continue work on these goals.

Excerpts from two of the family treatment interchanges—a family therapy session with a social worker and a session on compliance with the doctor—are used to illustrate further the processes of family therapy

TABLE 6.1. Family Treatment Plan for Mrs. G.: Treatment Team Assignments

Goal	Family therapist	Physician	Nurse	Occupational therapist
1. Educate family about depression	1. Family therapy; review reading assignments	1. Meet with family to discuss depression, treatment, prognosis	1. Discuss depression during initial assessment; assign readings about depression; lead "Family Night" psychoeducational series	1. —
2. Identify and modify maladaptive assumptions	2. Family therapy; use CT procedures	2. Address family issues in individual therapy sessions with Mrs. G.	2. Identify "hot" cognitions during family visits; brief CT interventions if possible	2. Individual OT sessions; question distorted assumptions
3. Reduce number and intensity of critical comments	3. Family therapy; identify automatic thoughts; use role-play exercises	3. Work on increasing Mrs. G.'s empathy toward children; coach on using less critical language	3. Coach Mrs. G. on effective communication	3. —
4. Reduce dependent and retributive behavior	4. Family therapy; behavioral rehearsal, graded-task assignment	4. Treat depression with pharmacotherapy; use activity schedules and graded tasks to promote independence	4. Assist with behavioral assignments	4. Individual OT sessions; meet with family before discharge
5. Reduce family burden	5. Family therapy; give support	5. Empathic and supportive responses to family	5. Empathic and supportive responses to family	5. Empathic and supportive responses to family
6. Improve treatment compliance after discharge	6. Family therapy; work in concert with physician	6. Session with family before discharge to work on compliance issues	6. Review compliance issues during discharge conference	6. —

on a CTU. During the second family therapy session, one of the agenda items was excessive criticism.

THERAPIST: We've decided to talk about the issue of criticism today. Who would like to start off?

SON: It's been going on so long, I've just tuned it out.

DAUGHTER: Well, I can't do that. Mother's comments really hit me hard—just like they're arrows that always find their mark.

MRS. G.: You make me sound like some kind of monster—always criticizing. I don't mean to do it. I'm just trying to give you encouragement to do your best.

DAUGHTER-IN-LAW: Well, my best is never good enough. I don't know what I could ever do to make you really accept me. And then you keep calling the house all hours of the day and night. It's like we never do anything to help you.

MRS. G.: If you would listen to me and understand me, I wouldn't need to call. It seems like you're always too busy for me. You have a party, or a concert, or have to work late—and I'm all alone.

THERAPIST: This would be a good place to stop to try to identify the assumptions that you have about one another. We started to do this the last session. Phyllis, you were talking about the arrows always hitting their mark. What are your assumptions about your mother's attitude toward you?

DAUGHTER: I'm never good enough for her. I've never pleased her, and I never will. She wants me to be married with children—and to be rich. I'm not any of those things.

MRS. G.: That's not true, Phyllis. I'm proud of you just the way you are.

THERAPIST: We'll have to explore the accuracy of Phyllis's assumption a little later, but for now let's find out some of the other assumptions. *(Therapist goes on to elicit assumptions from Michael and Sarah and then turns back to Mrs. G.)* Mrs. G., you've been silent for a while. What are you thinking?

MRS. G.: *(Starts to cry)* That I've been a pretty terrible mother. Nothing I've done has turned out right. My children don't even like me; I just seem to be a burden for them.

SON: Mother that's not true. We love you, but we can't handle the way you've been acting.

THERAPIST: Michael has just stated the problem in another way. What we might do now is to examine each of the assumptions to see how accurate they are and then to restate them in a way that will help us to begin to solve the problem. Let's stick with Mrs. G.'s beliefs for now. I hear you saying, "I've been a terrible mother; no one likes me; I'm just a burden." What's the evidence either for or against the accuracy of these statements?

DAUGHTER: Mother always put pressure on us to do our best, but she meant well. I guess we all need to have some expectations from our parents. I'm so down on myself that any little criticism really gets to me.

SON: It never bothered me till after Dad died and Mother got so depressed. It was as if nothing was ever right after he died. Both of them had high expectations. In a way that helped me get through college and get a good job. Mom's depression has been a burden on everybody, including her—but *she's* not a burden. We love her and just want her to get well.

DAUGHTER-IN-LAW: Michael tries to be good to his mother. I have to say, though that she really does criticize us a lot—especially me.

THERAPIST: What are you hearing them say Mrs. G.?

MRS. G.: I guess there's some truth to the idea that I criticize too much. They really seem to care about me, though. I need to cut down on the criticism and start to get better so I'm not dragging everybody down.

The therapist then outlined a series of behavioral exercises to practice less critical ways of communicating in the family system, after which the group examined the assumptions of other family members. The session ended with a specific homework assignment for Mrs. G. to write thought records in which she identified and changed hypercritical automatic thoughts and for the children also to examine and alter, if possible, their automatic thoughts when their mother requested help.

The issue of treatment compliance was explored in a family session with the psychiatrist. Mrs. G. had taken medication irregularly prior to admission, and family members thought this was one of the reasons she remained depressed.

DOCTOR: We decided to get together to talk about taking medications after discharge. Let's start by seeing if there are any questions or problems.

DAUGHTER: Mother just doesn't seem to want to take medicines like they're prescribed. It's like she knows better. The doctor has either prescribed too much or too little, so she does what she wants.

DAUGHTER-IN-LAW: We get real uncomfortable with this. She lives alone, and we're afraid she'll overdose or something.

MRS. G.: I'd never do *that*.

DOCTOR: There does seem to be a problem here. It would help if we could find out what each of you think about the idea of taking medication for depression.

SON: I hate to admit it, but . . . I think you should be able to get better on your own. Taking a medicine for depression seems like a sign of weakness. If Mother has to take a drug, it even makes me feel weak. Maybe I've been undermining the drug treatment.

DAUGHTER: Well, I wish I would have known that. I've been giving Mother just the opposite message. I think she has a biochemical problem.

DOCTOR: Mrs. G., what do you think?

MRS. G.: I guess I see it both ways. I'm sort of mixed up about it. My husband would never have wanted me to take drugs. He'd be just like Michael—you know, just tough it out.

The psychiatrist proceeded to elicit additional thoughts about taking medication. He then helped the family to examine the validity of their cognitions. A balanced, cognitive–biological model of depression (see Chapter 7) was presented to help the family change their either/or thinking about medication. Finally, a behavioral reinforcement system for treatment compliance (as described in Chapter 7) was introduced after the family joined together to support pharmacotherapy.

Additional family therapy was provided throughout the hospital stay. The majority of the treatment was provided by the social worker, who had received specialty training in both family therapy and cognitive therapy. However, other professionals with cognitive therapy expertise (e.g., psychiatrist, nursing staff, and occupational therapist) were able to support the family treatment effort. By the time of discharge, Mrs. G.'s level of depression was substantially improved. She was able to function independently in the home setting, the amount of criticism in family communications was diminished considerably, and the children were able to offer genuine support to their mother. Further family therapy was planned for the aftercare phase of treatment.

REFERENCES

Baucom, D., & Epstein, N. (1990). *Cognitive behavioral marital therapy*. New York: Brunner/Mazel.

Beach, S. R. H., Sandeen, E. E., & O'Leary, K. D. (1990). *Depression in marriage: A model for etiology and treatment*. New York: Guilford Press.

Beck, A. T. (1988). *Love is never enough.* New York: Harper & Row.

Beck, A. T., & Greenberg, R. L. (1974). Coping with depression. (Available from the Institute for Rational Emotive Therapy, 45 East 65th Street, New York, NY 10021.)

Beck, A. T., Rush, A. J., Shaw, B. F., & Emery, G. (1979). *Cognitive therapy of depression.* New York: Guilford Press.

Burns, D. D. (1980). *Feeling good.* New York: William Morrow.

Burns, D. D. (1985). *Intimate connections.* New York: William Morrow.

Epstein, N. (1980). Social consequences of assertion, aggression, passive aggression, and submission: Situational and dispositional determinants. *Behavior Therapy, 11,* 662–669.

Epstein, N. (1981). Assertiveness training in marital treatment. In G. P. Sholevar (Ed.), *The handbook of marriage and marital therapy* (pp. 287–336). New York: Spectrum.

Epstein, N. (1982). Cognitive therapy with couples. *The American Journal of Family Therapy, 10*(1), 5–16.

Epstein, N., & Bishop, D. S. (1981). Problem centered systems therapy of the family. In A. Gurman & D. Kniskern (Eds.), *Handbook of family therapy* (pp. 444–482). New York: Brunner/Mazel.

Epstein, N., & Eidelson, R. J. (1981). Unrealistic beliefs of clinical couples: Their relationship to expectations, goals, and satisfaction. *The American Journal of Family Therapy, 9*(4), 13–22.

Epstein, N., & Jackson, E. (1978). An outcome study of short-term communication training with married couples. *Journal of Consulting and Clinical Psychology, 46*(2), 207–212.

Epstein, N., Schlesinger, S. E., & Dryden, W. (1988). *Cognitive–behavioral therapy with families.* New York: Brunner/Mazel.

Epstein, N., & Williams, A. M. (1981). Behavioral approaches to the treatment of marital discord. In G. P. Sholevar (Ed.), *The handbook of marriage and marital therapy* (pp. 219–285). New York: Spectrum.

Gotlib, I., & Colby, C. (1987). *Treatment of depression: An interpersonal systems approach.* New York: Pergamon Press.

Jacobsen, N., & Margolin, G. (1979). *Marital therapy.* New York: Brunner/Mazel.

Schmaling, K. B., Fruzzetti, A. E., & Jacobson, N. S. (1989). Marital problems. In K. Hawton, P. M. Salkovskis, J. Kirk, & D. M. Clark (Eds.), *Cognitive behaviour therapy for psychiatric problems: A practical guide* (pp. 338–369). New York: Oxford University Press.

Teichman, Y. (1984). Cognitive family therapy. *British Journal of Cognitive Psychotherapy, 2*(1), 1–10.

Weiss, R. L. (1975). Contracts, cognition, and change: A behavioral approach to marriage therapy. *The Counseling Psychologist, 5*(3), 15–26.

Part III

THE BIOMEDICAL INTERFACE

Chapter 7

Cognitive and Biological Therapies: A Combined Approach

Jesse H. Wright, M.D., Ph.D.,
Michael E. Thase, M.D.,
and Tom Sensky, Ph.D., M.B., M.R.C.Psych.

The roots of cognitive therapy (CT) are embedded in a long tradition of psychological explanations for mental disorders, whereas somatic therapies are based on biochemical or physiological explanations for psychopathology. Differences between the two approaches abound. Theoretical constructs and treatment methods are dissimilar. Aside from a small number of psychiatrists, the professional orientations of cognitive therapists and pharmacotherapists also typically vary. Nevertheless, cognitive and somatic treatments are often used together in hospital settings, and even in the most conceptually pure cognitive therapy unit (CTU), various types of somatic therapy are typically integrated into the patients' overall treatment plan (Wright, Thase, & Beck, 1992). This chapter explores theories, procedures, and issues related to combining CT and pharmacotherapy. We present a psychobiological treatment model that capitalizes on a productive interchange between cognitive and biological therapies.

COMPREHENSIVE THEORIES

There are several comprehensive theories that can provide a framework for combining psychotherapy and somatic therapy. Engel's (1977) biopsychosocial theory is the most easily understood and widely used formulation. He argues that all illnesses have biological, psychological, and social influences. Thus, treatment interventions may be directed at a wide range of etiological variables.

Akiskal and McKinney (1975) offer a similar but more specific integrative theory for understanding the diversity of findings from research on depression. They suggest that depression is the result of a "psychobiological final common pathway" in which multiple factors (e.g., cognitive, behavioral, social, biomedical, genetic, and/or psychodynamic) coalesce in disease expression. From this perspective, competing theories offer different windows from which to observe the process of depression. The most sophisticated and potentially beneficial application of this approach would involve a thorough knowledge of all pertinent research data and an ability to synthesize this information together in an integrated approach to treatment.

General systems theory (Von Bertalanffy, 1956) also encourages an inclusive view of etiology and therapy. This theoretical construct has been used to understand complex living systems ranging from individual cells to families and multinational organizations (Murray, 1975; Rizzo, 1976; Miller, 1978; Chase, Wright, & Ragade, 1981a, 1981b). The advantage of general systems theory is that it provides a detailed explanation of how living systems are organized and regulated. This approach shares the position of the biopsychosocial theory that all interrelated systems have far-reaching influences on one another. Applications in psychiatry have included studies of decision making, family structure, drug abuse, and inpatient psychiatric units (Schlenger, 1973; Murray, 1975; Chase et al., 1981a, 1981b).

All of these theoretical viewpoints offer an acceptable general framework for combining psychotherapy and pharmacotherapy. However, none of them incorporate data from studies of cognitive therapy and pharmacotherapy (reviewed later in this chapter), nor do they provide any specific guidelines for treatment. Furthermore, the relationships among the various factors that may be involved in psychiatric disorders are not spelled out.

We have developed a working model for combined therapy (Figure 7.1) that is a fusion of the theoretical perspectives of Engel (1977) and Akiskal and McInney (1975) and the cognitive model for depression and anxiety (Wright, 1988; Wright & Borden, 1991). The primary features of this cognitive–biological model are that cognitive processes are viewed as the mediator between the environment (e.g., stressful events, interpersonal relations, or memories of events) and any biological response. Similarly, biological processes are seen as the bridge between cognition and any behavioral response to the environment.

Emotional reactions are an important part of the model. We consider emotions to be stereotypic or patterned psychobiological phenomena that may be triggered by environmental events (via cognitive

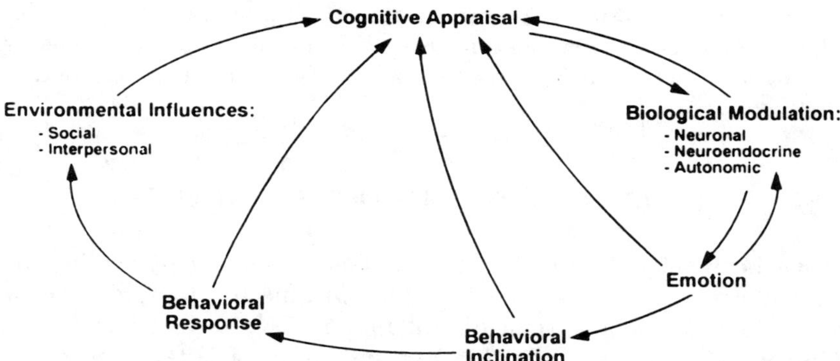

FIGURE 7.1. The cognitive–biological model for combined pharmacotherapy and psychotherapy.

appraisal) and/or biological (e.g., CNS regulation, neuroendocrine processes, drugs, or other chemical agents) mechanisms. For example, an emotion (anxiety) might be stimulated in a panic-disorder patient by (1) a misinterpretation of the danger or risk in a situation, (2) a genetically determined biological dysregulation, or (3) an exogenously administered biological agent such as an infusion of sodium lactate (Clark, 1986; Gorman et al., 1989; Klosko, Barlow, Tassinari, & Cerney, 1990). The emotional reaction, including neurophysiological arousal and activation of neuroendocrine cascades, is interpreted cognitively and leads to further biological responses until behavior (or a series of behaviors) results.

The clinical implications of the cognitive–biological model are that it (1) provides a working formula for understanding how environmental and social influences are mediated through a linked, cognitive–biological pathway, (2) suggests that biological processes may be influenced by cognitive interventions, and (3) recognizes that cognition is influenced by social, biochemical, emotional, and behavioral factors. Although the cognitive therapist may direct his or her attention primarily at modifying disordered information processing (and associated maladaptive behavior), the actions of the treatment may be translated throughout the entire system described in Figure 7.1. It is possible that similar results could be obtained through another portal of entry (e.g., interpersonal, biochemical) to the system.

We suggest that a theoretical position that considers the interrelationships among environment–cognition–biology–emotion–behavior should be utilized in the cognitive milieu. In many, if not most, cases treated in an inpatient setting, this approach will lead to the use of combined pharmacotherapy–psychotherapy treatment regimens. A full review of research on the reciprocal relationship among cognition, biological processes, and related factors is beyond the scope of this chapter. However, a clinical rationale for combined treatment is presented in the next section.

RATIONALE FOR COMBINED TREATMENT

It has been suggested for many years that combining psychotherapy with pharmacotherapy could facilitate outcome through additive or synergistic interactions (Uhlenhuth, Lippman, & Covi, 1969; Conte, Plutchik, Wild, & Karasu, 1986). Examples of possible favorable interactions include a positive placebo effect of medication on the response rate to psychotherapy; pharmacological enhancement of accessibility to psychotherapy (via reduced arousal or enhanced learning and memory functioning); pharmacotherapy and psychotherapy exerting significant effects on different types of target symptoms (e.g., relief of insomnia or loss of appetite via pharmacotherapy versus reduction of hopelessness and suicidal ideation in the early sessions of cognitive therapy); and improved drug compliance as a result of progress in psychotherapy (Group for the Advancement of Psychiatry, 1975; Wright & Schrodt, 1989). Psychotherapy may also have direct physiological effects including acute alterations of synaptic transmission (Kandel, 1979) and reversal of state-dependent neurobiological abnormalities (Shear et al., 1991; Thase & Simons, 1992). Moreover, psychotherapy could work in concert or synergistically with medication to reverse neurophysiological or chemical abnormalities of the disorder (Kandel & Schwarz, 1983; Mohl, 1987).

Negative interactions between psychotherapy and pharmacotherapy also have been hypothesized, although they generally have not been confirmed (Group for the Advancement of Psychiatry, 1975; Wright, 1987; Wright & Schrodt, 1989). One negative interaction could result if pharmacotherapy prematurely reduces levels of anxiety or depression, thus diminishing the patient's motivation for psychotherapy (Group for the Advancement of Psychiatry, 1975). Conversely, it has been proposed that patients may "act out" transference issues in therapy via medication noncompliance (Group for Advancement of Psychiatry, 1975). Also, cognitive therapy procedures, if ill-timed and/or too demanding for seriously ill patients, might heighten arousal or increase demoralization, thus interfering with the response to medication (Wright & Schrodt, 1989).

A number of outcome studies have examined pharmacotherapy–psychotherapy interactions in depression. Early reports studying interpersonal, group, and marital therapies were reviewed by Hollon and Beck (1978). They noted that outcome studies have been designed primarily to compare the efficacy of pharmacotherapy versus psychotherapy and, therefore, have not revealed much about interactions between treatments. Unfortunately, even more recent outpatient studies investigating cognitive and behavioral therapies, alone and in combination with pharmacotherapy, have continued to use similar designs (e.g., Blackburn, Bishop, Glen, Whalley, & Christie, 1981; Hersen, Bellack, Himmelhoch, & Thase, 1984; Murphy, Simons, Wetzel, & Lustman, 1984). Specific hypotheses about proposed mechanisms or synergistic or additive effects have thus received only minimal attention (Wright & Schrodt, 1989; Simons & Thase, 1990). Early reports suggesting differential target symptom effects for psychotherapy vis-à-vis pharmacotherapy (Rush, Kovacs, Beck, Weissenburger, & Hollon, 1981; Rush, Beck, Kovacs, Weissenburger, & Hollon, 1982; DiMascio et al., 1979) typically have not been replicated by other groups (Hollon, 1990; Sotsky et al., 1990; Simons, Garfield, & Murphy, 1984). In summary, the overall results of these comparative, outpatient studies suggest that, in some cases, cognitive therapy and pharmacotherapy studies have shown either a modest additive effect in producing symptom relief or a more rapid onset of action (Conte et al., 1986; Simons & Thase, 1990), and there is little well-replicated evidence of synergy or symptom specificity between CT and pharmacotherapy (Simons & Thase, 1990). Conversely, there is no evidence that the therapies detract from one another (Conte et al., 1986; Wright, 1987; Wright & Schrodt, 1989).

Both Wright and Schrodt (1989) and Simons and Thase (1990) have discussed the limitations of such comparative outcome research. In particular, rigid requirements of controlled studies may result in treatment procedures that are quite different from those used in regular clinical practice. For example, research protocols often call for patients to receive "fixed doses" of psychotherapy and medication, and the pharmacotherapist and cognitive therapist may not be able to function as a team (e.g., Hersen et al., 1984). Therapy outcome studies also have used rather homogeneous groups of mildly to moderately depressed outpatients as subjects and, as a result, may be limited in their ability to detect additive effects by the so-called "ceiling effect" (Simons & Thase, 1990). Further, research comparing two or three forms of active treatment (i.e., each modality alone and their combination) requires double the sample sizes typically employed in single-site clinical trials comparing a single active treatment and placebo, as do those studies using a factorial design to test for hypothesized interactions. Therefore, even the most rigorously designed, controlled clinical trial with sample sizes of 15 to 25 subjects per cell may not have adequate statistical power to identify additive or interactive effects.

By contrast, hospitalized patients often have multiple diagnoses, more severe psychopathology (including suicidal ideation and behavior), and impaired social support systems. Thus, maximum treatment efforts are required. As such, there may be much more room to demonstrate an additive effect between CT and pharmacotherapy. The findings of Miller, Norman, and Keitner (1989), Miller, Norman, Keitner, Bishop, and Dow (1989), and Bowers (1990) that suggest such additive effects when cognitive and behavioral therapies are used to augment standard inpatient treatment plans support this notion. Parallel findings have been reported concerning the addition of psychoeducational marital or family interventions (Clarkin et al., 1990; Hogarty et al., 1986). Perhaps of greatest relevance, in subsequent analyses of Miller, Norman, and Keitner's (1989) study of hospitalized depressives, patients with high levels of dysfunctional attitudes or cognitive distortions at pretreatment responded significantly better to combined treatment than to standard pharmacotherapy, whereas patients with lower levels of cognitive disturbances received no differential benefit when CT was added to standard inpatient care (Miller, Norman, & Keitner, 1990; Whisman, Miller, Norman, & Keitner, 1991). In routine practice, it therefore seems likely that the inpatient treatment team may provide an array of CT procedures in addition to pharmacotherapy with a reasonable expectation of additive therapeutic effects.

CASE SELECTION

A combination of CT and pharmacotherapy is used for most inpatients treated on a CTU. However, decisions can be made by the treatment team about the emphasis of the therapies. Table 7.1 lists disorders for which CT can be considered as a primary treatment as well as those for which CT is best used in a supportive or auxiliary role. These recommendations are based on our clinical experience (Wright & Schrodt, 1989; Thase & Wright, 1991) as well as a review of data from CT outcome studies (see Chapter 1) and psychopharmacological research (e.g., Baldessarini, 1977; Meltzer & Coyle, 1987; Wright & Lippmann, 1988).

Both CT and pharmacotherapy are viewed as primary interventions for conditions in which their treatment efficacy is well established (e.g., nonpsychotic unipolar depression or panic disorders) or in which an extensive clinical literature describes detailed treatment methods, but standards of treatment efficacy have not yet been documented (e.g.,

TABLE 7.1. Indications for Cognitive Therapy

Cognitive therapy as a primary treatment
- Major depression
- Anxiety disorders
- Personality disorders
- Substance abuse
- Eating disorders
- Adjustment disorders

Cognitive therapy as an adjunctive treatment
- Bipolar disorder
- Major depression with psychotic features
- Organic affective disorder
- Schizophrenia
- Other psychotic disorders

personality disorders). Although the efficacy of antidepressant pharmacotherapy has been established unequivocally for the most severely impaired, hospitalized patients with major depression, the empirical investigation of CT as the primary treatment of unmedicated depressed patients is still in its infancy (Thase, Bowler, & Harden, 1991). Thus, until further evidence is available, we typically do not recommend CT in lieu of pharmacotherapy (outside of a research setting) unless patients cannot take antidepressant medication safely (e.g., first trimester pregnancy), have not responded to multiple medications (and will not accept ECT), or refuse to take medication (Thase & Wright, 1991).

Electroconvulsive therapy or intensive pharmacotherapy regimens (i.e., an antidepressant plus an antipsychotic medication) remain the treatments of choice for major depression with psychotic features such as delusions and/or hallucinations. Likewise, lithium carbonate or an alternate mood-stabilizing chemotherapy regimen is the standard treatment for the depressed phase of bipolar affective disorder. Cognitive therapy may be used to augment somatic therapies for the affective psychoses by enhancing treatment adherence (Cochran, 1986; Rush, 1988) or improving coping strategies (Wright, 1987; Wright & Schrodt, 1989). Further, although ECT and psychotherapy are sometimes considered to be mutually exclusive, patients who receive unilateral electroconvulsive therapy usually do not suffer from memory disturbances that preclude participation in cognitive therapy, particularly when sessions are held on the days alternating between ECT treatments. Indeed, many patients have an improved ability to remember and concentrate following effective somatic treatment and, thus, can begin to benefit from cognitive therapy after starting a course of ECT (Wright, 1987). As described in Chapters 4 and 14, CT has also been used to enhance the response to pharmacotherapy in psychosocial rehabilitation programs for even more severely ill patients, including schizophrenics (Perris, 1989; Wright & Schrodt, 1989) and in medication-refractory, psychotic depressions (Bishop, Miller, Norman, Buda, & Foulke, 1986).

Beyond its applications in major depression, CT may be used alone when the admission diagnosis does not support pharmacotherapy. Patients admitted in acute situational crises (e.g., DSM-III-R diagnoses of adjustment disorder with depressed mood) are the most common examples of this potential indication. Although most patients in such crises can be treated on an outpatient basis, the severity of the patient's acute dysphoria, the presence of significant hopelessness, or an unsuccessful suicide attempt may necessitate hospitalization. Cognitive therapy can be useful in helping the patient to resolve crises in a short period of time and preparing to return to the home setting.

When a severely depressed patient adamantly refuses to accept recommended pharmacotherapy, the individual cognitive therapist may be able to address this rift in the treatment alliance. In such a circumstance, the therapist and patient may negotiate an initial contract for therapy with an understanding that failure to respond to CT may be viewed as evidence that pharmacotherapy could be reconsidered as a worthwhile treatment. We have found this pragmatic application of collaborative empiricism to be quite successful in selected cases of "resistant" depression. Moreover, we recommend this approach (rather than discharge against medical advice or "forced" prescription of medication) because it respects the possibility that there may be a rational basis underlying a nonpsychotic patient's decision to reject pharmacotherapy.

If a patient who refuses medication does not respond to an "adequate" course of inpatient CT (e.g., 10 inpatient sessions; Thase & Wright, 1991), the cognitive therapist may help the patient to examine automatic negative thoughts and dysfunctional attitudes that may be related to the decision not to take medications. Often, in such cases, rigid "anti-antidepressant" attitudes are part of a broader pattern of stoicism or dysfunctional beliefs about loss of control. Despite the use of such cognitive therapy interventions, some individuals may continue to elect not to receive medication. The vigor of the therapist's efforts to continue to challenge such negative attitudes about medication needs to be related to the severity of the patient's symptoms and the degree of response to inpatient CT. For example, a patient with nonpsychotic depression who is showing signs of a partial response to CT would probably continue with this form of therapy, coupled with occasional queries from the therapist about the patient's attitudes concerning medications. However, a severely depressed inpatient with persistent suicidal ideation or delusions who is not improving would warrant more intensive and protracted therapy interventions directed at the issue of medication refusal.

Even on units offering well-integrated CT programs, pharmacotherapy may be used without adjunctive therapy in some instances. This approach is indicated for patients who have severe psychoses with marked delusions and hallucinations, catatonia, moderate or severe mental retardation, or profound behavioral regression. Nevertheless, CT often may be added after somatic treatment has ameliorated the most florid symptoms of psychosis or regression. Another possible reason for using medication alone is when the patient or family adamantly rejects the use of psychotherapy. We have not, however, encountered this particular problem on our inpatient units. Indeed, following the guidelines for treatment selection described earlier, CT has been almost universally welcomed by the patients on our units and their families as an important part of their therapeutic program.

THE THERAPEUTIC RELATIONSHIP

The least complex form of therapeutic relationship in combined cognitive therapy and pharmacotherapy occurs in outpatient treatment, when a psychiatrist who is an expert in both treatment approaches delivers these therapies in a highly integrated manner. The psychiatrist can present a unified model for treatment based on one of the comprehensive theories discussed earlier in this chapter. Outpatient therapy with a physician pharmacotherapist and a nonphysician cognitive therapist is somewhat more complicated, especially if the therapists have not articulated a common treatment philosophy. The situation becomes even more convoluted when the patient enters the hospital and is confronted by a host of therapists who may or may not have shared goals and procedures.

Development of collaborative relationships for combined CT and pharmacotherapy in the inpatient setting is illustrated in the following case vignette.

Mrs. A. was a 42-year-old woman admitted to the hospital after taking an overdose of 90 alprazolam (Xanax®) tablets. She had received the medication from her family doctor the previous week because of anxiety and depression. Mrs. A.'s outpatient psychotherapist had been against the prescription of medication because she believed that pharmacotherapy would undercut the patient's motivation for treatment.

Moreover, the therapist also was concerned about Mrs. A.'s risk for suicide.

Mrs. A. was admitted to a psychiatric inpatient unit that provided a cognitive therapy program. As described in Chapter 3, the unit used the primary therapist model of inpatient CT. Mrs. A. was evaluated by a psychiatrist who diagnosed major depression. He recommended treatment with a combination of imipramine and individual CT, with the hospital psychologist serving as the cognitive therapist. Mrs. A. also joined an inpatient cognitive therapy group led by the unit's chief nurse. Family cognitive therapy was initiated by Mrs. A.'s social worker during the second week of hospitalization.

Admission to the hospital and development of a multifaceted treatment plan centered around CT and pharmacotherapy placed Mrs. A. and her therapists in an intricate web of relationships. This network is diagrammed in Figure 7.2. There were six patient–therapist relationships and 16 therapist–therapist relationships identified for this case. All of these had the potential for either facilitation or inhibition of therapeutic progress.

Ideally, the team of therapists shares a common treatment philosophy, understands and respects one another, has a good working knowledge of each other's field of interest, communicates on a regular basis, and presents themselves as a team to the patient (Wright, 1987). Unfortunately, this was not the case early in Mrs. A.'s treatment, as described below.

The outpatient therapist was psychodynamically oriented. She thought that Mrs. A.'s main problem was difficulty in developing trusting and gratifying relationships. This therapist believed that medication would be of little value. The family doctor had been treating Mrs. A.

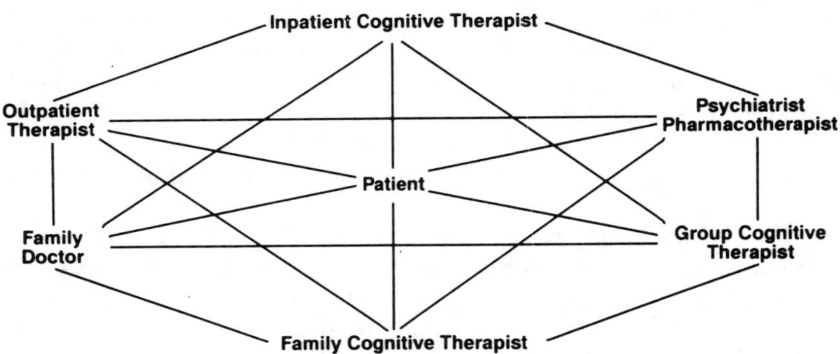

FIGURE 7.2. Therapeutic relationships in combined cognitive therapy and pharmacotherapy.

since she was a child. He knew that Mrs. A. had been under a great deal of stress because her alcoholic husband had lost his job and her mother had developed cancer. The family doctor had prescribed alprazolam to help her to cope better with this understandably difficult situation. However, her family doctor became somewhat angry and more distant after the patient attempted suicide. The psychiatrist believed that both the outpatient therapist and the family doctor had not recognized a classic, major depression. His top priority was to begin vigorous antidepressant pharmacotherapy as soon as possible. The inpatient cognitive therapist saw the situation somewhat differently. She recognized profound hopelessness, superimposed on a base line characterized by low self-esteem and basic assumptions regarding personal inadequacy and the untrustworthiness of loved ones. These symptoms seemed to be appropriate targets for cognitive therapy.

Mrs. A. was confused by these varied presentations and recommendations. She had a close relationship with her family doctor and trusted him very much. Yet, following the suicide attempt, her doctor was telling her that he could no longer help her. Moreover, a new doctor (her inpatient psychiatrist) was recommending a very different type of medication. The outpatient therapist had been very supportive but had not been clear in explaining how their therapy was supposed to work. On the other hand, the inpatient psychotherapist talked a great deal more and seemed to be telling Mrs. A. that there was something wrong with the way she was thinking.

These conflicts were articulated and reviewed by the inpatient treatment team at a case conference held during the first week of hospitalization. Team members were concerned that Mrs. A.'s treatment would be seriously compromised unless a broad collaboration between the therapists and the patient could be achieved. Thus, a remedy was designed that followed the steps outlined in Table 7.2. First,

TABLE 7.2. Formation of Collaborative Relationships in Combined Cognitive Therapy and Pharmacotherapy

Identify all combinations of patient–therapist and therapist–therapist relationships
Examine these relationships for strengths and weaknesses
Articulate therapist's case conceptualizations
Identify areas of conflict and mutual agreement
Discuss relationship analysis with all members of treatment team
Strive for maximum agreement in treatment philosophy and procedures
Present an integrated and cohesive treatment philosophy to patient
Reevaluate therapeutic relationships at regular intervals

the team invited the outpatient therapist and the family practitioner to attend a treatment planning conference designed to develop a comprehensive therapy plan that could be endorsed by all involved. Concurrently, psychoeducational procedures were initiated to help Mrs. A. understand the rationale for the shift in goals for the psychotherapy and the role of both CT and pharmacotherapy as a combined treatment regimen.

At the treatment planning conference, each of the therapists briefly described his or her formulation of the case and therapeutic goals. The family doctor was able to ventilate his anger about Mrs. A.'s suicide attempt. He was able then to reengage by "handing over" the psychotropic medication prescription responsibilities to the attending psychiatrist. The outpatient therapist seemed more accepting of the severity of the episode of depression and agreed to defer further psychodynamic therapy until after Mrs. A. had stabilized. Finally, the triad of inpatient therapists established a coordinated plan of therapy with an appropriate division of labor.

Of course, not all conflicts regarding the management of such cases have clear-cut resolutions. As discussed in Chapters 3 and 15, "power plays" between various team members and hospital "political" struggles between professional disciplines may surface during the treatment team process. For example, the public discussion of the relative merits (or worth) of CT and pharmacotherapy during a treatment team meeting could serve as a conduit for venting long-standing tensions between disciplines such as clinical psychology and psychiatry. When such conflicts arise, we consider it to be the team leader's or unit director's responsibility to recognize the problem and serve as a moderator in order to achieve an acceptable solution. In extreme cases, this may require a private meeting to "clear the air" and reinstill a spirit of collaboration. In our experience, patients with severe personality disorders are the most likely to provoke splits or disputes among their treatment team's members. Effective and expeditious solution of such problems is one of the significant challenges for inpatient cognitive therapy.

TREATMENT PROCEDURES

A unified conceptualization of CT and pharmacotherapy is most easily understood by the patient when it is presented from the outset of treatment. We use the cognitive–biological model for mood disorders described earlier to help patients and families understand the rationale for combined therapy. This model builds on evidence from various lines of research that a diverse group of risk factors (e.g., genetic, acquired defects secondary to early trauma or abuse, dysfunctional attitudes that have resulted from maladaptive social learning, or the effects of various illnesses or medications) may interact in reactions to life stress. In explaining depression, the therapist might use the analogy of a duodenal ulcer or hypertension to describe the roles of risk (or diathesis) and stress (Simons & Thase, 1990). Adverse events and the way the individual copes with environmental change may be involved in producing the symptoms, but underlying biological processes also play a role. Combined therapy thus can be directed both at helping the individual manage stress more effectively and at reversing the somatic pathology.

Setting an Agenda

This integrative model for therapy can be reinforced by one of the most basic cognitive therapy techniques—agenda setting. If issues pertaining to both cognitive and pharmacological therapies are placed on each day's agenda and are treated as equal partners in the recovery process, the likelihood of competition between or among treatments is diminished considerably. The hospital environment offers rich opportunities for using agenda-setting techniques to join the cognitive and pharmacological approaches to treatment. Table 7.3 lists sample therapy agendas for a hospitalized patient. This illustrates how an agenda can be used to link together a diverse set of treatment initiatives. Clear communication between therapists and patients is crucial for the success of this approach.

Psychoeducational Techniques

Psychoeducational procedures can be used to improve the patient's understanding of how both treatments work. Also, the value of both modes of treatment can be emphasized during various psychoeducational activities. There are several advantages to encouraging the patient to be an informed consumer. First, collaboration is promoted when the treatments are demystified and the roles of patient and therapists are made specific. Hopeful expectations for the effects of therapies also can be made explicit. The patient is provided with information that can prevent misunderstandings and clarify points of confusion, thus increasing the chances of a favorable treatment outcome. For example, a well-informed patient who experiences a common medication side effect will be prepared for potential problems and will probably continue taking the medication, at least until he or she has the opportunity to discuss the problem with a doctor (Simons & Thase, 1990). In contrast,

TABLE 7.3. Interlocking Agendas for Combined Cognitive Therapy and Pharmacotherapy

Individual therapy	Group therapy	Family therapy	Medication group
1. Homework	1. Homework	1. Conflict about finances	1. Information about medication
2. Coping with wife's criticism	2. Handling criticism	2. Questions about medication	2. Attitudes about medication
3. Medication issues (i.e., side effects, expectations, signs of response, overcoming stigma)	3. Medication issues	3. Homework (i.e., thoughts/feelings about the patient's condition and treatment)	3. Family reactions (i.e., to the hospitalization, medication, and therapy)
4. Fear of returning to work		4. Upcoming home visit	4. Side effects

when patients are surprised by the development of an unexpected side effect, they may become discouraged, anxious, or angry and, as a result, refuse to take the medication. Although such disputes may be resolved during a subsequent doctor's rounds, they may erode the patient's trust in the competence or forthrightness of the treatment team. In this regard, the cliche "forewarned is forearmed" is axiomatic.

One of the distinguishing features of cognitive therapy is its emphasis on psychoeducational procedures as a routine treatment component (Beck, Rush, Shaw, & Emery, 1979; Wright & Beck, 1983; Wright, 1988). If pharmacotherapy is added, specific information about this approach is also needed. Methods for psychoeducational interventions for patients with affective disorders and their families have been developed (Holder & Anderson, 1990; Frank, Prien, Kupfer, & Alberts, 1985) and are now frequently included as part of comprehensive inpatient treatment programs. At a minimum, the patient and family need to be provided with an explanation of the presumed mechanisms or targets of drug action, common or likely side effects, methods of managing these reactions, and a projection for length of treatment. This information may be presented during individual therapy sessions, physician ward rounds, family meetings, and specific psychoeducational groups designed to discuss pharmacotherapy. Psychoeducational materials should be reviewed carefully before they are approved for use in the hospital settings (see Chapter 15).

Enhancing Compliance

The prescription of a drug for emotional symptoms often has a powerful meaning for the patient. Many of the standard CT interventions such as guided discovery (Socratic questioning), eliciting and testing automatic thoughts, and schema modification may help facilitate the compliance with pharmacotherapy. For example, guided discovery can be used to identify and question the patient's attitudes about taking medication, as illustrated in the following vignette.

Mr. B. was hospitalized after reporting to his outpatient therapist that he was considering suicide. At the conclusion of Dr. J.'s admission interview the following discussion took place.

Dr. J.: You've described the kind of symptoms that usually respond to medication.

Mr. B.: I've never really considered taking drugs.

Dr. J.: What do you think of the idea?

Mr. B.: I don't know, I'm not a big fan of drug therapy.

Dr. J.: I'd like to hear more about your views of medication. What came into your mind when I suggested that a medicine might help.

Mr. B.: I guess I was mixed up. Part of me was glad to hear that something could be done, but some other bells were going off.

Dr. J.: What were the other bells warning you about?

Mr. B.: *(Pause)* You should be able to do this on your own. Taking a drug would be a cop-out.

Further questioning revealed a plethora of dysfunctional automatic thoughts about pharmacotherapy. These were centered around several major themes that are commonly involved in cognitive responses to prescription of medication: personal weakness, fear of medication effects, fear of the opinions of others, problems with the therapeutic alliance, and misunderstandings about the illness (Wright & Schrodt, 1989). Typical automatic thoughts in each of these areas are described in Table 7.4.

In many inpatient settings, the attending psychiatrist has not received training in CT. However, in the case of Mr. B., the physician was an experienced cognitive therapist. In another setting, a nonmedical cognitive therapist could work in conjunction with the psychiatrist to accomplish the same goal.

A variety of procedures can be used to modify distorted cognitions in combined pharmacotherapy and psychotherapy. Thought recording was used in subsequent sessions with Mr. B. During an early therapy session, Mr. B. wrote "medications are just a crutch" in the automatic thoughts column in the Daily Record of Dysfunctional Thoughts (see Chapter 1). The therapist asked Mr. B. to examine the validity of this cognition by generating evidence that would support or refute the statement. A more adaptive viewpoint was then recorded in the rational thoughts column. "Medication has helped many people recover from depression. If you use a 'crutch' for a legitimate reason and it helps with recovery, it doesn't mean you are weak. There is nothing wrong with getting assistance when you need it." The therapist also helped Mr. B. to identify and label cognitive errors such as absolutistic thinking, selective abstraction, and arbitrary inference (see Chapter 1).

As noted earlier, repetitive themes or patterns of automatic thoughts about medication usually indicate the presence of an underlying schema. Therapeutic work on identifying and testing schemas can be helpful in promoting the patient's acceptance of pharmacotherapy. Such work also may be of benefit in modifying related maladaptive

TABLE 7.4. Common Cognitions about Medications

Personal strength and self-control	Fear of medication effects	Fear of others' opinions	Problems with the therapeutic alliance	Misunderstanding about the illness
"I should be able to get better on my own."	"I won't be able to function."	"If my boss finds out, I'll get fired."	"I'm just a guinea pig."	"My problems are real—how could drugs help?"
"Medications are just a crutch."	"I'm the one that always gets the side effects."	"I don't want my children to know."	"Can I trust this doctor?"	"If there is something wrong with my brain, I'm doomed."
"I shouldn't give in."	"I'll get hooked."	"If I get better, they'll give the credit to the drug."	"Doctors give pills to avoid their patients."	"I'm just a loser. Medication won't change that."

Adapted from Wright & Schrodt (1989).

attitudes that have a negative influence on other areas of functioning. Mr. B.'s automatic thoughts regarding self-control suggested the underlying basic assumption: "I must be strong at all times." Although this schema had been adaptive in many ways (e.g., a hard-working life style had helped Mr. B. become economically successful and hold powerful positions in the community), it also had significant liabilities. He was extremely guarded and was virtually unable to accept support from his family or co-workers. At times, his behavior was overbearing and insensitive. Furthermore, treatment for his episode of depression had been delayed significantly by his dysfunctional attitudes, and even after hospitalization, he was reluctant to begin pharmacotherapy.

Some patients also have positive distortions about pharmacotherapy. In extreme cases, they may endow medication with quasimagical powers, believing that it will cure them without any effort on their part. These patients often have significant problems in the hospital milieu when they decline or denigrate participation in therapeutic activities and when they behave listlessly in psychotherapy. In a cognitive milieu, concerted efforts will be made to modify automatic negative thoughts and schemas that perpetuate this behavior. We have found that a consistent and repetitive treatment program geared at developing increased self-awareness, enhanced coping skills, and use of self-help methods is the best way to counter such attitudes within the overall treatment program. In particular, receipt of feedback from other patients (in a group therapy or during focus or "wrap-up" groups) seems to be a particularly powerful aid in helping a patient become aware of the impact of passive behavior or magical expectations.

Benign positive distortions about biological treatments are not usually addressed. For example, a patient who is genuinely hopeful about the prospects of pharmacotherapy might, if questioned, estimate a 90% chance of recovery. Although this may be an inflated expectation, we would not typically suggest a homework assignment aimed at development of a more sober (realistic) estimation, such as a recommendation that the patient complete a careful reading of the literature in order to determine the actual response rate (i.e., approximately 60–70%). Instead, we would allow this mildly positive distortion to go unchallenged because it is likely to promote recovery by assisting with a positive placebo effect, and there is little chance that it will do harm. In the event of nonresponse, a multitude of alternate treatments are available (e.g., Simons & Thase, 1990).

Family members can also have a wide variety of negative and positive distortions about medications. Family attitudes can have profound effects on the patient's response to pharmacotherapy. A well-informed family that is supportive of somatic treatment will encourage hopefulness and treatment adherence (Frank et al., 1985). In contrast, the family with limited information and conflicting or hostile attitudes can derail a treatment program rapidly (see Chapter 6). Thus, working with the family provides another valuable element of the combined treatment approach with inpatients. Our inpatient programs include a series of "family nights" where psychoeducational materials on pharmacotherapy and cognitive therapy are presented in a group format.

Attitudes of staff members about both pharmacotherapy and cognitive therapy can also have a significant effect on outcome. Ideally, all staff members should be highly knowledgeable about the indications, dosages, and side effects of psychotropic medications. Consistency of information provided to patients and a positive attitude about both modalities of therapy are essential (Thase & Wright, 1991). Evidence of problems with staff attitudes or expertise should be addressed vigorously and repeatedly in staff meetings, retreats, and inservice educational programs.

Behavioral techniques such as activity scheduling, graded-task assignments, and rehearsal are another major component of the combined CT and pharmacotherapy approach. Mastery and pleasure ratings from the Daily Activity Schedule (see Chapters 1 and 3 for detailed explanations of the use of the Daily Activity Schedule) can give valuable data about how the patient views taking medication. For example, a self-rating mastery score of 2 (on a 10-point scale) following attendance at a medication information group would indicate potential problems. The treatment team may ask pertinent questions on reviewing this information. "Was the patient asked to attend this group prematurely? Would other, more circumscribed psychoeducational procedures be better suited to the patient's level of functioning? What thoughts about medication may have triggered this low rating?"

Changes in behavioral ratings after medication doses also can be indicative of significant side effects or negative attitudes about medication. One patient became considerably less active each day after receiving a dose of 1.0 mg of clonazepam (Klonopin®) at 1:00 p.m. Her mastery ratings typically fell, and for several days she declined to participate in scheduled afternoon groups. In this case, the patient was experiencing an adverse sedative response to medication. The problem was relieved promptly by discontinuation of the midday dose. Another patient became much more energetic after nortriptyline was started. She began to sleep through the night, and she had increased interest and higher pleasure ratings. These positive medication effects were detected on the Daily Activity Schedule.

Graded-task assignments are used when patients are markedly fearful of taking medication. In extreme cases, such fears may reach phobic proportions. Instead of "pushing" a patient to begin pharmacotherapy immediately, a stepwise approach can help introduce the patient to medication gradually. Mrs. C., who suffered from both major depression and panic disorder, agreed that medication would benefit her, but she was terrified of side effects. Each time she visualized taking medication she became anxious and tremulous, and she reported feeling as if her throat were constricting. A graded-task assignment was developed in collaboration with the patient, as follows: (1) read a pamphlet on tricyclic antidepressants; (2) discuss fears and concerns with nurse and doctor; (3) talk with another patient who is taking a tricyclic antidepressant and record a summary of this conversation in a notebook; (4) attend medication group; (5) look at picture of antidepressant pills; (6) write out a two-column list of common side effects and their countermeasures; (7) hold an imipramine pill in hand; (8) imagine anticipated reactions to taking an initial dose of medication and rehearse coping with a mild level of distress; (9) take one test dose of imipramine 25 mg; and (10) discuss responses with nurse and doctor. After these tasks were successfully accomplished, Mrs. C. agreed to begin a regular nightly dose of medication.

Lack of adherence to treatment recommendations is one of the primary reasons for failure of pharmacotherapy (Thase & Kupfer, 1987). It has been estimated that between 30% and 70% of outpatients fail to comply with their pharmacotherapy regimen (Blackwell, 1982). Although problems with noncompliance are minimized during inpatient treatment, a vigorous attempt should be made to help patients develop positive attitudes about medication in order to improve the chances of optimal adherence following discharge. Even the best-intentioned patient may have difficulty in sustaining a complicated schedule of medication when it is prescribed over a protracted period of time. Behavioral techniques can be especially useful in promoting long-term medication compliance (Wright, 1987; Wright & Schrodt, 1989; Rush, 1988).

Positive reinforcers for medication adherence should be identified and promoted where possible. As described elsewhere (Beck et al., 1979), the cognitive therapist has sufficient flexibility to choose from a wide menu of potential reinforcers, although we suggest that the use of penalties (or other forms of punishment) should generally be avoided and that the choice of reinforcement should be arrived at collaboratively. These reinforcers can be found in both intra- and interpersonal spheres. The patient's daily activities can be examined to develop a schedule that facilitates or reinforces medication taking. A morning medication dose might be paired with breakfast if this is a convenient or pleasurable activity. The family system should also be examined for potential reinforcers. For example, a favorite meal or family outing might be used to reward one week's compliance for a patient who has had a problem with treatment nonadherence.

Note should also be made of the effect of the therapist's attitudes and behavior on medication adherence (Barrett & Wright, 1984; Wright & Schrodt, 1989). Does the therapist seem positive about the medication? Are medication issues placed consistently on the agenda, or does the therapist seem disinterested in medication and treat it as having minimal significance? We strongly suggest that nonmedical primary therapists regularly ask how other aspects of a patient's treatment are going. The importance of medication (and other therapeutic modalities) is subtly reinforced in this manner, and, when pertinent, problems can be addressed. Consultation and ongoing supervision can be used when it appears that the therapist is either actively or unwittingly discouraging treatment adherence.

Other interventions that can help promote full compliance include reminder systems (e.g., divided pill boxes, wristwatch alarms, or medication logs) and behavioral rehearsal. Reminders are especially useful for geriatric patients and other individuals with impaired memory and concentration. Behavioral rehearsal helps to identify automatic negative thoughts and interpersonal barriers to taking medication (e.g., embarrassment at taking pills at work, interference by social activities, or negative family responses) and provides a mechanism for practicing ways of continuing the medication schedule. The array of cognitive and behavioral techniques described here can play an important role in encouraging treatment adherence and therefore decreasing the risk of relapse.

SUMMARY

Cognitive and biological therapies are two of the major forces in contemporary psychiatric treatment. In this chapter, we describe a cognitive–biological theoretical model that can guide those who wish to integrate the two approaches in clinical practice. In outpatient settings, cognitive therapy is used commonly without accompanying pharmacotherapy. However, adequate therapy of hospitalized patients, who have higher levels of psychopathology, usually necessitates a combined approach.

One of the major features of the cognitive milieu is the joining of psychotherapeutic and biological interventions in a comprehensive treatment plan. A collaborative therapeutic relationship, in which cognitive therapists, psychopharmacologists, adjunctive therapists, nurses, and the patient share a common treatment philosophy, is strongly encouraged. Other therapeutic procedures that help unite the two approaches include agenda setting, psychoeducational interventions, and therapeutic work on enhancing compliance with pharmacotherapy.

We conclude that a cognitive–biological treatment model can serve as an organizing general theory for the cognitive milieu. Although much work remains to be done on understanding the reciprocal relationships among the environment, cognition, biological processes, emotion, and behavior, there is little doubt that all of these factors can be involved in psychopathology. The challenge for the future is to better understand treatment interactions and to use this information to develop more effective comprehensive therapies.

REFERENCES

Akiskal, H. S., & McKinney, W. T. (1975). Overview of recent research in depression. Integration of ten conceptual methods into a comprehensive clinical frame. *Archives of General Psychiatry, 32*, 285–305.

Baldessarini, R. J. (1977). *Chemotherapy in psychiatry*. Cambridge, MA: Harvard University Press.

Barrett, C. L., & Wright, J. H. (1984). Therapist variables. In M. Hersen, L. Michelson, & A. S. Bellack (Eds.), *Issues in psychotherapy research* (pp. 361–391). New York: Plenum Press.

Beck, A. T., Rush, A. J., Shaw, B. F., & Emery, G. (1979). *Cognitive therapy of depression*. New York: Guilford Press.

Bishop, S., Miller, I. N., Norman, W., Buda, M., & Foulke, M. (1986). Cognitive therapy of psychotic depression: A case report. *Psychotherapy, 23*, 167–173.

Blackburn, I. M., Bishop, S., Glen, A. I. M., Whalley, L. J., & Christie, J. E. (1981). The efficacy of cognitive therapy in depression. A treatment trial using cognitive therapy and pharmacotherapy, each alone and in combination. *British Journal of Psychiatry, 139*, 181–189.

Blackwell, B. (1982). Antidepressant drugs: Side effects and compliance. *Journal of Clinical Psychiatry, 43*, 14–21.

Bowers, W. A. (1990). Treatment of depressed inpatients. Cognitive therapy plus medication, relaxation plus medication, and medication alone. *British Journal of Psychiatry, 156*, 73–78.

Chase, S., Wright, J. H., & Ragade, R. (1981a). Decision making in an interdisciplinary team. *Behavioral Sciences, 26*, 206–215.

Chase, S., Wright, J. H., & Ragade, R. (1981b). The inpatient psychiatric unit as a system. *Behavioral Sciences, 26*, 197–205.

Clark, D. M. (1986). A cognitive approach to panic. *Behaviour Research and Therapy, 24*, 461–470.

Clarkin, J. S., Glick, I. D., Haas, G. L., Spender, J. H., Lewis, A. B., Peyser, J., DeMane, N., Good-Ellis, M., Harris, E., & Lestelle, V. (1990). A randomized clinical trial of inpatient family intervention verse results for affective disorders. *Journal of Affective Disorders, 18,* 17–28.

Cochran, S. D. (1986). Compliance with lithium regimens in the outpatient treatment of bipolar disorder. *Journal of Compliance Health Care, 1,* 151–169.

Conte, H. R., Plutchik, R., Wild, K. V., & Karasu, T. B. (1986). Combined psychotherapy and pharmacotherapy for depression. *Archives of General Psychiatry, 43,* 461–479.

DiMascio, A., Weissman, M. M., Pursoff, B. A., Neu, C., Zwilling, M., & Klerman, G. L. (1979). Differential symptom reduction by drugs and psychotherapy in acute depression. *Archives of General Psychiatry, 36,* 1450–1456.

Engel, G. L. (1977). The need for a new medical model: A challenge for biomedicine. *Science, 196,* 129–136.

Frank, E., Prien, R. F., Kupfer, D. J., & Alberts, L. (1985). Implications of noncompliance on research in affective disorders. *Psychopharmacology Bulletin, 21,* 37–42.

Gorman, J. M., Battista, M. D., Goetz, R. R, Dillon, D. J., Liebowitz, M. R., Fyer, A. J., Kahn, J. P., Sandberg, D., & Klein, D. F. (1989). A comparison of sodium bicarbonate and sodium lactate infusion in the induction of panic attacks. *Archives of General Psychiatry, 46,* 145–150.

Group for the Advancement of Psychiatry. (1975). *Pharmacotherapy and psychotherapy: Paradoxes, problems, and progress* (Vol. 9, Report 93). New York: Mental Health Materials Center.

Hersen, M., Bellack, A. S., Himmelhoch, J. M., & Thase, M. E. (1984). Effects of social skill training, amitriptyline, and psychotherapy in unipolar depressed woman. *Behavior Therapy, 15,* 21–40.

Hogarty, G. E., Anderson, C. M., Reiss, D. J., Kornblith, S. J., Greenwald, D. P., Jauna, C. D., & Madonia, M. J. (1986). Environmental/personal indicators in the course of schizophrenic research group: Family psychoeducational, social skills training, and maintenance chemotherapy in the aftercare treatment of schizophrenia: One year effects of a controlled study on relapse and expressed emotion. *Archives of General Psychiatry, 43,* 633–642.

Holder, D., & Anderson, C. M. (1990). Psychoeducational family intervention for depressed patients and their families. In G. I. Keitner (Ed.), *Depression and families impact and treatment* (pp. 159–184). Washington, DC: American Psychiatric Press.

Hollon, S. D. (1990). Cognitive therapy and pharmacotherapy for depression. *Psychiatric Annals, 20,* 249–258.

Hollon, S., & Beck, A. T. (1978). Psychotherapy and drug therapy: Comparisons and combinations. In S. L. Garfield & A. E. Bergin (Eds.), *Handbook of psychotherapy and behavior change* (2nd ed., pp. 437–490). New York: John Wiley & Sons.

Kandel, E. R. (1979). Psychotherapy and the single synapse: The impact of psychiatric thought on neurobiologic research. *The New England Journal of Medicine, 301*, 1028–1037.

Kandel, E. R., & Schwartz, J. H. (1983). Molecular biology of learning: Modulation of transmitter release. *Science, 218*, 433–443.

Klosko, J. S., Barlow, D. H., Tassinari, R., & Cerny, J. A. (1990). A comparison of alprazolam and behavior therapy in treatment of panic disorder. *Journal of Consulting and Clinical Psychology, 58*, 77–84.

Meltzer, H. Y., & Coyle, J. T. (Eds.). (1987). *Psychopharmacology: The third generation of progress, in association with the American College of Neuropsychopharmacology*. New York: Raven Press.

Miller, I. W., Norman, W. H., & Keitner, G. I. (1989). Cognitive-behavioral treatment of depressed inpatients: Six- and twelve-month follow-ups. *American Journal of Psychiatry, 146*, 1274–1279.

Miller, I. W., Norman, W. H., & Keitner, G. I. (1990). Treatment response of high cognitive dysfunction depressed inpatients. *Comprehensive Psychiatry, 30*, 62–71.

Miller, I. W., Norman, W. H., Keitner, G. I., Bishop, S. T., & Dow, M. G. (1989). Cognitive behavioral treatment of depressed inpatients. *Behavior Therapy, 20*, 25–47.

Miller, J. H., (1978). *Living systems*. New York: McGraw Hill.

Mohl, P. C. (1987). Should psychotherapy be considered a biological treatment? *Psychosomatics, 28*, 320–326.

Murphy, G. E., Simons, A. D., Wetzel, R. D., & Lustman, P. J. (1984). Cognitive therapy and pharmacotherapy, singly and together, in the treatment of depression. *Archives of General Psychiatry, 41*, 33–41.

Murray, M. E. (1975). A model for family therapy: Integrating system and subsystem dynamics. *Journal of Family Therapy, 2*, 187–197.

Perris, C. (1989) *Cognitive therapy with schizophrenic patients*. New York: Guilford Press.

Rizzo, N. D. (1976). General systems theories: It's impact in the health field. In W. H. Werley (Ed.), *Health research: The systems approach* (pp. 15–24). New York: Springer.

Rush, A. J. (1988). Cognitive approaches to adherence. In A. J. Frances, & R. E. Hales (Eds.), *American Psychiatric Press review of psychiatry* (Vol. 7, pp. 627–642). Washington, DC: American Psychiatric Press.

Rush, A. J., Beck, A. T., Kovacs, M., Weissenburger, J., & Hollan, S. D. (1982). Comparison of the effects of cognitive therapy and pharmacotherapy on hopelessness and self-concept. *American Journal of Psychiatry, 139*, 862–866.

Rush, A. J., Kovacs, M., Beck, A. T., Weissenburger, J., & Hollon, S. D. (1981). Differential effects of cognitive therapy and pharmacotherapy on depressive symptoms. *Journal of Affective Disorders, 3*, 221–229.

Schlenger, W. E. (1973). Systems approach to drug users services. *Behavioral Science, 18*, 137–147.

Shear, M. K., Fyer, A. J., Ball, G., Josephson, S., Fitzpatrick, M., Gitlin, B.,

Frances, A., Gorman, J., Liebowitz, M., & Klein, D. F. (1991). Vulnerability to sodium lactate in panic disorder patients given cognitive–behavioral therapy. *American Journal of Psychiatry, 148*(6), 795–797.

Simons, A. D., Garfield, S. L., & Murphy, G. E. (1984). The process of change in cognitive therapy and pharmacotherapy in depression: Changes in mood and cognition. *Archives of General Psychiatry, 41,* 45–51.

Simons, A. D., & Thase, M. E. (1990). Mood disorders. In M. E. Thase, M. Hersen, & B. A. Edelstein (Eds.), *Handbook of outpatient treatment of adults* (pp. 91–138). New York: Plenum Press.

Sotsky, S. M., Glass, D. R., Shea, M. T., Pilkonis, P. A., Collins, J. F., Elkin, I., Watkins, J. T., Imber, S. D., Leber, W. R., Moyer, J., & Oliveri, N. E. (1991). Patient predictors of response to psychotherapy and pharmacotherapy: Findings in the NIMH treatment of depression collaborative research program. *American Journal of Psychiatry, 148,* 997–1008.

Thase, M. E., Bowler, K., & Harden, T. (1991). Cognitive behavior therapy of endogenous depression: Part 2: Preliminary findings in 16 unmedicated inpatients. *Behavior Therapy, 22,* 469–477.

Thase, M. E., & Kupfer, D. J. (1987). Characteristics of treatment resistant depression. In J. Zohar & R. H. Belmaker (Eds.), *Treating resistant depression* (pp. 23–45). New York: PMA Publishing.

Thase, M. E., & Simons A. D. (1992). The applied use of psychotherapy in the study of the psychobiology of depression. *The Journal of Psychotherapy Practice and Research, 1,* 72–80.

Thase, M. E., & Wright, J. H. (1991). Cognitive behavior therapy with depressed inpatients: An abridged treatment manual. *Behavior Therapy, 22,* 579–595.

Uhlenhuth, E. H., Lippman, R. S., & Covi, L. (1969). Combined pharmacotherapy and psychotherapy. *Journal of Nervous and Mental Disease, 148,* 52–64.

Von Bertalanffy, L. V. (1956). General systems theory. *General Systems, 1,* 3.

Whisman, M. A., Miller, I. W., Norman, W. H., & Keitner, G. I. (1991). Cognitive therapy with depressed inpatients: Side effects on dysfunctional cognitions. *Journal of Consulting and Clinical Psychology, 59,* 282–288.

Wright, J. H. (1987). Cognitive therapy and medication as combined treatment. In A. Freeman & V. Greenwood (Eds.), *Cognitive therapy: Applications in psychiatric and medical settings* (pp. 36–50). New York: Human Sciences Press.

Wright, J. H. (1988). Cognitive therapy of depression. In A. J. Frances, & R. E. Hales (Eds.), *American Psychiatric Press review of psychiatry,* Vol. 7 (pp. 554–570). Washington, DC: American Psychiatric Press.

Wright, J. H., & Beck, A. T. (1983). Cognitive therapy of depression: Theory and practice. *Hospital Community Psychiatry, 34,* 1119–1127.

Wright, J. H., & Borden, J. (1991). Cognitive therapy of depression and anxiety. *Psychiatric Annals, 21,* 424–428.

Wright, J. H., & Lippmann, S. B. (1988). Use of antipsychotic drugs in depression: Problems and opportunities. *Postgraduate Medical Journal, 82*, 61–67.

Wright, J. H., & Schrodt, G. R. (1989). Combined cognitive therapy and pharmacotherapy. In A. Freeman, K. M. Simon, L. E. Beutler, & H. Arkowitz (Eds.), *Comprehensive handbook of cognitive therapy* (pp. 267–282). New York: Plenum Press.

Wright, J. H., Thase, M. E., & Beck, A. T. (1992). *Survey of inpatient cognitive therapy treatment programs*. Unpublished manuscript.

Chapter 8

Cognitive Therapy with Medical Patients

Tom Sensky, Ph.D., M.B., M.R.C.Psych., and
Jesse H. Wright, M.D., Ph.D.

There are two principal reasons why cognitive therapy should be effective in the management of emotional disturbances in persons with physical disease. First, there is good evidence that individual responses to illness are related more closely to cognitive factors than to variables such as the severity or symptoms of the disorder (Sensky, 1990). Secondly, there is a high prevalence of psychiatric symptoms among physically ill people. The most common problems are depression and anxiety (Wright et al., 1980; Kamerow, 1988; Zung, Magruder-Habib, Velez, & Alling, 1990). These are the types of emotional reactions for which cognitive therapy was initially developed (Beck, 1976; Wright & Borden, 1991).

The practice of cognitive therapy with patients who have medical disorders uses many of the standard techniques that have been described elsewhere in this book. Thus, what follows is not intended as an account of the full range of cognitive therapy procedures that are used with the physically ill. We instead focus on describing the cognitive and behavioral impact of medical illness and on illustrating adaptations of cognitive therapy for this patient group.

The chapter begins with a brief review of studies of the efficacy of cognitive interventions for persons suffering from physical illness. This serves as an introduction to some of the medical applications of cognitive therapy. We then turn to a description of several aspects of practice in which cognitive therapy with those who are physically ill may differ from the treatment of other patients. Special emphasis is given to theoretical constructs that can assist with case conceptualization. The final section of the chapter discusses treatment of medically ill patients in the cognitive milieu.

EFFICACY OF COGNITIVE THERAPY WITH MEDICAL PATIENTS

Treatment manuals or descriptions of cognitive approaches to treatment are available for the management of pain (Turk, Meichenbaum, & Genest, 1983; Phillips, 1987a), the emotional aspects of cancer (Moorey & Greer, 1989; Scott, 1989), and somatization or hypochondriasis (Barsky, Geringer, & Wool, 1988; Salkovskis, 1989; Warwick & Salkovskis, 1989). Outcome studies using these cognitive methods have already been published or are currently being undertaken.

A number of investigators who have used cognitive therapy with medical patients have reported encouraging results. Atkins, Kaplan, Timms, Reinsch, and Lofback (1984) observed that six sessions of cognitive therapy (involving both cognitive and behavioral techniques) for patients with chronic obstructive airway disease led to a significant increase in mobility, exercise tolerance, and subjective "well-being" as compared to a no-treatment control group. Further evidence of the usefulness of cognitive therapy in pulmonary diseases came from a study of asthma patients who received 10 sessions of cognitive therapy (Maes & Schlosser, 1988). Subjects in this investigation became less anxious, required less corticosteroid medication, and were not as preoccupied with their asthma after treatment. Larcombe and Wilson (1984) found a significant improvement in depressed multiple sclerosis patients who were treated with cognitive therapy as compared to control subjects placed on a waiting list. Also, individual therapy that included cognitive and behavioral components led to symptomatic improvement in a sample of patients with inflammatory bowel disease (Schwarz & Blanchard, 1991).

A cognitive approach has been found to be effective in reducing psychological distress associated with mastectomy for cancer (Tarrier & Maguire, 1984). In other studies, cognitive interventions have been demonstrated to be effective in the management of chronic pain (Turner & Clancy, 1986; Phillips, 1987b; Skinner et al., 1990) and migraine headache (Richardson & McGrath, 1989). Cognitive techniques reduced morbidity and mortality in selected patients who suffered myocardial infarction (Friedman et al., 1986), and preliminary evidence has been gathered of the likely efficacy of cognitive therapy in atopic eczema (Horne, White, & Varigos, 1989) and epilepsy (Goldstein, 1990).

Further work will clarify which cognitive techniques are most useful for particular types of problems among medical or surgical patients, although it is likely that many commonly used techniques will be widely applicable. The next section of this chapter examines modifications of cognitive therapy for patients with significant medical disorders. These observations apply to both hospitalized patients and those who are treated on an outpatient basis. However, individuals with severe illnesses often are encountered in the hospital setting.

ADAPTATIONS OF COGNITIVE THERAPY FOR MEDICAL PATIENTS

Referral of Patients with Physical Illness

Patients with medical illnesses come to psychiatric treatment through different routes. One direction is taken by those who recognize that they have a significant psychiatric disorder, such as depression. These individuals may request a referral through their primary care physician or may contact the psychiatric service directly. For these patients, the psychiatric symptoms are the predominant issues for which they wish to be treated. Medical issues play a secondary but important role.

Other patients with medical illnesses are referred for psychiatric treatment through a more complicated process. They may not recognize or admit the presence of psychiatric symptoms or the possibility of a psychological component to their disorder. The primary physician's suggestion of a psychiatric consultation may come as a shock or as an unwanted intrusion. In this case, the therapist must recognize, and usually modify, the patient's cognitions about his referral before proceeding with treatment. For these patients, medical problems such as chronic pain, obstructive pulmonary disease, or diabetes may remain their major concern.

Examples of common patient beliefs regarding psychiatric referral are listed in Table 8.1. Cognitions about not being believed or being abandoned by the primary physician are particularly troublesome. For example, Mrs. A., a 38-year-old woman with recurrent migraine-like headaches, had been seen in the emergency room or admitted to the medical service seven times in the previous 3 months for severe headache, nausea, and vomiting. She was a highly anxious woman who reported that she had been unable to continue with her job as computer programmer or to complete household chores. When her neurologist finally recommended psychiatric treatment after telling her that all her x-rays and laboratory tests were normal and that she was using excessive medication, Mrs. A. reacted with markedly dysfunctional cognitions and intense anger. The cognitions included thoughts such as: "Nobody believes me. . . . They think I'm faking it. . . . They've given up on me. . . . I can't make it without pain killers."

Other patients will be dissatisfied with the referring doctor for not

TABLE 8.1. Common Themes of Cognitions about Psychiatric Referral

If the doctor tells me that there is no physical cause for my symptoms, he/she is saying that I'm imagining it.
My doctor must be giving up.
My doctors have been wrong in the past; how can I be certain that they're correct this time?
Symptoms as severe as mine must have a real (that is, physical) cause.
To subject me to all the tests I've had, the doctor must have considered that my symptoms have a physical cause; my symptoms are unchanged, but now the doctor has changed his/her mind about them.
If I experience any bodily symptoms, that's a sure sign that I'm becoming ill (again).
I'm the only person on this medical ward who has been referred for therapy. That means I'm not coping as well as everyone else (or as the doctors expect).
My referral for therapy indicates that the doctors think I'm losing my mind.
If I'm very ill, the doctors won't be honest with me.
If I fall ill (or relapse), nothing in life can be worthwhile.

having managed to "cure" their problems. For such individuals, a suggested psychiatric consultation is just another example of the doctor's inadequate skills and judgment. Even among patients who are apparently coping well, it is possible to elicit "evidence" they have collected of medical inadequacy or even incompetence (Sensky, 1989). Mr. M., a retired engineer, was referred to a psychiatrist because he had become depressed after the diagnosis of prostatic cancer. Although he reported considerable respect for the internist who had treated him for many years, he had other cognitions that had the potential of undermining the treatment process. These included thoughts such as: "What's wrong with the medical profession that they can't pick these things up in time? He must be getting rid of me; he can't face me since this happened." Among outpatients, such dysfunctional beliefs might lead the patient to reject referral and decline the assessment interview. However, patients who are hospitalized on a medical ward are less likely to be "selected out" in this way because the therapist comes to visit them rather than the other way around. Still, the presence of distorted cognitions about the referral can lead to significant problems with initiating therapy.

The First Interview: Engaging the Patient

From what has been said, it is evident that during the first session the therapist must consider the patients' beliefs and assumptions about the previous medical interventions and the expectations of the referral for psychiatric treatment—especially if inpatient hospitalization is being considered. As discussed in Chapter 7, patients often come to the hospital with a complex network of doctors and other therapists. For example, someone with low back pain may have consulted an orthopedic surgeon, a neurologist, a neurosurgeon, a specialist in a pain clinic, a chiropractor, an osteopath, and an acupuncturist as well as a family doctor. It is important to understand the patient's view of the role of each of the professionals and how each has contributed to the patient's "model" of his problems.

The patient's perception of symptoms, including the explanations he or she offers for them, must be reviewed in detail. It is worth emphasizing to the patient that, whatever the reasons behind the referral for treatment, the therapist will keep an open mind until they have together formed a complete picture of the patient's illness and problems. For many patients, the opportunity to review the illness thoroughly may prove therapeutic in itself and may also help to engage the patient in therapy by demonstrating that the patient's problems are being taken seriously. Some patients, for example those who show prominent hypochondriacal features, are likely to have been told what their problem *isn't* but remain mystified as to what it actually *is*.

The therapist should also attempt to understand the patient's beliefs regarding the antecedents and consequences of his medical condition. Because such beliefs are likely to be highly idiosyncratic (Sensky, 1990), the patient may not previously have had the opportunity to explore them in depth. For example, Mr. P., a 72-year-old man, developed persistent headaches 2 weeks after his wife's death from a stroke. Both he and his wife had always prided themselves on having "stoical" characters. They regarded showing emotions as a sign of weakness. In her husband's eyes, Mrs. P. had borne her stroke with great fortitude until she "broke down" and cried; a few days later, she was dead. For Mr. P., this was clear evidence that showing emotions was extremely dangerous.

Medical staff reported problems in the rehabilitation of a middle-aged man, Mr. R., who was admitted after he developed incapacitating anxiety subsequent to a second myocardial infarction. Socratic questioning revealed that Mr. R. believed that his first heart attack was caused by straining to pass urine (the symptoms had started while he was urinating). Not surprisingly, he attempted to avoid all forms of stress and subsequently was unable to use any toilet with the door closed.

Development of a comprehensive, cognitive–biological model for treatment is one of the most useful strategies for engaging the medical patient in therapy. We usually present such a model during the first interview because it helps the patient understand and accept the importance of cognitive processes in coping with physical illness. To illustrate, Mrs. A., the woman with migraine headaches described earlier, had the following interchange with the consulting psychiatrist:

Mrs. A.: So now I don't know what I can possibly do. My doctor says she can't find anything wrong, and yet I still have these terrible headaches. I'm not imagining them!

Dr. W.: I've talked with your doctor about the situation, and I got a different impression about what she thinks. You said she told you, "nothing was wrong." Could she have said it in a different way? What did she actually tell you?

Mrs. A.: Well, she said the MRI scan and EEG were completely normal.

Dr. W.: And what else?

Mrs. A.: That's about it . . . except she didn't know what else to do, and I was starting to use too much medication.

Dr. W.: Then the statement, "nothing's wrong with me" was your interpretation of what you thought your doctor meant.

Mrs. A.: Yes, I guess it was.

Dr. W.: You've had a very common reaction to being referred to a psychiatrist. Many people jump to the conclusion that the doctor believes that there is no physical illness or no reason for the symptoms. When you step back from it, what do you really think is happening?

Mrs. A.: I know I have a headache that won't go away, and I've been under a lot of stress. I'm just not coping very well anymore. I guess Dr. S. never told me she didn't think the headaches were real.

Dr. W.: That sounds more accurate. I don't think that anyone doubts that you are in pain. Dr. S. asked me to see you to find out whether we could help you manage the stress and cope better with the problem. Would you like to hear how I view the interaction between problems like headaches and stress?

Mrs. A.: Yes, I would.

The therapist went on to explain a cognitive–biological model of illness (see Chapter 7) and to illustrate the model with actual stressful events and emotional and cognitive responses from the patient's own experience (including her dysfunctional cognitions about the referral). This played a significant role in decreasing the patient's hesitancy to enter into psychiatric treatment and gave her an initial glimpse of the potential benefits of cognitive therapy.

The Therapeutic Contract

Whenever possible, patient and therapist should agree on a shared formulation for treatment (as in the case of Mrs. A. described above). They can then plan the work they will undertake together. However, this may not always be feasible at the outset of therapy. For example, hypochondriacal patients are often very reluctant to view their problems in psychological terms, even if they have been offered a detailed account of likely psychological mechanisms (Salkovskis, 1989; Warwick & Salkovskis, 1989). In such instances, it is appropriate for the therapist to emphasize the empirical nature of cognitive therapy. If, during a time-limited collaboration, patient and therapist find no evidence that cognitive therapy is helpful, the therapist will help arrange other treatment options. Continued follow-up by the referring physician or surgeon will also help to insure that the medical aspects of treatment will not be overlooked. As a prelude, it also is helpful to examine the advantages and disadvantages of trying a different therapeutic method. The patient's lack of progress to date in seeking satisfactory relief of the symptoms can be seen as one reason for trying a new approach.

The therapeutic contract should include all components of the treatment program. With medical patients it is especially important to recognize the need for ongoing physical treatment(s), reevaluation of symptoms, and integration of care with the medical team (e.g., physicians, technicians, physical therapists, and others). If the patient requires hemodialysis, is undergoing chemotherapy, or is due to have surgery in a week's time, the cognitive therapy should be planned to help the patient receive necessary care and learn to cope with the medical illness to the greatest extent possible.

Assessment

Quantitative assessment of target physical symptoms or problems, as well as cognitions, is essential. The chief purpose of this is to establish appropriate baselines and to measure change. In some cases, standard biochemical or other laboratory test results will be important dependent variables in therapy—for example, blood glucose, glycated hemoglobin, or serum electrolytes. Symptoms might also be quantified according to established norms with instruments such as the McGill Pain Questionnaire (Melzack, 1975). However, bearing in mind that the problems of individual patients may be highly idiosyncratic, such previously validated assessments may not be specific enough to measure pertinent change. Another purpose of such instruments is to provide "model" items for individual assessments. Even if it is inappropriate to use the whole instrument, the patient and therapist may agree that particular items are relevant measures of progress in therapy.

Other scales utilized routinely in cognitive therapy (particularly those that focus exclusively on cognitions) can be used with physically ill people. The Hopelessness Scale is a good example (Beck, Weissman, Lester, & Trexler, 1974). However, physical illness may confound interpretation of other measures—particularly scales that assess depression or anxiety. Commonly used rating scales include somatic symptoms (e.g., weight loss, insomnia, appetite disturbance, and fatigue or lethargy) that can be caused by the physical illness rather than an affective disturbance. Although the Beck Depression Inventory (BDI) has been used often with people with physical illness, ratings must be interpreted with caution (see, for example, Kathol & Petty, 1981; House, 1988). The Hospital Anxiety and Depression Scales (Zigmond & Snaith, 1983) have been developed and validated for use with people who are medically ill.

A number of other measures are available. Some are intended to be generally applicable to people with physical illness, such as health locus of control scales (Wallston, Wallston, & DeVellis, 1978), whereas other instruments are more specific. Examples are shown in Table 8.2. The assessment of somatization and illness behavior has been thoroughly reviewed by Kellner (1987).

Choosing appropriate assessment measures can be difficult, particularly because the relationships between psychological and physical states are complex and may not follow the direction predicted by intuition. For instance, blood glucose control would appear to be an appropriate measure to gauge therapeutic effects in individuals with diabetes. However, there is suggestive evidence that good blood glucose control may be associated with erroneous and potentially dysfunctional beliefs in the families of diabetic adolescents (Sensky, Stevenson, Magrill, & Petty, 1991) and in some adults with diabetes (Sensky, 1992; Sensky & Petty, 1992). It is possible that these beliefs may sustain good glucose control at the expense of raised anxiety or depression. Focusing too narrowly on either blood sugar or affective disturbance would, under such circumstances, lead to an inadequate and flawed case formulation.

TABLE 8.2. Examples of Self-Administered Rating Scales to Measure Cognitions of People with Physical Illness

Scale	Reference
General cognitive scales	
Cognitive Errors Questionnaire	Lefebvre (1981)
Illness Attitude Scale	Kellner (1981)
Illness Beliefs Questionnaire	Pilowsky & Spence (1981)
Implicit Models of Illness Questionnaire	Turk, Rudy, & Salovey (1986)
Multidimensional Health Locus of Control	Wallston, Wallston, & DeVellis (1978)
Self-Control Schedule	Rosenbaum & Smira (1986)
Scales to rate coping	
COPE Inventory	Carver, Scheier, & Weintraub (1989)
Coping Strategies Questionnaire	Rosenstiel & Keefe (1983)
Medical Coping Modes Questionnaire	Feifel, Strack, & Nagy (1987)
Ways of Coping Scale	Folkman & Lazarus (1980)
Scales to measure specific cognitive parameters	
Amplification Scale	Barsky et al. (1988)
Cognitive Orientation Questionnaire	Drechsler, Bruner, & Kreitler (1987)
Cognitive–Somatic Anxiety Questionnaire	Schwartz, Davidson, & Coleman (1978)
Mental Adjustment to Cancer Scale	Watson et al. (1988)
Pain Cognitions Questionnaire	Boston, Pearce, & Richardson (1990)
Pain-Related Control Scale	Flor & Turk (1988)
Pain-Related Self-Statements Scale	Flor & Turk (1988)
Symptom Interpretation Questionnaire	Robbins & Kirmayer (1991)

Conceptualization

The case conceptualization links the patient's symptoms with underlying mechanisms, allows the patient and therapist to construct a detailed model to explain the problems, and suggests possible experiments and therapeutic directions (Persons, 1989). Each individual patient's situation, of course, requires a unique formulation. However, some themes are common, if not universal, and should be considered in every conceptualization. These include hopelessness, uncertainty regarding the future in general and the illness in particular, threatened loss of control, and fears of diminished autonomy. Expectations of changes in significant relationships are also observed frequently in patients with significant medical illness. For example, a woman who is scheduled for a mastectomy may forecast that she will be viewed as less desirable or worthwhile after surgery. It is helpful as a first step in therapy to disentangle the different themes or components and work on them separately. The distinction suggested by Moorey and Greer (1989) between threats to survival and threats to body image may be useful in this regard.

Physical illness commonly leads people to evaluate themselves in a negatively distorted manner. Conversely, depression or anxiety can lead to distorted appraisal of somatic symptoms (Fava, Pilowsky, Pierfederici, Bernardi, & Pathak, 1982; Barsky, Goodson, Lane, & Cleary, 1988; Croyle & Uretsky, 1987). Cognitive formulations described by Beck and others (see Chapters 1 and 4) can be quite helpful in managing these situations. Mrs. E., a patient with multiple sclerosis, was developing progressively worsening muscle weakness and sensory loss. She had been recently confined to a wheelchair. Her husband reported that she was morose, withdrawn, and very negativistic. As her depression deepened, Mrs. E. reached the point where she was unable to function in the home.

After admission to the hospital, Mrs. E. began to articulate thoughts that she had not communicated to her husband, such as: "I'm ugly. . . . How could he want to touch me? . . . I'm useless in bed. . . . I'm disgusting." Her therapist helped Mrs. E. to recognize that her negatively distorted automatic thoughts were worsening the depression and were interfering with her ability to function at the maximum level possible. Thought records were used to modify these cognitions and to devise alternate behaviors. These included discussions on how she could resume a meaningful sexual relationship with her husband. An example of one of Mrs. E.'s thought records is presented in Table 8.3.

It is essential in most cases, if not all, to identify the patient's preferred coping strategies and those that may have been neglected. Assessment of the flexibility of problem-solving mechanisms is also important. Instruments available to measure coping (some of which are noted in Table 8.2) may be used to offer clues. Comprehensive scales, such as one developed by Heim and his colleagues (Heim et al., 1987) may be particularly helpful. However, the utility of coping scales is limited if they are used only to get a cross-sectional perspective of present coping modes.

The treatment of Mrs. W., a woman who had been a champion athlete in her younger days, illustrates the importance of understanding how a person has managed stress in the past and what barriers there may be to using these strategies to manage current problems. Mrs. W. was admitted to the hospital in a coma. This proved to be caused by

TABLE 8.3. Daily Record of Dysfunctional Thoughts: Mrs. E.

Situation	Automatic thoughts	Emotion	Rational response
I went to the family buffet and thought people were staring at me.	I'm like a sideshow.	Depression	I have a handicap, but I'm not a freak.
	I'm a sorry excuse for a person, and I wish I never had been born.	Anxiety	I do many useful things.
		Self-hate	I have worthwhile traits.
	I'm useless.		This is personalization.
	I used to be pretty; now I'm ugly.		It takes courage to fight a handicap.
	I'm not even worth anything in bed.		I'm not useless: I can pay the bills, straighten the house, help the children with homework.
			I haven't been taking care of myself, but I can look pretty good if I fix myself up. I can give my husband pleasure (and enjoy it myself too).

end-stage renal failure. She recovered from the effects of the organic brain syndrome to face the prospect of starting peritoneal dialysis. Severe depression with profound hopelessness and helplessness ensued.

On one occasion, Mrs. W. fell to the floor in a dramatic fashion while a nurse was demonstrating to her how she was to prepare her dialysis bags. The physician ascertained that Mrs. W. was unharmed and conscious. However, she was unwilling to open her eyes and sit up. After he eventually coaxed her into "waking," further discussion revealed that she was afraid that she would never succeed in getting her dialysis technique to the standard of the nurse who demonstrated it. She had formed the belief that "unless I get this 100% correct, I'll die."

In the past, Mrs. W. had usually coped with difficult problems by setting them aside for others to tackle, while she had concentrated on her sporting or social skills. This was the first time she had been confronted with a situation in which she was unable to do this. Mrs. W. acknowledged to the therapist that she felt trapped and helpless. In this case, the therapist needed to help the patient recognize "forgotten" or partially developed coping strategies that could be built up through the therapy process. One of these attributes was Mrs. W.'s ability to dedicate herself to repeated practice as she had done as an athlete during her school years. This skill was brought to bear on the problem of learning to cope with the sequelae of severe physical illness.

Experimentally tested concepts derived from cognitive psychology offer frameworks that may be useful in understanding cognitive responses of individuals who have physical illnesses or somatic symptoms (Sensky, 1990; Sensky, in press). Although a comprehensive review of such formulations is beyond the scope of this chapter, their application can be illustrated by brief descriptions of the health belief and *self-complexity* models.

The *health belief* model (Becker, 1974) suggests that how an individual responds to illness or its threat will depend on an appraisal of several key areas. The person must first see herself or himself as susceptible to the disease (or a complication of the disease) for which treatment is being advised. In addition, the disease (or complication) must be regarded as serious. Also, the perceived benefits of treatment should outweigh the risks or costs. The case vignette below illustrates how the health belief model can be used to guide treatment interventions.

DR. S.: I understand from the nurses that you told them you were surprised that Dr. B. decided to admit you from the clinic. Why were you admitted?

MR. G.: I have no idea. The dialysis used to make me sick, but I've been feeling quite well for some time. I've had some difficulty sticking to my diet, and Dr. B. has been nagging me about that.

DR. S.: Do you mean that Dr. B. admitted you because you weren't keeping to your diet? Was that all?

MR. G.: Well, she told me that my potassium was rather high.

DR. S.: What does that mean, as far as you are concerned?

MR. G.: She told me that my potassium was high because I wasn't sticking to the diet and that I could drop dead from a heart attack.

DR. S.: Would that be a good enough reason to admit you to the hospital?

MR. G.: I can't really believe it. I think Dr. B. is exaggerating to scare me into keeping to my diet. I've messed about with the diet before and didn't even have any symptoms, let alone have a heart attack. If a man can't have a good time eating and drinking once in a while, what's the sense in going on?

DR. S.: Your last point is important, and we should return to it later. Getting back to the diet though, can you tell me some more about what you understand about the possible dangers of having a high serum potassium level and how this might affect you?

Another useful strategy for case conceptualization, the self-complexity model, has been described by Linville (1987). This formulation suggests that an individual's vulnerability to emotional distress in the face of a noxious environmental event is inversely related to the complexity of the person's view of himself. Self-complexity is based on the number of distinct important facets of self (including social roles, skills, relationships, activities, goals, and others) identified by the individual. The fewer the number and narrower the range of such aspects of self, the more likely it is that an adverse event will be appraised as threatening and will lead to depression or anxiety. Conversely, the more multifaceted the representation of self, the less likely it is for a stressor to cause an adverse emotional response.

Mr. C., a married engineer who developed a degenerative neurological disorder, offers an illustration of the application of the self-complexity model. He was admitted to the psychiatric unit after telling his neurologist that he couldn't "go on." Although Mr. C. didn't have vegetative symptoms of depression, he expressed intense guilt and hopelessness. He told his therapist that his only real achievement in life had been success at work. Mr. C. had just accepted a disability determination because he could no longer meet the physical demands of his job. One therapeutic approach in such a case is to work toward increasing the person's self-complexity. For example, Mr. C.'s therapist encouraged him to recall other interests and experiences:

DR. D.: You've told me that your work meant everything to you.

MR. C.: That's right. I was a "workaholic" and didn't really pay much attention to anything else.

DR. D.: Sometimes people tend to forget other parts of their lives when they get consumed by something that seems very important. It might help to think for a while about some of your other dimensions.

MR. C.: I guess it won't hurt to try.

DR. D.: Okay, let's make a list of some other things that have interested you or that you have done.

MR. C.: One thing that comes to mind is working for my undergraduate school. I really loved my college years, and I've tried to help out a bit with fund raising. Of course, there's my family; but the kids are all grown up and living in other cities. I need to figure out how to relate to them without feeling like a fifth wheel.

DR. D.: You've already brought up several possibilities. We can explore these further as we go on. But, for now, let's see if we can add to the list. What we want to do is to get a broad picture of all the parts of you that you might want to develop now that you have more time.

MR. C.: Okay, it sounds like a good idea.

Other concepts derived from applications of cognitive therapy may be useful in understanding individual responses to physical illness. For example, a common cognitive feature of posttraumatic stress disorder is the assumption that the world (or certain aspects of it) is fundamentally unsafe and unreliable. When illness starts suddenly and is unheralded (as, for example, with many heart attacks), the patient may develop a firm belief that any minor bodily change is likely to be disastrous. For example, Mr. G. had coronary artery bypass surgery following three myocardial infarctions but was repeatedly admitted to the hospital for further investigations after complaining of a variety of new symptoms. He revealed that he was terrified that he might pass out. His belief was that this would lead to another heart attack. Consequently, he became increasingly vigilant about signs that might presage a fainting spell. Any suspicion that he was losing touch with his surroundings would make him anxious, and his symptoms would then escalate.

Mr. G.'s therapist used the posttraumatic stress concept to help the patient understand what was happening to him. Examples of other people who had been traumatized were used to show Mr. G. how improved coping and increased well-being were possible. Mr. G. and his therapist were then able to begin testing the validity of the unrealistic fears. This is another example of how the case conceptualization can point the way to a successful intervention for a patient who has significant physical illness.

Therapist's Cognitions

Therapists with limited experience in working with the physically ill may have difficulty collaborating with the patient because of their own beliefs or attitudes. Also, therapists who are not medically qualified may be wary of embarking on a detailed exploration of the patient's illness. How will it be possible to judge whether or not the patient's beliefs are accurate? In fact, this question is a trap. The cognitive therapist is not the "expert" regarding the patient's medical illness. However, some patients try hard to cast their therapist in this role—not only as expert but also as advocate. This potential problem can be avoided by adequate collaboration in defining the patient's problems, precise agenda setting in the therapy, and effective interchanges with the referring physician.

Another assumption that the therapist might make is that it is always desirable or helpful to fill gaps in the patient's knowledge or understanding. In the cognitive treatment of depression or anxiety, it is usually accepted that a key task is to gather and evaluate evidence to help the patient gain a more realistic perspective. If the therapist practices the techniques that are taught to patients, he or she is likely to approach physical illness in the same way—gather sufficient data to appraise the threats to well-being and/or life. However, for medical patients, this process of acquiring and using information is considerably more complex. For some individuals who are attempting to cope with a serious or life-threatening illness, there may be a short-term advantage in preserving inaccurate or unrealistic beliefs (Taylor, 1983; Sensky, 1989).

If therapy reveals that the patient's knowledge or understanding about a medical problem is vague or inconsistent, the first question to answer is whether he or she wants to know more and what the advantages and disadvantages might be of doing so. Thus, it might be appropriate to ask someone who is denying that he has cancer: "To help me understand things better, let's assume for the moment that a person has a serious illness. If this did happen, what information would the person want to have? What advantages would there be in learning about the illness? Do you think that there are any risks involved in getting or not getting information?"

In some instances, the therapist may be tempted to condone or even share some of the patient's dysfunctional cognitions. If the therapist were in the patient's place (having just had both arms amputated, for example), would he or she not feel just as miserable or hopeless as the patient? Even if the therapist is able to empathize accurately with the patient's feelings, this does not mean that the patient's cognitions should be endorsed automatically. These need to be explored and tested as in cognitive therapy of other disorders.

Problems are especially likely to arise in working with terminally ill or dying patients. Mrs. L., a divorcee in her 60s, was admitted because of depression following a relapse of chronic leukemia. The oncologists were pessimistic regarding her prognosis. Nevertheless, they had offered Mrs. L. further chemotherapy. One of her problems was her difficulty in deciding whether to undergo another course of chemotherapy. Previous courses had been very uncomfortable for her. During her first therapeutic interview, it emerged that she had an accurate impression of her prognosis and was overwhelmed by it. The therapist was also deeply saddened, but he was able to identify several opportunities to use cognitive therapy procedures to help Mrs. L. Making a problem list was very helpful to Mrs. L. She identified several tasks that were important to her that she could expect to complete, even though she was quite ill. Succeeding at these not only increased her sense of self-control but also lifted her mood. In addition, Mrs. L. felt very guilty about "leaving" her two children, a daughter who was currently ending a difficult relationship and a son who was in his late 20s and had never really left home. Mrs. L. had divorced their father when both children were very young. She subsequently came to believe that if she had worked harder at the marriage the children would have had a father and would thereby have been spared all their current difficulties. She and her therapist explored the validity of this belief and were able to put her children's difficulties into a different perspective. This helped Mrs. L. to make the most she could from the few months she had left to live.

There is a danger that the therapist may overreact in another direction if he or she regards any dysphoria as evidence that there must still be dysfunctional cognitions to be found and corrected. Sometimes, this reflects the therapist's own cognitions about physical disability or decline. A careful examination of the therapist's thoughts and feelings (i.e., a cognitive therapy equivalent to analyzing countertransference) may be required. Techniques might include the therapist writing a personal thought record or discussing a case with a colleague. The goal is to allow appropriate expression of grief over what the patient has lost, or is about to lose, while still keeping a focus on using cognitive therapy to enhance coping mechanisms.

MEDICAL PATIENTS IN THE COGNITIVE MILIEU

Indications for Psychiatric Hospitalization

The indications for psychiatric hospitalization of patients with serious physical illness may vary in different settings. Some units, particularly those located in general hospitals, may be fully equipped to treat patients with severe medical illnesses. Psychiatrists and nurses on such units are usually well accustomed to caring for patients with a mixture of medical and psychiatric symptoms. Also, there is ready availability of other medical specialists, ancillary personnel (e.g., respiratory therapists, physical therapists), and laboratory support. In contrast, free-standing psychiatric units that are located away from medical centers may be less well prepared to manage physically ill patients. Certain cognitive milieus such as those that use the staff model (see Chapter 3) may avoid taking patients with significant medical illness because the physical problems may limit the patient's ability to participate fully in the standard cognitive therapy program. Frequently, special adaptations or customization of the treatment program are required—especially for those patients with a significant disability or handicap.

Table 8.4 contains a list of indications for psychiatric hospitalization of patients with physical illness. Cognitive therapy units (CTUs) located in general hospitals or university settings may choose to admit a wide range of patients with these problems. The most common reason for hospitalization is the concurrence of psychiatric problems, particularly major depression. In many of these cases, the psychiatric symptoms

TABLE 8.4. Patients with Physical Illness: Indications for Psychiatric Hospitalization

Abuse or neglect
Chronic pain
Complex pharmacologic regimen
Concurrent psychiatric disorder
Danger to self or others
Diagnosis cannot be made
Family system breakdown
Inability to function
Substance abuse
Treatment resistance

such as suicidal ideation or psychosis are the major reasons for admission.

Another frequent precipitant to hospitalization is lack of response to conventional therapy, either medical interventions or outpatient psychiatric treatment. The University of Louisville CTU receives many patients who have had a host of laboratory tests and have been given trials of a wide variety of medical treatments without relief of symptoms. These individuals have usually ceased to function in an effective manner. They have chronic pain, inability to manage tasks of daily living, or have been overwhelmed by attempting to adapt to a major medical illness. Comorbidity of psychiatric and medical disorders has been shown to increase the frequency of treatment resistance (Mayou, Hawton, and Feldman, 1988; Keitner, Ryan, Miller, Kohn, & Epstein, 1991).

Other medically ill patients are hospitalized after substance abuse (alcohol, illicit drugs, or prescription medications) has been detected. Patients with chronic medical illness, especially illness associated with pain, are at a heightened risk for developing substance abuse. At times, admission to the psychiatric unit is recommended when a conclusive diagnosis cannot be made on the medical or surgical unit. Individuals with suspected conversion disorders may require careful observation on a psychiatry service before an accurate diagnosis can be made and effective treatment can be initiated. Patients who have medical disorders also may be hospitalized for institution of pharmacotherapy for psychiatric symptoms. This is needed when there is a high vulnerability for significant drug reactions or interactions.

Severe disruptions in the family system are another common antecedent of psychiatric admission. This can occur when the family support system becomes exhausted by the burdens of a devastating medical illness or where a dysfunctional family becomes more pathological under the stress of a physical disorder. In extreme cases, the medical patient can be the target of abuse or neglect. This is seen with a wide variety of medical illnesses. However, elderly persons and women with chronic disorders appear to be at the greatest risk of mistreatment by their families.

The Treatment Team

One of the important advantages of inpatient hospitalization is the ability to draw on the resources of a large number of professionals who can concentrate their efforts on developing treatment interventions that will address both psychiatric and medical issues. Effective collaborative relationships and careful treatment planning are necessary. This is illustrated with the case of Mrs. J., a 42-year-old woman who was transferred to the CTU from the rehabilitation medicine service of a general hospital.

Mrs. J. had been diagnosed as having spinal stenosis at age 34. Several back operations and subsequent admissions to the rehabilitation unit had failed to stem a gradual deterioration in function. Finally, psychiatric hospitalization was arranged after Mrs. J.'s rehabilitation medicine physician and a consulting psychiatrist agreed that depression and anxiety were limiting Mrs. J.'s chance of reaching an optimally functional state. Trials of outpatient therapy and antidepressants had been unsuccessful.

The primary symptoms at the time of admission were chronic pain, profound weakness, lack of interest in the environment, and inability to ambulate or to manage any household chores. Mrs. J. had been, at one time, a rather robust woman who had been pleased with her ability to cook, "keep house," and to contribute to the family's welfare by working as a part-time secretary. Now she could hardly get out of bed. Everything she tried to do seemed like an overwhelming task. In the last few months, she had begun to give up hope of ever returning to her "old self."

On the day after admission, the treatment team discussed Mrs. J. at a planning conference. The rehabilitation medicine physician (Dr. M.), a physical therapist, and an occupational therapist were invited to join the team because it was thought that a joint effort would be required. Psychiatric staff needed to know Mrs. J.'s limitations and what she might be capable of doing if treatment were successful. Conversely, Dr. M. and the physical and occupational therapists thought that they could be more effective if they were aware of the psychiatric formulation and the plans for cognitive behavioral therapy. Mrs. J. joined the treatment conference after the first 15 minutes. The team believed that a strong collaboration among all parties would be needed to break through the therapeutic impasse.

The treating psychiatrist, Dr. W., chaired the meeting and facilitated development of a clearly specified treatment plan. Mrs. J. was asked to list her goals for the hospitalization. (She had prepared for this prior to the treatment conference.) Mrs. J. listed her goals as: (1) to be able to walk around the house without assistance; (2) to resume cooking for family; (3) to be able to attend son's basketball games; (4) to enjoy improved self-confidence. Dr. M., Dr. W., the physical therapist, the occupational therapist, and the psychiatric nurse articulated their goals, and a consensus was reached. The team then designated treatment interventions for each of the goals.

The overall case conceptualization shared by Mrs. J. and the treatment team was that she had become so discouraged and frightened by her back problems that she had essentially given up. Her hopeless and helpless thinking had led to a lack of effort. This had caused a further weakening of her physical strength because of lack of exercise. Inability to perform tasks had worsened her low self-esteem. Guilt and self-recrimination made her less able to break out of her downward spiral. Thus, the treatment program was designed to gradually build up physical functioning while promoting guilt reduction and improved self-confidence. Graded-task assignments were carried out both in the physical therapy department and on the inpatient unit. At the same time, the CTU staff helped Mrs. J. to identify and modify distorted cognitions. The occupational therapist worked with Mrs. J. on practicing activities of daily living.

After 20 days of hospitalization, Mrs. J. was able to walk 100 feet without assistance. She had also cooked several meals in the CTU's kitchen and had completed successful family outings. Mrs. J. had identified a number of positive personal attributes. Attention to these resources helped her make significant progress in recapturing some of her vitality. For example, she was able to knit sweaters for her children, spend time learning a word-processing program, and write several recipes for a church cookbook. The BDI score improved from a value of 28 on admission to 11 at the time of discharge.

Another patient, Mr. U., illustrates the problems that can result from having multiple individuals involved in medical care. This gentleman was a 47-year-old former truck driver who had received a heart transplant six months before admission to the psychiatry service. Much to the chagrin of the cardiac surgeon and the rehabilitation service, Mr. U. had resumed heavy cigarette smoking and alcohol consumption and was refusing to participate in cardiac rehabilitation. He reported that "it's no life; you wouldn't want to live like this either; why shouldn't I smoke and drink?"

The cardiology team had responded to Mr. U.'s behavior with exhortations and thinly veiled anger. "How could he do this after he got a new heart?" Exploration of the situation by the cognitive therapist revealed that Mr. U. had tried to participate in the rehabilitation program in the first few weeks after the transplant. However, it seemed as if everywhere he turned someone was telling him what to do. He had to change his diet, stop smoking and drinking, exercise daily, and manage stress differently. An underlying schema had emerged: "If someone tells me what to do, they must think I'm stupid." Early experiences with his father and other authority figures had reinforced this belief. At first, Mr. U. had felt angry and depressed. Then he just refused to do any of the biddings of his doctors.

Treatment of Mr. U. proceeded on several levels. Individual cognitive therapy helped him see how the maladaptive schema was having a very deleterious effect. He agreed to resume the cardiac rehabilitation program after he reconceptualized the situation and better understood the motivations of his physicians. The medical care team was also asked how they could improve their communications with Mr. U.

The Patient Group

Admission of patients with medical disorders usually has a significant impact on the entire patient group. This is particularly true when there are patients with obvious physical disabilities, such as those who receive hemodialysis, require oxygen for pulmonary disease, or have hair loss or other stigmata of chemotherapy for cancer. The number of medical patients on the unit can also make a difference. The CTU at the University of Louisville often has six to eight patients with severe medical problems on the 20-bed unit. This means that coping with medical illness is a common theme in the unit community meeting, group therapy, or other therapeutic sessions. Even patients who are not currently medically ill are touched by this because they are reminded of family members who have had similar problems or think of times in their own lives when they have faced physical illnesses.

Group leaders need to support rational empathic responses to the medically ill while, at the same time, they must observe for possible reinforcement of maladaptive illness behaviors. Mrs. J., the 42-year-old woman with spinal stenosis described earlier, is an example of a patient who can evoke considerable sympathy and support from the patient group. Just as family members had done at home, Mrs. J.'s fellow patients could fall into the trap of doing things for Mrs. J. that would reinforce her helplessness and functional incapacity. Encouragement of her attempts to complete graded-task assignments would be much more beneficial than completing the task for her. To give a specific illustration, Mrs. J. decided that one of her initiatives would be to attempt to carry her dinner tray from the serving cart to the table where she ate. Other patients had been carrying her tray during the first few days of hospitalization. However, inadvertent reinforcement of illness behavior was avoided when Mrs. J. told the patient group about her plan during a unit community meeting and asked them to help with the task only if she requested it.

Patients frequently comment that they are heartened by seeing that others have similar problems and that recovery is possible. Generally, an inpatient unit has a mixture of patients, some of whom have made substantial progress and are preparing for discharge. This can be used to build hopefulness in those who are facing formidable medical problems.

Mr. L. had recently been diagnosed as a diabetic. Insulin had been started, but blood glucose levels were still very labile. He was quite pessimistic about the future. What would his life be like when he had to fear hypoglycemic attacks, coronary artery disease, and blindness? Admission to the psychiatry unit had followed an overdose of sleeping medication. This patient was helped considerably by interchanges with other patients who also had medical problems but were further along with the cognitive therapy program. He was able to see how they had begun to cope better with their illness. Also, the other patients were able to apply what they were learning from cognitive therapy sessions *in vivo* to help Mr. L. learn to counter hopeless and helpless cognitions.

Mr. O., a 58-year-old man with chronic obstructive lung disease, stopped in to visit Mr. L. in his room: "I can see that you're still really down. Have you read *Coping with Depression* yet? It really helped me. I was focusing on my problems and not seeing any of my strengths or opportunities." They went on to discuss how the stress of severe physical illness put both of them into a tailspin in which they only saw the catastrophic side of their life situation. This case demonstrates how a cognitive milieu can benefit patients with medical disorders when the patient culture is supportive and is knowledgeable about the basic concepts of cognitive therapy.

The most dramatic and searching effects of medical illness on the milieu occur when a patient is dying. Although it is rare for a medical patient actually to die on the psychiatry unit, admissions of those with terminal cancer, end-stage cardiac disease, AIDS, or other advanced medical illness are possible. Mrs. K. was a 45-year-old woman with metastatic breast carcinoma. She had developed tumors in the liver, lung, and spine. Admission to the CTU followed a hypomanic episode in which she didn't sleep for 5 days, made unwise investments, and attempted to have affairs with several married men. After a few days of pharmacotherapy, the manic symptoms abated, and Mrs. K. was again facing a grim future. She became depressed and reported that she might as well die now because all she had ahead of her was pain.

This type of case stirs intense reactions from other patients. How would they react if they were in similar circumstances? Should you try to go on even if there is no hope? Can you really live one day at a time? It is important to deal with these existential issues in both individual and group therapy. This can help the patient respond to this situation in a responsible manner and also help others to learn more about their own attitudes and resources.

The Family

Many of a patient's dysfunctional cognitions may be shared by, or derived from, his or her family (Sensky, 1989). Even though the patient is admitted to the CTU, the family's cognitive responses remain highly relevant. This is illustrated by the case of Mrs. T., a 50-year-old depressed woman who tried to hang herself shortly after a family visit. Fortunately, a breakaway closet rod prevented a lethal outcome of this serious suicide attempt.

This patient had been admitted because of severe, debilitating back pain and depression. There had been a "nonfusion" of the lumbar vertebrae after a surgical procedure. Mrs. T. had denied suicidal ideation but had been kept on "close observation" status by the treatment team because she had a moderately severe degree of hopelessness. Her husband, a director of an industrial firm, visited the evening of the suicide attempt, ostensibly to give her support. However, his message triggered the emergence of a highly destructive underlying schema.

Mr. T. thought that he was being helpful when he told his wife that he had cancelled a business trip to Europe in order to be with her. He had not appeared to be outwardly angry or resentful. But, Mrs. T. recalled times in the past when her husband had made comments like: "You never want to go anywhere; how are we going to get ahead if you keep dragging me down?" Her conclusion on the night of the suicide attempt was: "I'm a burden. . . . He knows I'll never get well. . . . I'd be better off out of the way so he can go on with his life."

Another patient, Mr. V., demonstrates the utility of involving the family in treatment. This man had previously been a successful high school teacher and the leader of a YMCA youth group. Chronic renal disease had forced him to leave his job and give up most of his activities. Much of his time was spent with peritoneal dialysis, which he performed four times daily. Mr. V. had become profoundly depressed and like Mrs. T., believed that he was a burden on his family.

Cognitive therapy with Mr. V. was carried out in several formats: individual, group, milieu, and family. One of the critical features of the last component of treatment was an honest discussion in family therapy of the impact of physical illness on the entire family. There was no question that all had suffered. Mrs. V. had to take on another part-time job, the two teenagers had less money for clothes and entertainment; but most of all, the family missed Mr. V.'s previous high energy and fun-loving attitude. With the family's help, Mr. V. was able to rethink his distorted self-concept. He had a chronic illness that had had a large impact on all of them, but he was not a "burden." They began to separate the undeniable negative influences of renal disease from guilt and self-depreciation. This allowed them to begin to develop effective coping strategies for managing the physical illness.

SUMMARY

There is growing evidence that cognitive therapy procedures can be useful in the treatment of patients with medical disorders. Although this application of cognitive therapy is in an early stage of development, results of initial outcome studies are encouraging, and cognitive therapy units are gaining increased experience in treating patients with significant physical illness. Important adaptations of cognitive therapy procedures for medical patients include (1) awareness of idiosyncratic cognitions about the referral process, (2) assessment of cognitions about physical symptoms and medical treatments, (3) modifications in the therapy contract to include necessary medical interventions, (4) incorporation of a variety of theoretical constructs (including those derived from studies of physical illness) in case conceptualization, and (5) identification of the therapist's own cognitions about medical illness. Admission of a medical patient to the cognitive milieu has far-reaching effects on the treatment team, the patient group, and the family. These diverse arenas provide many opportunities for using cognitive therapy in the treatment of patients who are suffering from both psychiatric and physical disease.

REFERENCES

Atkins, C. J., Kaplan, R. M., Timms, R. M., Reinsch, S., & Lofback, K. (1984). Behavioral exercise programs in the management of chronic obstructive pulmonary disease. *Journal of Consulting and Clinical Psychology*, *52*, 591–603.

Barsky, A. J., Geringer, E., & Wool, C. (1988). A cognitive–educational treatment for hypochondriasis. *General Hospital Psychiatry*, *10*, 322–327.

Barsky, A. J., Goodson, J. D., Lane, R. S., & Cleary, P. D. (1988). The amplification of somatic symptoms. *Psychosomatic Medicine*, *50*, 510–519.

Beck, A. T. (1976). *Cognitive therapy and the emotional disorders*. New York: Meridian.

Beck, A. T., Weissman, A., Lester, D., & Trexler, L. (1974). The measurement of pessimism: The Hopelessness Scale. *Journal of Consulting and Clinical Psychology*, *42*, 861–865.

Becker, M. H. (Ed.). (1974). *The health belief model and personal health behavior*. Torofare, NJ: Slack.

Boston, K., Pearce, S. A., & Richardson, P. H. (1990). The pain cognitions questionnaire. *Journal of Psychosomatic Research, 34*, 103–109.

Carver, C. S., Scheier, M. F., & Weintraub, J. K. (1989). Assessing coping strategies: A theoretically based approach. *Journal of Personality and Social Psychology, 56*, 267–283.

Croyle, R. T., & Uretsky, M. B. (1987). Effects of mood on self-appraisal of health status. *Health Psychology, 6*, 239–253.

Drechsler, I., Bruner, D., & Kreitler, S. (1987). Cognitive antecedents of coronary heart disease. *Social Science and Medicine, 24*, 581–588.

Fava, G. A., Pilowsky, I., Pierfederici, A., Bernardi, M., & Pathak, D. (1982). Depressive symptoms and abnormal illness behavior in general hospital patients. *General Hospital Psychiatry, 4*, 171–178.

Feifel, H., Strack, S., & Nagy, V. T. (1987). Degree of life-threat and differential use of coping models. *Journal of Psychosomatic Research, 31*, 91–99.

Flor, H., & Turk, D. C. (1988). Chronic pain and rheumatoid arthritis: Predicting pain and disability from cognitive variables. *Journal of Behavioral Medicine, 11*, 251–265.

Folkman, S., & Lazarus, R. S. (1980). An analysis of coping in a middle-aged community sample. *Journal of Health and Social Behavior, 21*, 219–239.

Friedman, M., Thorensen, C. E., Gill, J. J., Ulmer, D., Powell, L. H., Price, V. A., Brown, B., Thompson, L., Rabin, D. D., Breall, W. S., Bourg, E., Levy, R., & Dixon, T. (1986). Alteration of type A behavior and its effect on cardiac recurrences in post myocardial infarct patients: Summary results of the recurrent coronary prevention project. *American Heart Journal, 112*, 653–665.

Goldstein, L. H. (1990). Behavioral and cognitive–behavioral treatments for epilepsy: A progress review. *British Journal of Clinical Psychology, 29*, 257–269.

Heim, E., Augustiny, K. F., Blaser, A., Burki, C., Kuhne, D., Rothenbuhler, M., Schaffner, L., & Valach, L. (1987). Coping with breast cancer—a longitudinal prospective study. *Psychotherapy and Psychosomatics, 48*, 44–59.

Horne, D. J., White, A. E., & Varigos, G. A. (1989). A preliminary study of psychological therapy in the management of atopic eczema. *British Journal of Medical Psychology, 62*, 241–248.

House, A. (1988). Mood disorders in the physically ill—problems of definition and measurement. *Journal of Psychosomatic Research, 32*, 345–353.

Kamerow, D. B. (1988). Anxiety and depression in the medical setting: An overview. *Medical Clinics of North America, 72*(4), 745–751.

Kathol, R. D., & Petty, F. (1981). Relationship of depression to medical illness: A critical review. *Journal of Affective Disorders, 3*, 111–121.

Keitner, G. I., Ryan, C. E., Miller, I. W., Kohn, R., & Epstein, N. B. (1991). Twelve-month outcome of patients with major depression and comorbid psychiatric or medical illness (compound depression). *American Journal of Psychiatry, 148*(3), 345–350.

Kellner, R. (1981). *Abridged manual for the illness attitude scales*. Albuquerque: University of New Mexico.

Kellner, R. (1987). Psychological measurements in somatization and abnormal illness behavior. In G. A. Fava, & T. N. Wise (Eds.), *Research paradigms in psychosomatic medicine* (pp. 101–118). Basel: Karger.

Larcombe, N. A., & Wilson, P. H. (1984). An evaluation of cognitive–behavior therapy for depression in patients with multiple sclerosis. *British Journal of Psychiatry, 145,* 366–371.

Lefebvre, M. F. (1981). Cognitive distortion and cognitive errors in depressed patients. *Journal of Consulting and Clinical Psychology, 49,* 517–525.

Linville, P. W. (1987). Self-complexity as a cognitive buffer against stress-related illness and depression. *Journal of Personality and Social Psychology, 52*(4), 663–676.

Maes, S., & Schlosser, M. (1988). Changing health behavior outcomes in asthmatic patients: A pilot study. *Social Science and Medicine, 26,* 359–364.

Mayou, R., Hawton, K., & Feldman, E. (1988). What happens to medical patients with psychiatric disorders? *Journal of Psychosomatic Research, 32*(4–5), 541–549.

Melzack, R. (1975). The McGill Pain Questionnaire: Major properties and scoring methods. *Pain, 1,* 277–299.

Moorey, S., & Greer, S. (1989). *Psychological therapy for patients with cancer.* London: Heinemann.

Persons, J. B. (1989). *Cognitive therapy in practice: A case formulation approach,* New York: W. W. Norton.

Philips, H. C. (1987a). *The psychological management of chronic pain: A treatment manual.* Champaign, IL: Springer.

Philips, H. C. (1987b). The effects of behavioral treatment on chronic pain. *Behavior Research and Therapy, 25,* 365–377.

Pilowsky, I., & Spence, N.D. (1981). *Manual for the illness behavior questionnaire.* Adelaide: University of Adelaide.

Richardson, G. M., & McGrath, P. J. (1989). Cognitive–behavioral therapy for migraine headaches: A minimal-therapist-contact approach versus a clinic-based approach. *Headache, 29,* 352–356.

Robbins, J. M., & Kirmayer, L. J. (1991). Attributions of common somatic symptoms. *Psychological Medicine, 21,* 1029–1045.

Rosenbaum, M., & Smira, K. B. A. (1986). Cognitive and personality factors in the delay of gratification of hemodialysis patients. *Journal of Personality and Social Psychology, 51,* 357–364.

Rosenstiel, A. K., & Keefe, F. J. (1983). The use of coping strategies in chronic low back pain patients: Relationship to patient characteristics and current adjustment. *Pain, 17,* 33–44.

Salkovskis, P. M. (1989). Somatic problems. In K. Hawton, P. M. Salkovskis, J. Kirk, & D. M. Clark (Eds.), *Cognitive behavior therapy for psychiatric problems* (pp. 235–276). Oxford: Oxford University Press.

Schwartz, G. E., Davidson, R. J., & Coleman, D. J. (1978). Patterning of cognitive and somatic processes in the self-regulation of anxiety: Effects of meditation versus exercise. *Psychosomatic Medicine, 40,* 321–328.

Schwarz, S. P., & Blanchard, E. B. (1991). Evaluation of a psychological treatment for inflammatory bowel disease. *Behavior Research and Therapy*, *29*, 167–177.

Scott, J. (1989). Cancer patients. In J. Scott, J. M. G. Williams, & A. T. Beck (Eds.), *Cognitive therapy in clinical practice: An illustrative casebook* (pp. 103–126). London: Routledge.

Sensky, T. (1989). Cognitive therapy with patients and chronic physical illness. *Psychotherapy and Psychosomatics*, *52*, 26–32.

Sensky, T. (1990). Patients' reactions to illness: Cognitive factors determine and are amenable to treatment. *British Medical Journal*, *300*, 622–623.

Sensky, T. (1992, June). *Cognitive factors relevant to diabetes and other chronic physical illnesses*. Paper presented at World Congress of Cognitive Therapy, Toronto, Ontario.

Sensky, T. (in press). Cognitive therapy in physical illness. In S. Moorey & M. Hodes (Eds.), *Psychological treatment in human disease and illness*. London: Gaskell Press.

Sensky, T., & Petty, R. (1992). *Psychosocial and cognitive correlates of metabolic control in Type I diabetes*. Manuscript in preparation.

Sensky, T., Stevenson, K., Magrill, L., & Petty, R. (1991). Family expressed emotion in non-psychiatric illness: Adaptation of the Camberwell Family Interview to the families of adolescents with diabetes. *International Journal of Methods in Psychiatric Research*, *1*, 39–51.

Skinner, J. B., Erskine, A., Pearce, S., Rubenstein, I., Taylor, M., & Foster, C. (1990). The evaluation of a cognitive–behavioral treatment program in outpatients with chronic pain. *Journal of Psychosomatic Research*, *34*, 13–19.

Tarrier, N., & Maguire, P. (1984). Treatment of psychological distress following mastectomy: An initial report. *Behaviour Research and Therapy*, *22*, 81–84.

Taylor, S. E. (1983). Adjustment to threatening events: A theory of cognitive adaptation. *American Psychologist*, *38*, 1161–1173.

Turk, D. C., Meichenbaum, D., & Genest, M. (1983). *Pain and behavioral medicine: A cognitive–behavioral perspective*. New York: Guilford Press.

Turk, D. C., Rudy, T. E., & Salovey, P. (1986). Implicit models of illness. *Journal of Behavioral Medicine*, *9*, 453–473.

Turner, J. A., & Clancy, S. (1986). Strategies for coping with chronic low back pain: Relationship to pain and disability. *Pain*, *24*, 355–364.

Wallston, K. A., Wallston, B. S., & DeVellis, R. (1978). Development of the multidimensional health locus of control scales. *Health Education Monographs*, *6*, 160–170.

Warwick, H. M. C., & Salkovskis, P. M. (1989). Hypochondriasis. In J. Scott, J. M. G. Williams, & A. T. Beck (Eds.), *Cognitive therapy in clinical practice: An illustrative casebook* (pp. 78–102). London: Routledge.

Watson, M., Greer, S., Young, J., Inayat, Q., Burgess, C., & Robertson, B. (1988). Development of a questionnaire measure of adjustment to cancer: The MAC scale. *Psychological Medicine*, *18*, 203–209.

Wright, J. H., Bell, R. A., Kuhn, C. C., Rush, E. A., Patel, N., & Redmon, J. E. (1980). Depression in family practice patients. *Southern Medical Journal, 73*(8), 1031–1034.

Wright, J. H., & Borden, J. (1991). Cognitive therapy of depression and anxiety. *Psychiatric Annals, 21*(7), 424–428.

Zigmond, A. S., & Snaith, R. P. (1983). The hospital anxiety and depression scale. *Acta Psychiatrica Scandinavica, 67*, 361–370.

Zung, W. W. K., Magruder-Habib, M. P. H., Velez, R., & Alling, W. (1990). The comorbidity of anxiety and depression in general medical patients: A longitudinal study. *Journal of Clinical Psychiatry, 51*, 77–80.

Chapter 9

The Role of the Nurse in the Cognitive Milieu

Kathleen A. Bowler, Ph.D., R.N., C.S.
Lisa J. Moonis, M.S.N., R.N., C.S.,
and Michael E. Thase, M.D.

The purpose of this chapter is to explore the role of the nurse in development and implementation of a cognitive milieu. The cognitive model offers an effective foundation for treatment of inpatients and provides cogent directions for educational and administrative activities with staff. After a brief overview of contemporary nursing practice, we discuss cognitive therapy (CT) applications by psychiatric nurses in individual and group therapy, program development, clinical assessment, planning, and supervision.

NURSING THEORY AND COGNITIVE THERAPY

The roles of nurses have changed dramatically over the past four decades—from "caretaker" to educator, leader, resource person, and therapist (Pothier, Stuart, Puskar, & Babich, 1990). Peplau's (1952) time-honored recommendation that nurses need to learn to use therapeutic techniques that help patients recognize and understand their situation is now widely accepted. A central tenet of this chapter is that the cognitive milieu offers nurses an ideal opportunity for development and application of therapeutic skills.

According to the American Nurses Association (1976), contemporary psychiatric and mental health nursing involves the following core elements: (1) the application of theories of human behavior as part of the science and art of specialized nursing practice; (2) use of these skills to achieve both corrective and preventative effects on mental disorders and their sequelae; and (3) promotion of optimal mental health for individuals, the community, and society.

Fawcett (1980) has emphasized the importance of developing a coherent theoretical model to guide nursing practice. We have found that the application of cognitive theory within a hospital milieu provides an effective framework for nursing practice. This experience has been supported by the results of several recent open (Scott, 1988; Thase, Bowler, & Harden, 1991) and controlled (Bowers, 1990; Miller, Norman, & Keitner, 1989; Miller, Norman, Keitner, Bishop, & Dow, 1989) clinical studies. Further, the cognitive model of treatment conforms with many widely held beliefs and assumptions of psychiatric nursing regarding the etiology and treatment of mental disorders. Eight key assumptions pertaining to the nursing application of cognitive theory and therapy are described below:

1. Psychiatric nursing is concerned with understanding psychopathological relationships between a patient's thoughts, feelings, and behavior as well as what actually has happened in a person's life and environment. The nurse works with the patient as part of a multidisciplinary team to address these problems in a collaborative and empirical manner.
2. The patient's thoughts and feelings represent responses to both internal and external prompts or stimuli. These cognitive and emotional responses tend to occur in repetitive patterns, shaping the person's behaviors.
3. The nurse's evaluation of a patient's mood and behavior on the ward can be expanded to include exploring, discussing, and recording what the person is thinking and/or perceiving. Helping the patient to put his or her conclusions or attributions about the meaning of events into words (i.e., articulating thoughts in terms of the cognitive triad: thoughts about self, world, and future) will strengthen this evaluation.
4. Cognitive therapy is an effective method to change dysfunctional patterns of thoughts, mood, and behaviors. Using this model of therapy, the nurse encourages successful adaption to stressful situations in the person's life. Like all effective therapists, the psychiatric nurse is most helpful when she or he is able to assist the patient to focus on understanding and modifying problem behaviors and emotional distress (rather than labeling the person as a "problem patient").
5. Although not effective in all cases of mental disorder, CT interventions have been proven to be effective for certain groups of

patients, particularly those suffering from depressive and anxiety disorders.
6. Cognitive therapy interventions can be used with benefit in both individual and group therapies.
7. Psychiatric nurses must receive specialized training in order to use this form of treatment effectively.
8. The principles of collaborative empiricism and guided discovery can also be applied to administrative and educational interventions.

Inpatient units offer nurses opportunities to work with patients who have numerous problems, including skill deficits, symptoms of Axis I disorders, and difficulties using healthy or adaptive coping behaviors in response to adversity. Nurses can help these individuals to begin to recognize and change maladaptive patterns of thinking and behavior. Various interventions can be used, including a combination of behavioral and cognitive techniques.

TREATMENT PROCEDURES

Behavioral Techniques

An example of the type of behavioral intervention frequently conducted by nurses in the inpatient unit is assertiveness training (e.g., Smith & Kirkpatrick, 1985). Many hospitalized patients have problems expressing strong feelings such as anger, and/or they have trouble resolving conflicts satisfactorily. Thus, assertiveness groups are employed in many inpatient milieu programs. On our unit at the Western Psychiatric Institute and Clinic, a nurse who has received advanced supervision in assertiveness training meets with a group of six to eight patients twice weekly to teach certain verbal and nonverbal behaviors that will help them learn to express themselves and resolve interpersonal conflict in a more effective fashion. Homework is assigned to be completed between sessions, and optional individual sessions may be used to supplement or reinforce newly acquired skills. The ward's milieu provides an ideal "arena" for patients to try out new skills learned in group sessions, and patients are encouraged to receive feedback from their peers. Subsequently, in concert with the multidisciplinary treatment team's overall assessment of the patient's progress, new assertiveness skills may be applied selectively in a family therapy session and/or during passes.

Sleep problems also have been treated by nurses using behavioral methods as an alternative to sleeping medication. A number of helpful and effective interventions have been described, ranging from having the patient keep a diary of sleep problems to the use of progressive deep-muscle relaxation techniques (Pawlicki & Heitkemper, 1985). In the latter case, a nurse can teach deep-muscle relaxation in a group setting, and its application for sleep induction or reduction of muscular tension can be addressed in focused individual sessions (Thase & Wright, 1991). Nurses also may help patients with sleep complaints by instructing them on ways to improve sleep hygiene. For example, patients may be educated on minimizing caffeine intake and stimulating evening activities, adhering to regular sleep and awakening times, and using stimulus-control strategies (e.g., removing the clock from sight or not lying awake in bed for more than 15 minutes).

Other behavioral strategies commonly used by psychiatric nurses include activity scheduling, graded-task assignments, self-monitoring procedures (such as Mastery and Pleasure ratings), and distraction or thought-stopping techniques (see Chapters 1 and 4). Although such behavioral techniques may have some specific short-term value when applied extemporaneously (i.e., helping to lessen dysphoria associated with inactivity and/or reducing the intensity of depressive ruminations), these strategies work best when they are incorporated into a comprehensive treatment plan. For example, Thase and Wright (1991) described a semistructured approach to inpatient CT in which psychiatric nurses function as cotherapists by supervising and assisting depressed patients with such behavioral homework assignments early in the course of individual therapy.

Cognitive Techniques

The wide variety of CT techniques employed in group and individual therapies have been considered in detail in Chapters 1, 4, and 5. In our experience, most psychiatric nurses have not received a sufficient level of training and supervision to formulate and implement an intensive CT treatment plan as primary or principal cognitive therapists. Nevertheless, all nurses working in a cognitive milieu need to acquire sufficient knowledge of the theories and methods of CT so that they can both support and reinforce the work of the primary therapist(s). Moreover, by virtue of their high level of accessibility to patients during evening, night, or weekend shifts, nurses may play a particularly valuable role in helping patients to recognize the relationship between cognitions and emotional reactions that arise in the hospital milieu.

Learning Cognitive Therapy

Much of the continuing education provided for nurses falls into the "in service" or single-session workshop categories (see Chapter 15). In our experience, as well as that of Reavley and Herdman (1985), such training exercises are insufficient to prepare nurses for working effectively within a cognitive milieu. Like Reavley and Herdman (1985), we recommend that more extended workshops or training modules be developed for this purpose. Novice cognitive therapists require didactic coursework, chances to observe skilled therapists at work, and clinical supervision in order to master CT (e.g., Chaisson, Beutler, Yost, & Allender, 1984).

Following a period of didactic instruction, in which *Feeling Good* (Burns, 1980) is used as a sourcebook, we utilize a training module based on the concept of the downward spiral (Beck, Rush, Shaw, & Emery, 1979) to help nurses understand the process of mood or behavior change in relation to automatic negative thoughts. As illustrated in Figure 9.1, the nurse may observe either a mood change (e.g., visible crying or sadness) or a problematic behavior (e.g., a patient's retiring to his or

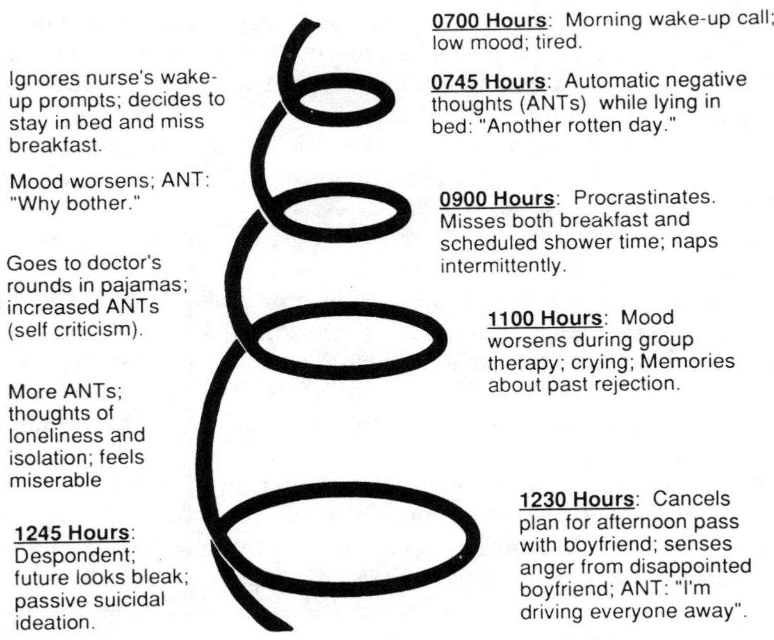

0700 Hours: Morning wake-up call; low mood; tired.
0745 Hours: Automatic negative thoughts (ANTs) while lying in bed: "Another rotten day."
Ignores nurse's wake-up prompts; decides to stay in bed and miss breakfast.
Mood worsens; ANT: "Why bother."
0900 Hours: Procrastinates. Misses both breakfast and scheduled shower time; naps intermittently.
Goes to doctor's rounds in pajamas; increased ANTs (self criticism).
1100 Hours: Mood worsens during group therapy; crying; Memories about past rejection.
More ANTs; thoughts of loneliness and isolation; feels miserable
1230 Hours: Cancels plan for afternoon pass with boyfriend; senses anger from disappointed boyfriend; ANT: "I'm driving everyone away".
1245 Hours: Despondent; future looks bleak; passive suicidal ideation.

FIGURE 9.1. The downward spiral: interaction of cognition, affect, and behavior.

her bedroom) during ward rounds. In a cognitive milieu, the nurse is taught to view such changes as evidence that "hot" or emotionally charged cognitions may be affecting the patient. This, in turn, is seen as an opportunity for therapeutic intervention. In practicum assignments, the nurse first learns to encourage or assist the patient to follow through with a relevant homework assignment or self-help intervention learned in group or individual therapy. For example, the nurse may help the patient with assignments such as documenting a mood change on a rating chart and recording coexisting automatic thoughts or self-directed application of thought testing and rational response techniques (Thase & Wright, 1991). With more experience and supervision, the nurse also can begin to initiate relevant CT interventions *de novo*. One of the gratifying aspects of learning to apply CT is to be able to use therapy techniques to help a patient forestall or reverse a "downward spiral."

In teaching nurses to use cognitive therapy methods that may help a patient counteract a downward spiral, we have found that elaboration of a technique initially described by Manderino and Bzdek (1986) is particularly useful. The following seven-step approach illustrates how this technique can be applied to a recalcitrant, underactive depressed patient.

1. If a patient refuses to participate in a certain activity, the nurse invites him or her to engage in an alternate therapeutic task, namely, an individual session devoted to using the thought-recording and testing technique.
2. If the patient agrees to participate, the nurse asks the patient to describe his or her thoughts and feelings about the decision not to participate in the activity.
3. The nurse and patient then collaborate to explore the evidence supporting this line of reasoning. If at all possible, the nurse encourages the patient to use a tablet or chalkboard to write his or her thoughts and responses "out loud."
4. Examples of thoughts illustrating particular types of cognitive distortions may be identified and highlighted. The nurse helps the patient to differentiate between factual and distorted automatic thoughts.
5. The patient is encouraged to reconsider his or her decision not to participate in the original activity (as a way of testing the validity of the automatic thoughts) or, if this is still unacceptable, to suggest an alternative activity of the patient's choosing.
6. After this exercise is completed, the nurse and patient discuss how its outcome either contradicted or confirmed his or her automatic negative thoughts.

7. The nurse and patient collaboratively discuss the "data" collected in this interchange. The nurse assists the patient to identify related patterns of thinking and/or behavior that may be helping to maintain or exacerbate the depressive episode. Whenever possible, the nurse encourages the patient to generalize what has been learned to areas of difficulty in the patient's life outside of the hospital. Thus, the process of intervention moves from addressing one particular situation (e.g., refusing to go to exercise group) to much broader and more important topics or themes (e.g., isolating oneself when depressed).

We have employed another useful strategy for nurse therapists who are beginning to work more directly with patients to test and modify automatic negative thoughts. This technique, derived from Burns's (1980) self-help book *Feeling Good*, is an alternative to the use of Daily Recording of Dysfunctional Thought logs (see Chapter 1). Using this approach, the nurse and patient agree to spend a one-to-one session (typically, 20 to 30 minutes in length) working on a problematic area. The nurse asks the patient to work through the following steps:

1. Identify the situation in which you (the patient) noticed the problem.
2. Describe your feelings at the time of the event (the nurse may need to help the patient learn to use words such as sadness, anger, anxiety, or embarrassment that describe dysphoric emotional states).
3. Try to recall and record your thoughts at the time of the emotional upset and write them down.
4. Examine your written statements for evidence of cognitive distortions or other logical errors.
5. Try to think of more positive or rational alternative statements and challenge the accuracy of each automatic thought. (The nurse often needs to assist the patient with developing alternative statements.)

As with any other group of novice therapists, nurses need professional supervision in order to learn to use Socratic questioning, rational response strategies, and behavioral interventions. We have found that having nursing staff rotate as cotherapists in group therapy (core or process groups) is an efficient means of enhancing skills of individual therapy as is the use of role playing during group or peer supervision. Strategies for staff education are discussed in detail in Chapter 15.

Group Therapy

Nurses may assume primary responsibility for psychoeducational and/or structured groups designed to support and reinforce the skills learned in individual and core group cognitive therapies (see Chapter 5). In our milieu, these specialized groups include a focus or goal-setting group, a depression education group that emphasizes the cognitive–biological model of this disorder and the value of combined treatment, and an evening group devoted to homework review (see Chapter 3). These groups have the advantage of being an efficient way to provide psychoeducation about common problems while offering patients the benefit of experiential learning and peer support. Chapter 5 discusses techniques for a wide variety of inpatient groups.

THE NURSE'S ROLE IN DEVELOPMENT OF THE COGNITIVE MILIEU

Most acute care inpatient units offer some form of specialized milieu in order to try to meet the needs of their patients. The inpatient milieu provides a setting in which the patient is likely to continue to experience maladaptive behaviors and symptomatology while, at the same time, to receive encouragement to test out more effective coping skills and behaviors. The milieu also insures protection of certain rights and privileges of the individual and provides a structured and controlled environment for therapeutic interventions (Pollard, Merkel, & Obermeir, 1986).

Development of a new or modified therapeutic milieu includes four tasks: assessment, planning, implementation, and evaluation. The assessment stage includes evaluating not only the patients' needs but the nursing staff's training requirements as well. Nurses are encouraged to discuss their concerns and reservations openly, and the unit's leadership team (e.g., the nurse clinical manager and the chiefs of psychiatry, psychology, and social work) must assess the nursing staff's level of interest and willingness to participate in the process of revising the milieu. Initiation of a new milieu is, of course, most problematic when nurses are ambivalent or unenthusiastic about the change.

At least some resistance to the change process will almost certainly occur and must be understood by the leadership team rather than be reflexively criticized as "acting out" or disloyal behavior (Rothstein & Robinson, 1991). In our experiences, as well as those of Kahn and Fredrick (1988), the use of a collaborative empirical approach and well-chosen cognitive interventions by the unit's leadership team help in the development of a high-functioning staff for the hospital milieu. For example, the chief nurse may conduct an ongoing training workshop in which staff are encouraged to examine their thoughts and feelings about anticipated changes. Staff can be encouraged to verbalize their concerns in exercises designed to identify and test-out distorted cognitions. It is helpful if the nursing leader initiates this process by disclosing his or her own automatic thoughts [e.g., "This new milieu may not work. . . . If it fails, I'll look like a fool. . . . They (staff nurses, the doctors, and/or nursing administration) will lose confidence in me. . . . Why can't I ever pull off an important accomplishment?"].

Defining the nurse's role in a structured cognitive milieu is particularly important in order to lessen the likelihood that patients will receive conflicting information from various staff members. For example, it should be determined whether nurses will function as primary therapists or if (and when) the nurses' interventions will be in support of another (primary) therapist. In the latter case, it is important to ensure that a method be in place to facilitate direct communication among all team members (Thase & Wright, 1991). Development of a written treatment plan that specifies nursing interventions is helpful in this regard, as is participation in weekly or twice-weekly multidisciplinary team meetings (see Chapter 3).

Nursing expectations for patients' behavior also should be clearly defined (Sebastian, Kuntz, & Shocks, 1990). Mechanisms to control boundaries are necessary when the unit's population includes patients with a general sampling of diagnoses, such as mania, schizophrenia, dementia, and severe Axis II disorders (Vallis, 1991). Junior staff need to learn how to ascertain the subtle and not-so-subtle cues that dictate when to use seclusion or a therapeutic "time-out" rather than a one-to-one session aimed at testing out cognitive distortions.

Attempting to understand the patients' perspective about being hospitalized is another consideration for nurses involved in developing a cognitive milieu. Common (and often unspoken) patient concerns about confidentiality, stigma, and the perceived indignity associated with losing basic civil liberties (for example, not being able to have a pack of matches or to determine one's own bedtime) can elicit feelings of shame or anger that, in turn, may interfere with the development of effective therapeutic alliances. Attention can be devoted to identifying and revamping ward procedures that are perceived by some patients as demeaning (e.g., a morning roll call or medication-call procedures) or countertherapeutic (methods of restriction or privileges that are unnecessarily punitive). In addition, efforts can be made to increase the clarity and utility of materials or booklets provided for orientation to an inpatient service.

ASSESSMENT STRATEGIES

Assessment

The nurse's assessment responsibilities within the cognitive milieu begin on the day of admission to the hospital, as in the following case example.

Ms. J. was a 32-year-old unmarried woman. She came to the Western Psychiatric Institute and Clinic's emergency room with her parents. Ms. J. had become increasingly depressed over the 3 months following a break-up with her fiancé. During this time, she experienced progressively worsening fatigue, hypersomnia, and diminished interest as well as frequent crying spells and thoughts of hopelessness. On the afternoon of the admission, she reported that she had tried to cut her wrist in a suicide attempt, but she had been stopped by a friend before she could inflict serious damage. After an emergency evaluation found that Ms. J. continued to have suicidal ideation she was admitted (voluntarily) to our cognitive therapy unit (CTU). Ms. J. had no prior history of psychiatric treatment, although she had taken an overdose of aspirin at age 18 following the end of her first serious love relationship.

The first responsibility of the primary psychiatric nurse assigned to work with Ms. J. was completion of the nursing assessment component of the multidisciplinary treatment plan. The focus of the nursing assessment was not only on Ms. J.'s history and current symptomatology but on physical, environmental, and psychosocial support issues as well.

Use of Guided Questioning

The nurse's assessment gains an added dimension when the cognitive perspective is used in framing questions. In Ms. J.'s case, the responses to several relatively simple assessment questions were as follows:

NURSE: How do you feel about yourself?

MS. J.: Miserable. Sometimes I feel like I am not worthy of being loved.

NURSE: What's your actual situation like? How would you describe it?

MS. J.: I feel like I have no one, like the whole world is against me.

NURSE: How does your future appear?

MS. J.: Bleak! Things never work out; they never get better. . . . it's hopeless.

Generally, when the nurse poses these types of questions during an admission assessment, the patient's automatic negative thoughts can be understood within the framework of the cognitive triad (Beck, 1976). Thoughts identified about the patient's view of self, world, and future thus help to shape the initial nursing-care plan. In the case of Ms. J., questions were asked in an open-ended format. When eliciting information, it is extremely important that the nurse allows ample opportunity for patients to describe their experiences fully. Assessment of the patient's view of self should give a detailed picture of self-concept (i.e., how the patient describes his or her level of confidence, self-efficacy, body image, or satisfaction). In order to clearly understand the patient's self-concept, the nurse may ask additional questions such as: "How would you describe yourself? What do you like about yourself? What thoughts come to mind when you think about yourself?"

Questions about the patient's view of the world provide an assessment of how he or she perceives the level of support or criticism from loved ones, employers, and others. Further, the nurse may want to inquire about the patient's sense of purpose in the world. The nature of such a "world view" differs widely from patient to patient. Therefore, it is useful to ask specific questions about work or school, family, friendships, and religious or spiritual matters.

The patient's view of the future is, in essence, a measure of hopefulness and morale. High levels of hopelessness have been associated with an increased risk of subsequent death by suicide (Beck, Steer, Kovacs, & Garrison, 1985). Predictions about the future are, of course, contingent partly on the patient's evaluation of self and the world. Patients who are able to recall past successes and accomplishments or who acknowledge having ample social supports typically are less likely to remain in a hopeless state than those who can recall few successes or who perceive their relationships as strained or unsupportive. To understand the phenomenology of a patient's apparent pessimism or hopelessness better, it is helpful to ask the following question: "What do you think the future holds for you?" For some individuals, the notion of future may be too abstract to be useful. In such cases, the nurse may ask more focused questions such as: "What do the next few months hold in store for you?" or "What are the chances that your situation will change over the next few months?"

Questions about the future should lead to discussion of the patient's plans or thoughts about escape, death, or suicide. In teaching nursing students to interview suicidal patients, we ask the student to try to consider the following: "What if you were suffering from a constant, almost unbearable pain for which there will surely be no cure. It is so intense that virtually all of your previously enjoyable activities have lost their meaning. Moreover, no one seems to really understand this pain. Could you understanding feeling suicidal?" Thus, we try to emphasize the distorted but compelling logic that may "justify" suicidal thoughts and behavior in a person who is convinced that his or her situation is hopeless. In the case of Ms. J., the following thoughts appeared to be intertwined with her persistent suicidal ideation: "I feel miserable. . . . I can't go on feeling this way. . . . Everything I've tried so far hasn't helped. . . . I'm a blight upon my friends and family. . . . I should muster up my courage and just end it all. . . . The world will be a better place without me."

We encourage the nurse who is learning CT techniques to resist the natural urge to try to rebut the patient's pessimism through persuasion. Rather, the nurse needs to learn to empathize with the patient's despair but also to look for evidence of cognitive distortions and to consider alternate, more hopeful views of the same situation. For example, the nurse may ask any of the following statements to initiate a dialogue aimed at reduction of the level of hopelessness. "I understand that you're feeling pretty hopeless right now. How certain are you that nothing can change (prompting, as necessary, a response using values such as 0%–25%–50%–75%–100%)? Do you see any hope of improvement, even for a little while, here in the hospital? Are you willing to try to change the way you feel?" If the patient responds affirmatively, the following step can be taken: "Let's identify, if we can, one thing (issue, thought) to work on right now that is part of your problem. If we can make some headway here, would you be willing to consider that as evidence against the idea of hopelessness?"

Another useful strategy involves asking patients to try to take a more objective or distant perspective of their problems (such as that held by another person). This approach is illustrated in the following questions: "Do others who know you agree that your situation is hopeless? If not, what is different between your position and theirs? What do you know about yourself that they don't seem to understand? What do they see in you (your situation) that you can't see? What does your doctor say about your level of hopelessness?"

Use of Feedback

The cognitive therapy approach differs from other modes of nursing assessment in that all information elicited during the interview should be reviewed with the patient. This allows the nurse to obtain feedback about the validity of the data or the impressions recorded and provides a rather specific way of condensing or restating material. Moreover, the provision and receipt of feedback throughout an assessment interview are very effective methods of establishing rapport (Beck et al., 1979).

Use of Objective Ratings

In addition to the interview mode of initial assessment, nursing staff may obtain further information by administering standardized ratings for depressive symptomatology such as the Hamilton Rating Scale for Depression (HRSD; Hamilton, 1960), the Beck Depression Inventory (BDI; Beck, Ward, Mendelson, Mock, & Erbaugh, 1961), and the Hopelessness Scale (Beck, Weissman, Lester, & Trexler, 1974). These forms provide a way of quantifying base-line symptomatology and may be used subsequently to measure change in symptoms during treatment. Standardized assessments also may help patients begin to understand how their thoughts and feelings fit into the more general pattern of signs and symptoms of a depressive syndrome.

TREATMENT PLANNING

The end-product of the assessment process is development of a treatment plan that is specific to the patient. An effective treatment plan clearly states the goals and expectations for the inpatient stay. On our unit, the results of the nursing assessment are combined in the case formulation with those of other disciplines (e.g., psychiatry, social work, psychology, recreational therapy, and expressive therapy) at a team meeting. The team meeting is usually held on the second or third day of hospitalization. Often, the primary nurse is the team member who meets with the patient to review the multidisciplinary treatment team's initial plan. This provides an opportunity for further discussion and feedback. Discrepancies between the team's formulation of the case and the patient's understanding of his or her condition may be promptly addressed in a one-to-one session or, if necessary, in a small group meeting with the entire treatment team.

In the primary nursing model, one member of the nursing staff is assigned to follow the patient from admission to discharge. Establishing continuity in the patient–nurse relationship is viewed as an important way to reach the goals of treatment. The primary nurse is responsible for monitoring the patient's progress, assessing the utility of the initial treatment plan, and ensuring that the team has the data necessary in order to fine-tune the plan to improve the match between the patient and therapy.

Not infrequently, a patient may inform the primary nurse about a problem that was not discussed at admission. For example, a patient may acknowledge the need for help with marital conflicts, excessive use of alcohol or other substances, or the sequelae of physical or sexual abuse only after building trust with the treatment team. In such cases, the primary nurse is able to provide immediate help (e.g., active listening, problem identification, and elicitation of pertinent thoughts and feelings) and propose a revision in the problem list for other members of the treatment team to consider.

An example of the initial nursing care plan for Ms. J. is presented in Table 9.1. In addition to the interventions described in the nursing care plan, Ms. J. was enrolled in a number of other therapeutic groups (see Table 9.2), and she was started on the antidepressant fluoxetine (Prozac®).

TABLE 9.1. Nursing Care Plan for Ms. J.: Week 1

Reported thoughts on admission	Goal	Intervention	Target date
I have nothing to live for.	Will not harm herself.	1. Attend "Introduction to Cognitive Therapy" on Monday 10–11 a.m. in group room.	1 week
I am a failure.			
Life is not worth living.	Will identify specific feelings she is having related to stressful events (i.e., work, loss of boyfriend).	2. Spend individual time with primary nurse; report suicidal thoughts.	Daily
		3. List specific feelings relating to the identified thoughts.	By Wednesday of week 1
		4. Review concepts of cognitive therapy.	Daily during week 1
		5. A beginning understanding of automatic negative thoughts will occur. Formulate a list of three items.	By Friday of week 1
		6. Attend group therapy daily 1–2 p.m.	Daily during week 1

TABLE 9.2. Sample of Ms. J.'s Group Schedule for Weekday Shifts

	Monday	Tuesday	Wednesday	Thursday	Friday
7:30 a.m.	Goal setting	Goal setting	Goal setting	Goal setting	Goal setting
8–9 a.m.	Breakfast	Breakfast	Breakfast	Breakfast	Breakfast
9–10 a.m.	Team rounds	Team rounds	Team rounds	Team rounds	Team rounds
10–11 a.m.	Intro to cognitive Tx	Homework review	Homework review	Homework review	Homework review
11–12 a.m.	Free time[a]	Free time	Free time	Free time	Free time
12–1 p.m.	Lunch	Lunch	Lunch	Lunch	Lunch
1–2 p.m.	Cognitive Tx	Cognitive Tx	Cognitive Tx	Cognitive Tx	Cognitive Tx
2–3 p.m.	Depression education	Women's issues	Medication education	Interpersonal relationships	Women's issues
3–4 p.m.	Relaxation Tx	Assertiveness	Anger management	Relaxation Tx	Assertiveness
4–5 p.m.	Free time	Free time	Free time	Free time	Free time
6–8 p.m.	Family time	Family time	Family time	Family time	Family time
8–9 p.m.	Wrap-up[b]	Wrap-up	Wrap-up	Wrap-up	Wrap-up

[a]Free time is used for individualized assignments, recreational therapy, exercise groups, or leisure activities.
[b]Wrap-up includes review of goals (attainment and revision) and each day's homework.

IMPLEMENTING MILIEU COGNITIVE THERAPY

During the first week of inpatient treatment, the focus of nursing interventions typically includes helping patients to learn the concepts of cognitive therapy and monitoring each patient's ongoing symptomatology and potential for self-harm. When necessary, a nurse may be assigned to observe the patient constantly in order to prevent suicidal or other self-injurious behavior. Although the primary goal of such observation is protection against self-directed violence, interactions at "close quarters" may afford additional opportunities for psychoeducational or therapeutic interventions.

Depending on the type of milieu program (see Chapter 3) and the level of therapeutic sophistication of the unit's nursing staff, the primary nurse may serve as either a principal therapist or a cotherapist. In the primary nursing model, an associate nurse also is assigned for work with the patients on shifts when the primary nurse is not on duty. The primary and associate nurses should discuss their patient's progress, difficulties, and treatment plans at change of shift or during peer supervision.

In this chapter, we focus on the role of the nurse as a cotherapist because those who are able to function as principal therapists will use the methods described at length in Chapters 4 and 5. It is important for the primary nurse to schedule individual sessions with patients each day in order to review homework and summarize progress made during the previous 24 to 48 hours. As a cotherapist, the nurse may play an integral role in assisting patients to begin to use the self-help assignments of CT. For example, patients often initially may report "I'm lost" or "I don't understand what is going on." The patient's confusion may be result from change in therapeutic focus and/or difficulties in concentration, attention, or learning. Some patients may be temporarily unable to engage productively in the new therapy because they perceive it as too demanding or complicated. At such times, the nurse may review or assist the patient in completion of a homework session and provide more basic or concrete instruction about the therapy. The nurse also may provide supplementary reading materials to highlight the central concepts of cognitive therapy.

Some progress usually is apparent by the end of the first week of treatment (Thase et al., 1991). Patients have gained an understanding of the methods of therapy, and they are better able to complete homework assignments. After the first week of therapy, Ms. J. was working well in both group and individual therapy. She could identify significant medication side effects, and her crying spells were limited to discussions of emotionally charged issues (such as when she discussed her recent break-up with her fiancé). Her BDI score after 1 week of therapy had dropped from 31 to 19, including a decrease from a score of 3 to 1 on the suicide item.

As patients begin to improve, it is important to remember that homework assignments need to be gauged to the individual's energy level as well as the ability to concentrate and use abstract thinking. The nurse can play an important role in this regard by reviewing the appropriateness of homework assignments and evaluating the patient's understanding and comfort with the treatment. Specifically, the nurse can provide the treatment team with direct observations of the patient's ability to use CT. The nurse also may be the only team member who can report on particular areas of difficulty that the patient may have in applying the therapy *in vivo*. Another component of the homework review process involves encouraging patients to disclose their thoughts and feelings of frustration, falling behind, or not being able to grasp the concepts of therapy. Patients may be helped to some degree by a supportive approach. However, an experienced nurse therapist will be able to combine "active listening" with a thought-recording or thought-testing exercise.

The nursing focus during the second week of treatment includes not only reinforcing the progress made in week 1 but also encouraging patients to take a more active part in their treatment. At this point, patients typically have begun to understand the integral association between thoughts and feelings. They have collected evidence that their moods are adversely influenced by distorted perceptions, biased recall, emotional reasoning, negative predictions, and other cognitive errors (see Chapter 1). Many patients who are at this level volunteer comments that are generally favorable (e.g., "I don't know why I haven't thought of this before. . . . It is so easy for me to think of things differently now. . . . I find this to be very helpful"), and attendance at milieu activities usually requires fewer prompts from the nursing staff. Also, it is common to observe patients holding "peer review" sessions and offering to help teach more recently admitted patients about this model of therapy. These changes have been likened to those observed during any intensive socialization or enculturation experience (Thase, in press). Ms. J.'s revised nursing care plan for the second week of treatment is summarized in Table 9.3.

In this current era of cost containment, it is common for depressed patients to be discharged after only 2 weeks of treatment at an acute-care facility. Nevertheless, third- and-fourth week treatment plans do

TABLE 9.3. Nursing Care Plan for Ms. J.: Week 2[a]

Goals	Intervention	Target date
Be able to recognize automatice negative thoughts and identify logical distortions embedded within the thoughts.	1. Record thoughts on a note card.	Daily
	2. Primary nurse will review list and teach Ms. J. how to recognize and name distortions.	Daily
	3. Complete homework assignments each evening.	Daily
	4. Homework will consist of above (1,2) plus reading material provided by primary nurse.	By the end of week 2
Begin testing the validity/accuracy of automatic each evening negative thoughts and use the rational response technique.	5. Identify the potential benefit in challenging and restating automatic negative thoughts.	By fourth day of week 2
	6. Attend all cognitive therapy groups; obtain feedback from her peers.	By the end of week 2

[a]BDI score 30.

need to be developed for patients who remain in the hospital because of a slow or incomplete response to therapy (see Thase & Wright, 1991), including most patients receiving combined treatment with pharmacotherapy or electroconvulsive therapy for severe depressive disorders (see Chapter 7). Ms. J. made a significant amount of improvement during the second week of inpatient treatment, leading to the treatment team's decision to plan a pass for that weekend. On the Friday before her pass, her BDI score had decreased to 11, and she seemed well stabilized on 20 mg per day of fluoxetine (Prozac®).

A final revision and updating of the nursing care plan is necessary when the patient has made sufficient progress to plan for discharge. As discussed in Chapter 16, it is important for the primary nurse to help the patient become actively involved in formulating the treatment goals necessary for the transition from the hospital to home. The preparation includes plans for predischarge passes or home visits and identification of ancillary services available outside of the hospital (e.g., support groups, church or common-interest groups, and referral agencies). Active participation by the patient's significant other(s) also is important to reinforce planning, and to address remaining interpersonal difficulties. For severely anxious or dependent patients, the nurse may be a stabilizing influence by helping the patient to perform preparatory homework assignments, such as completing an activity schedule for use during the first week after discharge. This plan may help carry over some of the structure of the inpatient setting to the patient's home environment.

Ms. J. reported that renewed thoughts about hopelessness were resurfacing on returning from her final weekend pass prior to discharge. During the hospitalization, Ms. J. had started to examine her schemas about being unattractive and unlovable. However, she had accidentally encountered her former fiancé while on the predischarge pass. That evening, she began to experience a slow but progressive downward shift in mood. Because Ms. J.'s primary nurse was not working that evening, another nurse covering as an "associate" noticed that Ms. J. seemed preoccupied and somewhat isolated. Ms. J. also acknowledged, with some embarrassment, that she had not yet had the chance to work through a Daily Record of Dysfunctional Thoughts sheet about her thoughts and feelings. A one-to-one meeting was held, during which Ms. J. described the circumstances of that afternoon. The associate nurse asked Ms. J. to record the event as the first step of the self-help exercise. Next, Ms. J. wrote down her feelings and thoughts, as illustrated in Table 9.4. During the subsequent discussion, Ms. J. identified her most negative thought (step 3) as "No one will ever really love me." Using Burns's (1980) list of mistakes in thinking, the nurse helped Sarah to identify "cognitive errors" that may have twisted or

TABLE 9.4. Five-Step Intervention

Five-step intervention		Ms. J.'s application of the intervention	
Step 1:	Identify event	Seeing former boyfriend	
Step 2:	Describe feelings relating to event	Depressed mood, crying	
Step 3:	List negative thoughts	"No one will ever really love me." "I really screwed up that relationship." "When I leave the hospital, I'll be all alone again."	
Step·4:	Identify cognitive distortions	Misfortunetelling, labeling, mental filtering, and catastrophizing	
Step 5:	Challenge thoughts and reformulate statement	Proposition "No one will ever really love me"	
		Pro	**Con**
		Recent breakup	My family and friends love me
		Absence of an enduring love relationship	I may fall in love again in the future
		Reformulation: "Life is a little unsettled at this point. . . . People do care."	

distorted her thoughts (step 4). They agreed that she had been using "fortune telling" (predicting situations negatively), "catastrophizing" (predicting the worst outcome), and "mental filtering" (focusing on a single negative event or thought to the exclusion of the positive). A discussion of these errors in thinking helped Ms. J. to understand how the event (i.e., seeing her ex-fiancé) had triggered the downturn. In order to challenge the specific automatic negative thoughts, Ms. J. made a chart listing the evidence that indicated that the negative thoughts were accurate as well as the evidence that the negative thoughts were inaccurate. Ms. J. listed:

"No one will ever really love me."

Evidence for	Evidence against
"I do not currently have a boyfriend."	"I have family who loves me." "I have friends who love me."

"I've never had a romantic love relationship that worked out."
"My fiancé dumped me for someone else."

"My pets love me."
"Even though I'm sensitive about this, I don't *really* need to be in a love relationship to be a worthwhile person."
"Just because no one's in love with me right now, it doesn't mean that it will never happen."
"I'm sad because I still miss Jim [fiancé]. It will take time to get over him."
"There is plenty of time to meet someone special in the future."

ADMINISTRATIVE INTERVENTIONS

In our experience, individual nurses can use CT interventions effectively without substantial administrative support, but a cognitive milieu requires both administrative and supervisory backing in order to achieve optimal results. The ward's chief nurse thus needs to set the tone for the remainder of the nursing staff. In this regard, the chief nurse must be able to "speak the language" of CT in ward and leadership group meetings and must be able to advocate the role of nursing within the milieu's multidisciplinary matrix.

Ideally, the chief nurse will have received training in CT before the unit is opened. Alternatively, he or she may be in an advanced stage of "off-site" training, concurrent with the unit's opening. When neither of these options is possible, we recommend that the chief nurse receive additional supervision and training while the milieu is being implemented. This will allow the chief nurse to function as a clinical manager (as well as administrative supervisor) as quickly as possible. We believe that this is important for two reasons: (1) supervision can be an ongoing and continuous process on the ward; and (2) staff are likely to give serious consideration to learning new therapeutic skills because their job performance evaluations are linked to skill acquisition. The chief nurse also should be in a position to explain the rationale and methods of the milieu to superiors in nursing or hospital administration.

The issues of supervision and evaluation of nursing staff performance deserve further comment. Whereas psychiatric nurses often agree that supervision and advanced training in CT are both beneficial and desirable, many are reluctant to expose their work to review via audio or videotaped sessions. Psychiatric nurses may be particularly sensitive about the supervisory process because, unlike many psychiatrists, psychologists, and social workers, the quality of their clinical work has never been subjected to this type of scrutiny.

Many nurses have talked with us during supervision about their insecurities as individual or group therapists. Applying the cognitive model in supervision is a useful way to approach these concerns. Examples of automatic thoughts verbalized by therapist trainees include the following: "I'm not helping this patient. . . . Other therapists seem to do better. . . . I should know this stuff already. . . . I'm not coming across well to the group." A confidential discussion of these statements in individual supervision often can assist the nurse therapist to be more tolerant of her or his imperfections and to decide if more intensive efforts are needed to master the therapy. Supervision sessions can lead to homework assignments, such as reading more advanced materials (e.g., Beck et al., 1979; Persons, 1989), a careful reexamination of basic books like Burns's (1980) *Feeling Good*, or reviewing the videotapes of experienced therapists. In rare cases, it is necessary for the supervisor to address possible alternative explanations for a nurse's difficulties in learning CT. For example, a nurse who is ideologically committed to a psychodynamic model of treatment may decide that he or she simply does not want to learn this model of therapy. In another case, an experienced nurse having trouble in the role of supervisee may assertively express the belief that advanced training in CT is not necessary in order to be an effective professional. A transfer to another unit may be the best option in such circumstances.

The chief nurse also can facilitate the staff's understanding of the cognitive model by using CT techniques for management of unit issues. When the cognitive model is actively practiced on a day-to-day basis on the unit, there are ample opportunities to reinforce concepts and enhance the skills of the staff. For example, during a time of turmoil on our unit, several staff members reported feeling overwhelmed by all the changes. At the next nursing staff meeting, the chief nurse established a problem-oriented agenda and, in the course of the discussion, the following potentially distorted thoughts were elicited: "We will never get all this work done. . . . This is never going to work." The supervisor was able to recognize both the maladaptive cognitions and the accompanying charged affect. She intervened in a supportive but constructive fashion. A cognitive approach to ward administration includes recognizing and acknowledging the feelings of staff members, identifying dysfunctional automatic thoughts and schemas, and working together to solve problems. As in individual therapy, exploration of distortions and implementation of thought testing are dependent on development of a collaborative alliance.

FUTURE DIRECTIONS

The nursing literature is replete with pleas for nurses to do research. Indeed, the importance of nursing research has been likened to a "social responsibility" (Sabol-Stevenson, 1988) and has been described as the "prime directive" for professional conduct (Fawcett, 1980). Yet, the literature on treatment research pertaining to inpatient practice contains very few publications by nurses about nursing practice.

The development of a cognitive milieu offers an opportunity for a renaissance of nursing research. Studies can range in scope from those investigating the acquisition of CT skills (e.g., Chaisson et al., 1984) to the efficacy of specific cognitive–behavioral interventions (e.g., McIntyre, Jeffrey, & McIntyre, 1984). Potential studies of particular interest would include cost–benefit analysis of training psychiatric nurses as primary therapists and trials evaluating the efficacy of nursing cotherapy when added to an "add-on" or primary therapist model of milieu treatment (see Chapter 3). Research addressing quality assurance aspects of program development also is important. For example collection of pre- and posttreatment depression ratings on all patients for 3 to 6 months before and after implementation of a cognitive milieu would provide crucial data concerning the impact of the new program.

SUMMARY

The cognitive milieu provides psychiatric nurses with stimulating and challenging opportunities for professional growth. With appropriate training and supervision, most nurses can learn to work effectively as cotherapists within a cognitive milieu, and a subgroup of nurses may become excellent primary cognitive therapists. In this chapter, we review the development and implementation of a cognitive milieu from the nurse's perspective. We also describe several useful training exercises and illustrate the responsibilities of a nurse on the multidisciplinary treatment team. The nurse may be asked to fill a variety of roles—clinician, educator, supervisor, administrator—in the rapidly changing environment of the psychiatric hospital. Cognitive therapy provides a theoretical background and pragmatic clinical tools for accomplishing these tasks. We look forward to the opportunities to refine and expand the role of the nurse within the cognitive milieu.

REFERENCES

American Nurses' Association Division of Psychiatric and Mental Health Nursing Practice. (1976). *Statement of Psychiatric and Mental Health Nursing Practice*. Kansas City, MO: American Nurses' Association.

Beck, A. T. (1976). *Cognitive therapy and the emotional disorders*. New York: International Universities Press.

Beck, A. T., Rush, A. J., Shaw, B. F., & Emery, G. (1979). *Cognitive therapy of depression*. New York: Guilford Press.

Beck, A. T., Steer, R. A., Kovacs, M., & Garrison, B. (1985). Hopelessness and eventual suicide: A 10-year prospective study of patients hospitalized with suicidal ideation. *American Journal of Psychiatry, 142*, 559–563.

Beck, A. T., Ward, C. H., Mendelson, M., Mock, J., & Erbaugh, J. (1961). An inventory for measuring depression. *Archives of General Psychiatry, 4*, 53–63.

Beck, A. T., Weissman, A., Lester, D., & Trexler, L. (1974). The measurement of pessimism: The hopelessness scale. *Journal of Consulting and Clinical Psychology, 42*, 861–865.

Bowers, W. A. (1990). Treatment of depressed inpatients. Cognitive therapy plus medication, relaxation plus medication, and medication alone. *British Journal of Psychiatry, 156*, 73–78.

Burns, D. D. (1980). *Feeling good: The new mood therapy*. New York: William Morrow.

Chaisson, M., Beutler, L., Yost, E., & Allender J. (1984). Treating the depressed elderly. *Journal of Psychosocial Nursing, 22*, 25–30.

Fawcett, J. (1980). On research and the professionalization of nursing. *Nursing Forum, 19*, 310–317.

Hamilton, M. (1960). A rating scale for depression. *Journal of Neurology, Neurosurgery, and Psychiatry, 23*, 56–62.

Kahn, E. M., & Fredrick, N. (1988). Milieu-oriented management strategies on acute care units for the chronically mentally ill. *Archives of Psychiatric Nursing, 2*, 134–140.

Manderino, M. A., & Bzdek, V. M. (1986). Mobilizing depressed patients. *Journal of Psychosocial Nursing, 24*, 23–28.

McIntyre, T. J., Jeffrey, D. B., & McIntyre, S. L. (1984). Assertion training: The effectiveness of a comprehensive cognitiven-behavioral treatment package with professional nurses. *Behaviour Research and Therapy, 22*, 311–318.

Miller, I. W., Norman, W. H., & Keitner, G. I. (1989). Cognitive–behavioral treatment of depressed inpatients: Six- and twelve-month follow-ups. *American Journal of Psychiatry, 146*, 1274–1279.

Miller, I. W., Norman, W. H., Keitner, G. I., Bishop, S. T., & Dow, M. G.

(1989). Cognitive behavioral treatment of depressed inpatients. *Behavior Therapy, 20,* 25–47.

Pawlicki, R. E., & Heitkemper, M. (1985). Behavioral management of insomnia. *Journal of Psychosocial Nursing, 23,* 14–17.

Peplau, H. E. (1952). *Interpersonal relations in nursing.* New York: G. P. Putnam's Sons.

Persons, J. B. (1989). *Cognitive therapy in practice: A case formulation approach.* New York: W. W. Norton.

Pollard, C. A., Merkel, W. T., & Obermeir, H. J. (1986). Inpatient behavior therapy: The St. Louis University model. *Journal of Behavior Therapy and Experimental Psychiatry, 17,* 233–243.

Pothier, P. C., Stuart, G. W., Puskar, K., & Babich, K. (1990). Dilemmas and directions for psychiatric nursing in the 1990's. *Archives of Psychiatric Nursing, 5,* 284–291.

Reavley, W., & Herdman, L.F. (1985). Training nurses in behavioral psychotherapy. *British Journal of Medical Psychology, 58,* 249–256.

Rothstein, M. M., & Robinson, P. J. (1991). The therapeutic relationship and resistance to change in cognitive therapy. In T. M. Vallis, J. L. Howes, & P. C. Miller (Eds.), *The challenge of cognitive therapy: Applications to nontraditional populations* (pp. 43–54). New York: Plenum Press.

Sabol-Stevenson, J. (1988). Nursing knowledge development: Into era II. *Journal of Professional Nursing, 4,* 152–162.

Scott, J. (1988). Chronic depression. *British Journal of Psychiatry, 153,* 287–297.

Sebastian, L., Kuntz, G., & Shocks, D. (1990). Whose structure is it anyway? *Perspectives in Psychiatric Care, 26,* 25–27.

Smith, S. L., & Kirkpatrick, M. (1985). Changing attitudes of disabled female through assertiveness training. *Rehabilitation Nursing, Nov–Dec,* 19–21.

Thase, M. E. (In press). Inpatient cognitive behavior therapy of depression. In L. Leibenluft (Ed.), *Psychotherapy on the short-term inpatient unit.* Washington, DC: American Psychiatric Press.

Thase, M. E., Bowler, K., & Harden, T. (1991). Cognitive behavior therapy of endogenous depression. Part 2: Preliminary findings in 16 unmedicated inpatients. *Behavior Therapy, 22,* 469–477.

Thase, M. E., & Wright, J. H. (1991). Cognitive behavior therapy with depressed inpatients: An abridged treatment manual. *Behavior Therapy, 22,* 579–595.

Vallis, T. M. (1991). Theoretical and conceptual bases of cognitive therapy. In T. M. Vallis, J. L. Howes, & P. C. Miller (Eds.), *The challenge of cognitive therapy: Applications to nontraditional populations* (pp. 3–24). New York: Plenum Press.

Part IV

SPECIAL APPLICATIONS

Chapter 10

Adolescent Inpatient Treatment

G. Randolph Schrodt, Jr., M.D.

The approach to psychiatric hospitalization of adolescents has undergone radical changes in the past decade. Previously, adolescents were hospitalized for months (and even years) on inpatient units that used treatment methods derived from psychoanalytic theory. Several factors have led to a reconceptualization of the goals and methods of inpatient treatment. First, serious questions have been raised regarding the relative efficacy of long- versus short-term hospitalization (Pfeiffer & Strzelecki, 1990). Lengthy hospitalization can cause traumatic disruption of normal family and social development, leading to "institutionalization" and difficulty with readjustment to life outside of the hospital. Another reason has been the emphasis on "least-restrictive" treatment modes, an outgrowth of the recognition that adolescents have legal rights with regard to their own medical and psychiatric care. Finally, concern about the cost of lengthy inpatient treatment has promoted the development of short-term, acute-care inpatient units for psychiatrically disturbed adolescents.

Recent epidemiologic studies have found that over 3 million adolescents have diagnosable psychiatric disturbances; most of these individuals do not receive any psychiatric care (Offer, 1987; National Institute of Medicine, 1989). Between 1968 and 1985, the suicide rate doubled among 15- to 19-year-olds and almost tripled among 10- to 14-year-olds (Fingerhut & Kleinman, 1989). The most serious health problems of adolescence (accidents, violence, drug and alcohol abuse, sexually transmitted diseases including HIV infection, suicide, and other psychiatric disorders) have been classified as "psychosocial morbidities" by the American Medical Association (Gans, Blyth, Elster, & Gaveras, 1990).

This background of psychological, social, and economic forces needs to be considered in designing adolescent inpatient units. Undoubtedly, there will continue to be a requirement for long-term residential treatment centers for some severely disturbed adolescents. However, the greatest need is for short-term diagnostic and acute-care units that are closely integrated with intensive outpatient programs for adolescents. This chapter is based, in part, on experiences in the development of such a short-term unit at the Norton Psychiatric Clinic, University of Louisville School of Medicine. This hospital-based treatment program for adolescents has been established with an organizational philosophy grounded in both biomedical and cognitive–behavioral approaches.

INDICATIONS FOR HOSPITALIZATION

In response to criticisms regarding an increase in the rate of psychiatric hospitalization of teenagers, and in an attempt to improve the quality of treatment, the American Academy of Child and Adolescent Psychiatry (AACAP, 1989) has established specific criteria for hospitalization. Contrary to popular beliefs, there are virtually no "elective" admissions to inpatient units. Admissions are generally precipitated by a crisis situation, clinical information is often incomplete, and emotions of the teenager, his or her family, and other concerned adults run high. In most cases, the adolescent does not directly initiate the request for hospitalization. Rather, some behavioral manifestation (e.g., suicide attempt, violence, truancy) is interpreted by concerned adults as an indication of psychiatric disturbance. Although behavioral disturbances such as running away, conflicts with parents, school failures, and other "acting-out" symptoms may be associated with psychiatric disorders, many "teenage problems" are neither psychiatric in origin nor indicators for inpatient treatment. Accordingly, many insurance companies will not authorize payment for treatment of primary conduct disorders or delinquency.

There is no psychiatric diagnosis (with the possible exception of delirium) that, in and of itself, is an indicator for hospitalization. With this in mind, the AACAP has established operational criteria for hospital admission.

1. *Risk of death or serious injury to self or others*. This is probably the most common reason for admission to an adolescent inpatient unit. A full description of assessment procedures for the suicidal adolescent is beyond the scope of this chapter. The interested reader is referred to reviews of this topic by Pfeiffer (1988) and Schrodt, Adams, and Siegel (1992).

2. *Significant pain or distress.* Severe depression, psychosis, anxiety, agitation, or psychosomatic impairment may require inpatient treatment.
3. *Severe disability or dysfunction.* An adolescent with bizarre, regressed, or agitated behavior may be incapable of functioning at home or in the school setting. Severe obsessive–compulsive behavior or loss of reality testing are potentially destructive to psychosocial development.
4. *Complex clinical condition.* A dual diagnosis (e.g., alcoholism and depression) or psychological complications from a concurrent medical condition such as diabetes may necessitate hospital care to provide evaluation and treatment.
5. *Failure of care at a lower level.* In some cases, the adolescent's condition may persist or deteriorate despite outpatient treatment. If disruptive behavior seriously impairs family life, arouses antagonism toward the patient, or makes evaluation and treatment ineffective, hospitalization is indicated. At times, a teenager may not have the community resources (e.g., partial hospital program) or support (e.g., involved family) to use a lower level of care.

INITIAL GOALS OF HOSPITALIZATION

The primary objectives of the first phase of hospitalization are (1) the establishment of a therapeutic alliance with the adolescent and his or her family, (2) a complete biopsychosocial evaluation, and (3) the identification of target problems and goals for hospitalization.

The Therapeutic Alliance

Participation in the evaluation process, engagement in therapeutic activities, and treatment outcome are in large measure related to the strength of the therapeutic alliance (Schrodt & Fitzgerald, 1987). However, the establishment and maintenance of a good working relationship with a hospitalized teenager and his or her family may be the single most difficult task that the clinician confronts on an adolescent inpatient unit. Teenagers often perceive that hospitalization is primarily for punitive reasons, and they usually anticipate a loss of personal freedom and autonomy. Although some older adolescents may have the maturity, from the beginning of hospitalization, to engage in a collaborative exploration of their problems, most adolescents have at least some dysfunctional attitudes and beliefs that must be identified and modified for effective treatment to proceed. Commonly, adolescents view themselves as victims and contend that they are not responsible for the problems that prompted hospitalization.

Even after a serious suicide attempt, many adolescents state simply that their behavior was "stupid" or "a mistake" and "won't happen again." In some cases, it is difficult to determine whether teenagers are minimizing their problems in order to be discharged, or whether they are incapable of recognizing that there are problems that need to be addressed. The minimization, denial, and bargaining of adolescents in the first days of hospitalization appear to be related to cognitive limitations such as poor problem-solving skills and immaturity (Schrodt & Wright, 1987). Egocentric "magical thinking" may lead some adolescents to believe that if they were discharged they could go home and "everything would be OK."

Teenagers may harbor overt or covert suspicions of the motives and intentions of the treatment team. The doctors and staff are seen commonly as malevolent authority figures or "wardens" who wish to control rather than help. Often the first question asked of the psychiatrist is "How long will I be here?" To compound this problem, the treatment team, at least initially, is believed to be in collusion with the parents. Hospitalization intensifies the extreme self-consciousness of normal teenagers, and it frequently creates overwhelming thoughts of powerlessness and helplessness. Also, the process of discussing problems, even if these difficulties are quite serious, can trigger fears of being criticized or labeled as "crazy."

It is important to recognize that many of these thoughts can be, to some extent, realistic. For example, some parents have the belief that the hospital will serve as a type of punishment. They can be dismayed to find later during hospitalization that their son or daughter is enjoying the experience or, in some cases, prefers the hospital to being at home. Although many problems are best formulated from a family systems perspective, some parents are resistant to involvement in family-oriented treatment. Hospitalization invariably requires some restriction of freedom and mobility—most notably in the early phase of treatment, when adolescents may be on suicide precautions, have limitations on phone calls and visitors, and have their belongings searched at the time of admission.

Laws regarding consent for admission vary among states, but younger adolescents are typically signed into the hospital by their parent or guardian. Even with older adolescents who voluntarily agree to hospitalization, the admission may at best be "pseudovoluntary." Inpatient treatment may seem at the time to be the best of the available options, all of which are bad. In cases of involuntary admission, the problem of establishing a therapeutic alliance is compounded significantly.

A cognitively oriented, problem-solving approach can facilitate the establishment of a therapeutic alliance (Schrodt & Fitzgerald, 1987). The initial step involves questioning the teenager to identify the issues that prompted admission, thoughts and feelings regarding hospitalization, and expectations of treatment. When distorted or dysfunctional attitudes or behaviors are uncovered, they can often be modified with explanations or "experiments" that include collecting data about the treatment program. Peers who have been on the unit longer and are further along in their treatment program are often the most powerful influences (for better or worse).

There are several helpful strategies in establishing a good working relationship with a teenager:

1. *The adolescent should be treated with dignity and respect*. At the time of admission, a search of belongings is necessary to prevent drugs, knives, and other contraband from being brought onto the unit. However, a full explanation of the purpose of the procedures is offered, the adolescent is present during the search, and the staff conducts this activity with considerable sensitivity. Careful attention is given to distorted labeling by patients, parents, or staff. No one is "crazy," "bad," or "worthless" because he or she is admitted to the hospital.

Issues of confidentiality need to be explained at the outset. Absolute confidentiality cannot be promised to any adolescent. For instance, state laws require the reporting of physical or sexual abuse. Threats of harm to others may require the involvement of outside agencies or notification of the intended victim. Nevertheless, the need for confidentiality with adolescents parallels that for adults (American Psychiatric Association Committee on Confidentiality, 1987). Most adolescents respond favorably to a therapeutic stance that all information received from parents and others will be shared with them. In addition, the therapist works with the adolescents to assist them in informing their parents about situations of which they need to be aware, such as pregnancy.

2. *The teenager and his or her family should be thoroughly oriented to the program at the time of admission*. Rules, regulations, and the overall treatment philosophy can be explained in several different ways: (1) by the admitting nursing staff; (2) by the primary therapist; (3) in a patient handbook; (4) in a videotaped orientation program; and (5) in small group orientation sessions that include patients who have been on the unit for a longer time. Many teenagers engage the staff in debates about the sensibility of certain rules (e.g., no smoking). Most of these issues can

be resolved by explanation of the utility of rules that make living closely together on an inpatient unit better for everyone involved.

3. *The adolescent should be encouraged to participate actively in treatment planning*. The treatment team and the adolescent almost always share one common objective—discharge from the hospital as soon as possible. The most efficient way to accomplish this is to work together to identify the problems that precipitated hospitalization and to develop a treatment plan that can be implemented on an outpatient basis.

4. *The therapeutic alliance requires ongoing monitoring and adjustment*. An emphasis on frequent feedback helps to insure that disruptions or problems in the working relationship are identified and corrected as soon as possible. The most powerful influence on the therapeutic alliance is the therapy itself. If teenagers come to find that engagement with a therapist leads to a more realistic and adaptive way of dealing with problems, they are much more likely to be open and active and to complete therapeutic assignments. A focus on here-and-now issues, clear definition of goals and objectives, and active development of the adolescent's sense of self-efficacy appear to enhance this type of alliance.

The Evaluation Process

Effective treatment is predicated on a thorough evaluation of the presenting problems. The primary goals of the evaluation process are (1) accurate psychiatric diagnosis, (2) a formulation of the significant medical, cognitive, behavioral, and social factors contributing to the disorder, (3) development of a problem list, with primary emphasis on those issues that necessitated hospitalization, (4) identification of treatment strategies, (5) assignment of therapeutic roles, and (6) establishment of short- and long-term goals and criteria for discharge. Adolescents, their families, and the members of the treatment team may have quite diverse opinions on what "the problem" actually involves. Depressed adolescents may relate that they are bored, misunderstood, and overwhelmed; the parent(s) may attribute the problem to bad friends, laziness, irresponsibility, or an ex-spouse; the staff may believe that the problem is inadequate parenting, a genetically determined neurochemical imbalance, or a characteristic negatively distorted way of thinking. Recognition of disparate thoughts and attitudes about the condition and its treatment is one of the objectives of the evaluation process.

Medical Assessment

For the most part, adolescents tend to have a lower incidence of medical problems than adult or geriatric inpatients. However, iron deficiency anemia, sexually transmitted diseases, pregnancy, medical sequelae of substance abuse, and neurological problems such as complex partial seizures are commonly found in hospitalized adolescents. A comprehensive medical history, review of systems, and a physical examination are indicated for all inpatients. Adolescents who have been sexually active should be tested for sexually transmitted diseases. Laboratory evaluation should include pregnancy tests and urine and/or serum drug screening. A sleep-deprived EEG, computerized tomography, or magnetic resonance imaging may be indicated, especially if a history of rage episodes, alterations of consciousness, or previous head trauma is elicited.

Psychiatric Evaluation

Adolescence is a peak decade for the onset of a number of "adult" psychiatric disturbances, including schizophrenia, bipolar disorder, obsessive–compulsive disorder, panic disorder, phobias, alcoholism and substance abuse, and sociopathy (Burke, Burke, Regier, & Rae, 1990). An accurate diagnostic assessment includes the correlation of information obtained from semistructured diagnostic interviews with the adolescent and his or her family, ward observation, self-report instruments, and psychological testing.

Adolescents can be more reliable historians regarding their own psychiatric symptoms than their parents. For instance, although a large percentage of high school students report serious suicidal ideation and past suicide attempts, usually their parents are unaware of these (Friedman, Asnis, Boeck, & Difiore, 1987). On the other hand, hospitalized teenagers may minimize or distort symptoms; their version of the history thus needs to be corroborated by interviews with family members, teachers and counselors, and close friends. Although unstructured interviewing may provide very important information, particularly when conducted by an experienced clinician, a thorough assessment, using a checklist of symptoms, can uncover previously unsuspected symptomatology such as phobias, obsessions, compulsions, panic attacks, and manic cycles.

Self-report measures such as the Child Depression Inventory (CDI; Kovacs, 1983) and the Hopelessness Scale (HS; Beck, Weissman, Lester, & Trexler, 1974) have been shown to be reliable and sensitive indicators of depressive symptoms in hospitalized adolescents (Kendall, Cantwell, & Kazdin, 1989). In addition to lending support for a diagnosis derived from interviewing, these scales provide a measure of severity of affective disturbance. Ratings can be followed on a weekly basis to monitor treatment outcome. Other useful self-report instruments include the Beck

Anxiety Inventory, (BAI; Beck, Epstein, Brown, & Steer, 1988), Drug Use Screening Inventory (DUSI; Tarter, 1990), and the Eating Attitudes Test (EAT; Garner & Garfinkel, 1979). A useful clinical scale for obsessive–compulsive disorder is the Yale–Brown Obsessive–Compulsive Scale (Y–BOCS; Goodman et al., 1989). Although the validity of these scales is dependent on the candor with which teenagers choose to respond, most adolescents appear to give an accurate evaluation of their symptoms (Kendall et al., 1989).

Psychological testing can serve a variety of purposes, including assessment of intellectual functioning, learning disabilities, attention span, level of cognitive maturity, personality characteristics (including impulse control), and reality testing. Observation of an adolescent on the unit, in daily interactions with peers and staff, also can provide a great deal of diagnostic information. A trained and experienced staff can generally make very accurate assessments of the psychopathology and interpersonal problems that precipitated hospitalization. For example, the first indication of cognitive limitations or functional illiteracy may be difficulty filling out a menu. The nursing staff may also observe sleep problems, enuresis, phobic avoidance, or intermittent alterations of sensorium or behavior.

Cognitive assessment is a critical prelude to beginning formal cognitive therapy. Many adolescents are incapable of formal operational thinking and find it difficult to reflect on their own thinking processes (Schrodt & Fitzgerald, 1987). The capacity to think "hypothetically," examine alternatives, and generate creative, adaptive solutions to problems is severely limited in many teenagers. Other adolescents have well-developed abilities to monitor their thoughts and behaviors. Cognitive–behavioral therapy, when geared appropriately to the cognitive maturity of the adolescent, appears to facilitate a more mature thinking style (Schrodt & Fitzgerald, 1987).

Basic attitudes or schemas can often be inferred from the adolescent's dress, choice of music, or manner of adapting to the inpatient unit. Common dysfunctional attitudes include the belief that "people are just trying to mess with me," intense dependency on the approval or affection of loved ones (especially peers), and a general sense of alienation and lack of commitment to anything except "sex, drugs, and rock and roll." Although a healthy sense of self-competence is a positive characteristic, some adolescents have an extreme, exaggerated notion of "independence" that makes collaboration difficult. The cognitive evaluation of hospitalized adolescents also includes an appraisal of their general sense of self-efficacy—a personal belief in one's ability to confront and deal effectively with problems (Bandura, 1977).

Depressed adolescents share many cognitive characteristics with adult depressives, including low self-esteem, a sense of personal inadequacy, helplessness, and hopelessness (Schrodt, 1992). However, adolescents tend to externalize the source of their problems and assume less personal responsibility than depressed adults (Schrodt, Fitzgerald, Wright, & Salmon, 1989). Anxious adolescents, like their adult counterparts, tend to have an exaggerated, generalized sense of vulnerability in response to threatening situations, often social in nature. Both teenagers and adults with eating disorders and obsessive–compulsive symptoms present with a dichotomous, perfectionistic thinking style.

TREATMENT PROCEDURES

Individual Therapy

Individual therapy with hospitalized adolescents presents certain problems and opportunities distinct from those encountered with outpatients. For example, early sessions tend to be focused on issues related directly to hospitalization and the anxiety associated with separation from home, school, and friends. Short (20 to 30 minutes), highly structured sessions are indicated for adolescents with severe symptomatology. Cognitive work on an inpatient basis also can be intensive. Daily individual therapy sessions provide frequent occasions to reinforce basic cognitive therapy concepts. On a unit with an integrated treatment philosophy other active components (e.g., family treatment, group therapy, activities therapies) can facilitate problem solving and provide an environment that is conducive to learning interpersonal skills (Schrodt & Wright, 1987).

The goals for individual therapy are established in the treatment-planning process and are defined by the specific problems that prompted hospitalization. There are also certain "generic" objectives that guide the individual therapist's actions (Schrodt, 1992):

1. Establish a collaborative therapeutic alliance.
2. Maintain a problem-oriented approach.
3. Identify negative automatic thoughts and their relationship to dysphoric mood and maladaptive behavior.
4. Pinpoint cognitive errors.
5. Test distorted automatic thoughts and underlying assumptions.
6. Replace or modify self-defeating cognitive styles with a more realistic and adaptive perspective.

7. Improve sense of self-efficacy by developing social skills and problem-solving abilities.
8. Develop strategies for relapse prevention.
9. Design therapeutic self-help assignments to be completed between therapy sessions.

Short-term therapeutic objectives include resolution of those symptoms that precipitated hospitalization. For instance, suicidal thoughts, hopelessness, and alienation from social supports are often on the agenda for individual cognitive therapy sessions. Some symptoms may not change substantially during short hospitalizations. Problems such as eating disorders, substance abuse, severe family dysfunction, and significant academic problems do not usually respond fully to brief interventions during the hospital stay. Likewise, sustained changes in self-esteem may be delayed until the patient can establish a more balanced self-appraisal, acquire interpersonal skills, and experience success in "real life" activities outside the hospital. The need for long-term treatment of these problems must be explained in order to foster realistic expectations. Nevertheless, individual therapy sessions can lay the groundwork and offer a "running start" for continued outpatient treatment. The reader is referred to reviews by Kendall and his colleagues (Kendall, 1991) and Schrodt (1992) for more specific discussions of cognitive therapy of particular disorders.

Family Therapy

The traditional nuclear family is almost a rarity among hospitalized adolescents. Divorce, remarriage, blended families, and multiple permutations of living arrangements are commonly observed. Hospitalized adolescents frequently have histories of family dysfunction, including substance abuse and psychiatric disturbances in the parents, physical and sexual abuse, poverty, and deficiencies of parental supervision and effective limit setting. Nevertheless, the lack of residential alternatives necessitates that most adolescents will return home after hospitalization.

Parental perceptions of the reasons for hospitalization, their formulation of "the problem," and their expectations of the treatment process vary greatly. Some families have the impression that the hospital should "fix" their child, with little or no involvement on their part. Other families are very suspicious of the treatment process and may fear the disclosure of abuse, neglect, marital problems, or psychopathology in other family members. Some parents are overinvolved with their teenager's problems and react negatively if they are not included in all therapeutic decisions. These "enmeshed" families often have difficulty respecting the confidentiality of their teenager's therapy.

Deficits in parenting skills are commonly observed and are often complicated by ineffective communication styles. Some parents have negative, absolutistic attitudes about their teenager and will tell them that they are "worthless," "hopeless," or "just like their father." In other cases, parents are self-conscious about being labeled as inadequate by the staff and may thus avoid dealing with important issues. Even under the best circumstances, parents of hospitalized adolescents are confused and upset. They require a great deal of support and guidance from the hospital staff. In recent years, the financial uncertainties and hardships secondary to insurance restrictions have added to the anxieties associated with the hospitalization of a family member.

Given the short length of stay in the hospital, the family therapist may have only two or three sessions with an adolescent and the family. As a result, the goals of family therapy primarily involve evaluation, crisis intervention, and, when indicated, referral for outpatient family treatment. However, in spite of time limitations, the cognitively oriented family therapist plays a critical role in the treatment process. The major objectives of family therapy are:

1. Establish a therapeutic alliance with the family.
2. Identify the reciprocal interaction of distorted perceptions and dysfunctional behavior patterns within the family system.
3. Modify the beliefs, attributions, and expectations that interfere with effective parenting.
4. Develop parenting skills, including communication, negotiation, conflict resolution, and ability to establish age-appropriate supervision and limits.

Family therapy sessions can be augmented with educational programs offered in the evening and by workshops designed to enhance parenting skills. Dinkmeyer and McKay's (1983) Systematic Training for Effective Parenting (STEP) program provides practical insights about adolescent development and offers specific techniques for building self-esteem, resolving conflicts, and promoting responsible independence.

Therapeutic out-of-unit passes offer an opportunity to practice adaptive coping skills outside of the hospital environment. Scheduled activities for a pass might include attending AA or Al-Anon, convening family meetings to discuss rules or other concerns, negotiating time to see friends, or simply spending time together with the family.

Homework

Adolescents vary greatly in their response to homework assignments. Past success or failure in school homework is often a good predictor of compliance with therapy assignments. Homework is most effective if it is perceived as pertinent, meaningful, and likely to reap predictable benefits. Some adolescents enjoy reading assignments and will find that pamphlets and books are very useful. However, for adolescents who have difficulty with reading, audio and video tapes may be a more readily accepted method of learning about cognitive therapy. Many adolescents, because of their early exposure to computers in school, are less intimidated than adults when they use cognitive therapy computer programs such as those produced by Selmi, Klein, Greist, Sorrell, and Erdman (1990). Most teenagers respond well to assignments such as making a list of negative thoughts, identifying cognitive distortions, and listing the pros and cons of different options. Other common assignments include activity scheduling for out-of-unit passes, graded-task assignments, practicing relaxation (often facilitated by biofeedback training and relaxation tapes), and preparing an agenda for family conferences. A regularly scheduled "reflection" time, spent alone in the teenager's room, provides an opportunity to complete assigned therapy homework.

Nursing Interventions

The nursing staff has a major role in hospital treatment. Nurses and psychiatric aides have multiple formal and informal interactions with teenagers and perform a variety of critical "front-line" therapeutic activities. Key therapeutic assignments include:

1. Assessment.
2. Orientation to the treatment program.
3. Management of the therapeutic activity schedule and level system for privileges.
4. Implementation of specific behavioral procedures.
5. Enforcement of ward rules, including assignment of room restriction for inappropriate behavior.
6. Patient and family education.
7. Assistance in completion of therapeutic homework.
8. Modeling of adaptive social skills, including communication, assertiveness, problem-solving, negotiation, and conflict resolution.

Inappropriate behavior such as breaking the therapeutic schedule, cursing, or property damage is generally managed by a room restriction or time-out. Restrictions allow time to "cool off," remove the "audience" that may be reinforcing the negative behavior, and provide a structure for the identification and testing of cognitions associated with the troublesome behavior. The length of the restriction is variable (usually 30 to 60 minutes) and is established after the staff member and teenager review the restriction form together.

The restriction form used on the Adolescent CTU at the Norton Psychiatric Clinic (University of Louisville) is a modified version of the Daily Record of Dysfunctional Thoughts (Beck, Rush, Shaw, & Emery, 1979). The use of this form by hospitalized adolescents is illustrated in the following example:

1. *What happened and how were you involved?* I was in Tom's room. He was smoking a cigarette.
2. *What were you feeling at the time?* (Rate feelings 1% to 100%. How strong were they?) Mad—95%.
3. *What were your first thoughts about what happened?* (Rate thoughts 1% to 100%. How strongly did you believe this?) It wasn't fair that I got restricted. I wasn't smoking. Everybody always dumps on me—100%.
4. *What made you believe this?* I don't smoke. I'm always getting in trouble.
5. *Are there any other ways to explain what happened?* Ed [psychiatric aide] told me I wasn't supposed to be in Tom's room without permission. He said that the staff didn't know which of us was smoking.
6. *What is so awful about what happened?* Tom didn't admit he was smoking.
7. *What could you have done differently in this situation?* Stay away from other kids who are breaking the rules. Also, instead of getting so mad, I could have appealed this decision to the nurse. She knows I don't smoke. It just seems like everybody criticizes me. Actually, lots of the staff treat me fairly.

The room reflection exercise helps teenagers to see that their perceptions of situations play a large part in shaping their reactions to environmental events. The process also reinforces the concepts that individuals are responsible for their own actions and that alternative responses are generally available.

Most adolescents do not receive room restrictions during their hospital stay. However, some adolescents have significant impulse control problems that become apparent on a highly structured inpatient unit. In some instances, the problem appears to be related to the absence of self-regulating cognitions rather than the presence of distorted thoughts. The impulsive adolescent usually has difficulty initiating reflective, information-processing activity (Kendall & Braswell, 1985). Many adolescents with anger control problems react almost automatically in situations where they are frustrated. Later they may be able to acknowledge that they tend to "act first, think later." Teenagers with impulse problems can benefit from structured cognitive–behavioral approaches that have been designed to improve self-monitoring. Examples include self-imposed time-outs to evaluate a situation, the practice of relaxation, and the use of more adaptive "self-statements" such as "I'm calm and in control. . . . I can deal with this situation" (Feindler & Ecton, 1986).

Nursing personnel assist adolescents with obsessive–compulsive disorder or anorexia nervosa to focus on behavior rather than respond to anxiety-producing thoughts. Behavioral approaches to OCD, such as thought stopping and response prevention, have been shown to be effective adjuncts to pharmacotherapy (Baer, 1991). Patients being treated for eating disorders are requested not to discuss food or "getting fat" during meals. Attempts to engage staff in these discussions are managed by redirecting the teenager with a statement such as: "Now is the time to focus on finishing the meal that has been prescribed by your doctor and dietician. After the meal, you can write down your thoughts and anxieties to discuss with your therapist tomorrow." Chapter 13 of this volume, as well as Garner and Garfinkel (1985), can be consulted for a more detailed description of the inpatient cognitive–behavioral treatment of eating disorders.

Group Therapies

Group therapy is a major component of most adolescent inpatient treatment programs. Teenagers tend to work well in groups because adolescence is a period of intense peer relationships. This form of therapy thus provides a sense of security and familiarity that may be lacking in individual or family therapies. Berkowitz and Sugar (1975) have identified general goals for adolescent group therapy: (1) obtain support and feedback from peers; (2) provide a miniature real-life situation for study and change of behavior; (3) stimulate new ways of dealing with situations and developing new relationship skills; (4) develop new concepts of self; (5) reduce the sense of isolation; (6) provide a feeling of protection from adults; (7) encourage self-examination; and (8) uncover relationship problems not evident in individual therapy.

Adolescents from several outpatient clinical settings were surveyed with a Q-sort technique to determine their perceptions of the relative value of different group experiences (Corder, Whiteside, & Hazelip, 1981). They ranked items related to group cohesiveness, diminished sense of isolation, expression of feelings, and feedback about interpersonal behavior as the most helpful experiences in group therapy. Interestingly, the adolescents consistently ranked direct advice and psychodynamic interpretations as the least helpful. The results also suggested that the use of techniques that actively structure the therapy sessions are likely to produce positive movement toward change.

Cognitive–behavioral group therapy sessions are generally structured by an agenda (Grossman & Freet, 1987). An agenda serves several purposes. It emphasizes the collaborative aspect of therapy because both group members and leaders play an active role. The agenda also provides specific, focused topics for discussion, supports logical problem-solving efforts, and promotes judicious use of time. At the end of a session, the agenda is reviewed to promote feedback and enhance the group member's sense of accomplishment.

Inpatient adolescent programs generally provide multiple group therapy experiences that vary in composition, focus, and degree of structure. This is consistent with the rationale that hospitalized teenagers have unique problems and learning styles and, therefore, can benefit from an individualized educational program.

Most adolescents (unless acutely psychotic or severely disruptive) who are admitted to the Adolescent CTU at the University of Louisville attend the "open-ended" group, which meets three times a week. The agenda of this group tends to be very similar to that of individual and family sessions. Attention is directed toward issues that led to hospitalization. The group therapists employ the techniques previously described for individual therapy, including the identification and testing of automatic thoughts, behavioral analysis, cognitive rehearsal, and training in problem solving.

A five-step problem-solving approach is taught that can enhance an adolescent's sense of self-control and interpersonal effectiveness. When a problem situation is encountered, the group works to: (1) accurately define the problem; (2) generate a list of possible solutions; (3) weigh advantages and disadvantages of each alternative; (4) develop an action plan; and (5) evaluate the outcome. A group format appears to facilitate the acquisition of problem-solving skills. Feedback from peers in the group provides different perspectives of the problem and possible solutions. Frequently, very creative action plans are formulated.

In conjunction with the open-ended group, highly structured or focused groups may be prescribed for teenagers with special problems such as chemical dependency or an eating disorder. The agenda and format of these diagnostically homogeneous groups can be more specialized than those of the open-ended groups. For instance, an eating disorders group can devote adequate time to discuss the biology of starvation, correct distorted beliefs about weight management, explore the psychology of body image distortions, and design behavioral approaches to disrupt binge–purge cycles. An attempt to accomplish these tasks in a more heterogeneous group would likely be met with boredom or resentment about taking the group's time for topics that do not have general applicability.

Some groups are highly didactic and closely resemble a classroom situation in which active participation is encouraged. Assertiveness training and stress management are well suited to this format. Basic information can be presented by group leaders verbally and can be reinforced by readings and audio or videotapes. Structured exercises, such as the analysis of certain communications (e.g., assertive versus aggressive) or the practice of progressive muscle relaxation and imagery make up the core of these group sessions.

Clarke, Lewinsohn, and Hops (1990) have developed a programmed 16-session "Adolescent Coping with Depression Course" that has been demonstrated to be effective in the treatment of depressed high school students. A parallel group program is available for their parents. Based on cognitive–behavioral principles, the course focuses on social skills, mood monitoring, constructive thinking, relaxation, communications, pleasant events, negotiation and problem-solving skills, and maintaining gains. A leader's manual is available, and group participants complete workbook assignments such as mood monitoring and activity records. On a short-term inpatient unit, it is generally impractical to run the "course" in its entirety because of rapid turnover of group membership. However, selected sessions are often well-suited to hospitalized adolescents, including those with problems other than depression. A particularly useful exercise involves the completion of the Pleasant Events Survey—Adolescent Version, an assessment of the frequency of involvement and sense of enjoyment experienced from several hundred different activities. The results can be used to design more enjoyable and productive activities after discharge.

School Program

With a few notable exceptions (e.g., teenagers with anorexia nervosa), most adolescents who require hospitalization have experienced difficulty with academic adjustment. School represents the primary structured and supervised activity of most teenagers; it is also a major arena for self-assessment of competence and performance. For this reason, problems such as learning disabilities can have profound consequences on the development of attitudes about self-worth and future aspirations.

A hospital-based special education program can provide a "second chance" for adolescents who have not received the individualized educational program they need for optimum performance. Many adolescents approach schoolwork with the expectation of frustration and failure, and they respond with poor effort, lack of persistence, and at times overt resistance or disruptive behavior. A school staff with specialized training, including a practical knowledge of cognitive–behavioral approaches, can work closely with the rest of the treatment team to enhance the adolescent's sense of self-esteem and accomplishment.

Pharmacotherapy

Although the principles and techniques of combined treatment with cognitive therapy and pharmacotherapy are discussed in a separate chapter in this volume, some comments regarding adolescent pharmacotherapy are offered here. Medications are indicated for a variety of psychiatric conditions of adolescents, including mood disorders, psychosis, obsessive–compulsive disorder, attention deficit hyperactivity disorder, bulimia nervosa, intermittent explosive disorder, and neuropsychiatric conditions such as Tourette syndrome. Some adolescents, particularly those who know a friend or family member who was helped by medication, have positive attitudes about pharmacotherapy. However, the prescription of psychotropic drugs generally evokes intense reactions from teenagers and their families.

Long-term compliance with medication is a major problem in the treatment of adolescents. For example, Strober, Morrell, Lampert, and Burroughs (1990) found that nearly a third of their adolescent patients with bipolar disorder discontinued lithium within 6 months of discharge from the hospital despite extensive education about the illness and its treatment. The group who discontinued prophylactic medication had a relapse rate three times higher than those who remained on lithium.

Cognitive and behavioral strategies can be employed in an attempt to enhance compliance (Wright & Schrodt, 1989). The initial strategy with adolescents is to anticipate and acknowledge problems with taking medication on a regular basis. Honest discussions about pharmacotherapy are encouraged by a collaborative doctor–patient relationship. Thorough explanations about the mental disorder and risks, side effects, and expected benefits of pharmacotherapy need to be provided for the adolescent and his or her family. Except in rare emergency situations, consent for medication should involve both parties. Clinical experience suggests that parents often have more reservations about medication than the teenager. However, in most cases, unfounded fears about psychotropic drugs (e.g., addictive potential or effects on future fertility) can be allayed by educational discussions and appropriate reading materials.

More extensive cognitive work may be required in individual therapy to deal with the insult to self-esteem associated with the diagnosis of an "illness," the "need" to take medicine, and the fear of being labeled as "crazy." Attitudes about medication may significantly change over the course of time. Beliefs and expectations prior to starting medication are likely to be modified by subsequent side effects or positive therapeutic benefits. Side effects such as acne, tremor, or weight gain may be seen as catastrophic to adolescents, particularly those with low self-esteem.

Medication also can become a focus of conflict between parents and the teenager. Family therapy sessions may be necessary to clarify the role of the parents in monitoring medication compliance. In their struggle for independence and autonomy, many teenagers will inform their parents that the medication is "none of your business." In most situations, especially with older, more mature adolescents, assuming primary responsibility for taking medication is a reasonable therapeutic objective. In cases where the risk of misuse or overdose is high, or when the adolescent fails to demonstrate the ability or willingness to take medication as prescribed, greater parental involvement is indicated.

Behavioral strategies to improve medication adherence can be initiated on the inpatient unit and continued on an outpatient basis. One important strategy is a simple dosage regimen. Teenagers often "forget" medication doses during the day because they may feel self-conscious about taking pills at school. A once- or twice-a-day dosage is effective in most cases, especially if it can be linked to other routine behaviors such as brushing teeth or meals. Daily dosage containers are well accepted by many teenagers, and they are particularly useful if patients are taking multiple medications several times a day. Recently, pill containers that have an electronic timer have become available. These devices can be used as a further memory prompt.

On the inpatient unit, patients can be placed on a self-monitoring program in which they approach the nursing staff at the time they are to take their medication. This strategy is also useful for adolescents who have adherence problems with treatment for medical conditions such as diabetes or epilepsy. The procedure is often coupled with some form of record keeping, such as a weekly medication chart. After discharge, a review of these records can provide an excellent means of regular compliance checks.

SUMMARY

Cognitive therapy was initially developed for the treatment of adult outpatients with mood disorders. However, this treatment approach has been expanded to cover other age groups, diagnostic categories, treatment formats, and clinical settings. Cognitive therapy techniques are suggested here for the treatment of hospitalized adolescents. Special attention is paid to the development of the therapeutic alliance—one of the fundamental requirements for the treatment of adolescent inpatients.

The responsibility for inpatient cognitive therapy is distributed among the multiple disciplines that work in the psychiatric hospital, the patient, and his or her family. This chapter highlights the processes involved in individual treatment, family therapy, nursing care, and group therapy. Ideally, these different venues for therapy are linked closely together by a strongly held cognitive–behavioral treatment philosophy. In many cases, pharmacological interventions are also important. Cognitive and biological viewpoints can be integrated at several phases of the inpatient experience, including diagnostic assessment, problem identification, treatment planning, and compliance monitoring.

Cognitive therapy procedures appear to be well suited for use with hospitalized adolescents. The collaborative and empirical nature of cognitive therapy minimizes struggles over power or control in the adolescent inpatient milieu. Standard cognitive therapy procedures can reduce many of the symptoms that precipitate admission, such as hopelessness, suicidal ideation, or oppositional behavior. The cognitive approach also can encourage development of adaptive problem-solving strategies that will lead to improved self-efficacy after discharge. Controlled research with adolescent inpatients remains a goal for the future. Economic strictures on adolescent inpatient care will present formidable obstacles to the completion of randomized treatment outcome studies.

ACKNOWLEDGMENTS

The author wishes to express appreciation to Barbara Fitzgerald, M.D., and Steve Burton, M.D. for helpful suggestions in the preparation of this manuscript.

REFERENCES

American Academy of Child and Adolescent Psychiatry. (1989). *Child and adolescent psychiatric illness: Guidelines for treatment resources, quality assurance, peer review, and reimbursement*, Washington, DC: American Academy of Child and Adolescent Psychiatry.

American Psychiatric Association Committee on Confidentiality. (1987). Guidelines on confidentiality. *American Journal of Psychiatry, 144*, 1522–1526.

Baer, L. (1991). *Getting control: Overcoming your obsessions and compulsions*. Boston: Little Brown.

Bandura, A. (1977). Self-efficacy: Toward a unifying theory of behavioral change. *Psychological Review, 84*, 191–215.

Beck, A. T., Epstein, N., Brown, G., & Steer, R. A. (1988). An inventory for measuring clinical anxiety: Psychometric properties. *Journal of Consulting and Clinical Psychology, 56*, 893–897.

Beck, A. T., Rush, A. J., Shaw, B. F., & Emery, G. (1979). *Cognitive therapy of depression*. New York: Guilford Press.

Beck, A. T., Weissman, A., Lester, D., & Trexler, L. (1974). The measurement of pessimism: The hopelessness scale. *Journal of Consulting and Clinical Psychology, 42*, 861–865.

Berkowitz, I. H., & Sugar, M. (1975). Indications and contraindications for adolescent group psychotherapy. In M. Sugar (Ed.), *The adolescent in group and family therapy* (pp. 3–26). New York: Brunner/Mazel.

Burke, K. C., Burke, J. D., Jr., Regier, D. A., & Rae, D. S. (1990). Age of onset of selected mental disorders in five community populations. *Archives of General Psychiatry, 47*, 511–518.

Clark, G., Lewinsohn, P., & Hops, H. (1990). *Leader's manual for adolescent groups: Adolescent coping with depression course*. Eugene, OR: Castalia.

Corder, B. F., Whiteside, L., & Hazelip, T. M. (1981). A study of curative factors in group psychotherapy with adolescents. *International Journal of Group Psychotherapy, 31*(3), 345–354.

Dinkmeyer, D., & McKay, G. D. (1983). *STEP/Teen: Systematic training for effective parenting of teens*. Circle Pines, MN: American Guidance Service.

Feindler, E. L., & Ecton, R. B. (1986). *Adolescent anger control: Cognitive–behavioral techniques*. New York: Pergamon Press.

Fingerhut, L. A., & Kleinman, J. C. (1989). *Trends and current status in childhood mortality, United States, 1900–85*. Vital and Health Statistics, Series 3, No. 26 (DHHS Publication No. PHS 89-1410). Hyattsville, MD: National Center for Health Statistics.

Friedman, J. M. H., Asnis, G. M., Boeck, M., & DiFiore, J. (1987). Prevalence of specific suicidal behaviors in a high school sample. *American Journal of Psychiatry, 144*, 1203–1206.

Gans, J. E., Blyth, D. A., Elster, A. B., & Gaveras, L. L. (1990). *America's adolescents: How healthy are they?* Chicago: American Medical Association.

Garner, D. M., & Garfinkel, P. E. (1979). The eating attitudes test: An index of the symptoms of anorexia nervosa. *Psychological Medicine, 9*, 273–279.

Garner, D. M., & Garfinkel, P. E. (Eds.). (1985). *Handbook of psychotherapy for anorexia nervosa and bulimia*. New York: Guilford Press.

Goodman, W. K., Price, L. H., Rasmussen, S. A., Mazure, C., Fleishmann, R. L., Hill, C. L., Heninger, G. R., & Charney, D. S. (1989). The Yale–Brown Obsessive–Compulsive Scale (Y–BOCS): Part I: Development, use, and reliability. *Archives of General Psychiatry, 46*, 1006–1011.

Grossman, R. W., & Freet, B. (1987). A cognitive approach to group therapy with hospitalized adolescents. In A. Freeman & V. Greenwood, (Eds.), *Cognitive therapy: Applications in psychiatric and medical settings* (pp. 132–151). New York: Human Sciences Press.

Kendall, P. C. (Ed.). (1991). *Child and adolescent therapy: Cognitive–behavioral procedures*. New York: Guilford Press.

Kendall, P. C., & Braswell, L. (1985). *Cognitive–behavioral therapy for impulsive children*. New York: Guilford Press.

Kendall, P. C., Cantwell, D. P., & Kazdin, A. E. (1989). Depression in children and adolescents: Assessment issues and recommendations. *Cognitive Therapy and Research, 13*, 109–146.

Kovacs, M. (1983). *The children's depression inventory: A self-rated depression scale for school-aged youngsters*. Unpublished manuscript, University of Pittsburgh School of Medicine, Pittsburgh.

National Institute of Medicine. (1989): Research on children and adolescents with mental, behavioral, and developmental disorders. Report of a study by a committee of the Institute of Medicine, Washington, DC: National Academy Press.

Offer, D. (1987). In defense of adolescents. *Journal of the American Medical Association, 257*, 3407–3408.

Pfeiffer, C. R. (1988). Risk factors associated with youth suicide: A clinical perspective. *Psychiatric Annals, 18*, 652–656.

Pfeiffer, S. I., & Strzelecki, S. C. (1990). Inpatient psychiatric treatment of children and adolescents: A review of outcome studies. *Journal of the American Academy of Child and Adolescent Psychiatry, 29*(6), 847–853.

Schrodt, G. R., Jr. (1992). Cognitive therapy of depression. In M. Shafii & S. L. Shafii (Eds.), *Clinical guide to depression in children and adolescents* (pp. 197–217). Washington, DC: American Psychiatric Press.

Schrodt, G. R., Jr., Adams, C. E., & Siegel, A. J. (1992). Pragmatic approaches to the treatment of depressed adolescents. In H. S. Koplewicz & E. Klass (Eds.), *Depression in children and adolescents* (pp. 219–234). New York: Harwood Academic Publishers.

Schrodt, G. R., Jr., & Fitzgerald, B. A. (1987). Cognitive therapy with adolescents. *American Journal of Psychotherapy, 41*, 402–408.

Schrodt, G. R., Jr., Fitzgerald, B. A., Wright, J. H., & Salmon, P. (1989). *The negative cognitive triad in depressed adolescents*. Paper presented at World Congress of Cognitive Therapy, Oxford, England.

Schrodt, G. R., Jr., & Wright, J. H. (1987). Inpatient treatment of adolescents. In A. Freeman & V. Greenwood (Eds.), *Cognitive therapy: Applications in psychiatric and medical settings* (pp. 69–82). New York: Human Sciences Press.

Selmi, P. M., Klein, M. H., Greist, J. H., Sorrell, S. P., & Erdman, H. P. (1990). Computer-administered cognitive-behavioral therapy for depression. *American Journal of Psychiatry, 147*, 51–56.

Strober, M., Morrell, W., Lampert, C., & Burroughs, J. (1990). Relapse following discontinuation of lithium maintenance therapy in adolescents with bipolar I illness: A naturalistic study. *American Journal of Psychiatry, 147*, 457–461.

Tarter, R. E. (1990). Evaluation and treatment of adolescent substance abuse: A decision tree method. *American Journal of Drug and Alcohol Abuse, 16*, 1–46.

Wright, J. H., & Schrodt, G. R., Jr. (1989). Combined cognitive therapy and pharmacotherapy. In A. Freeman, K. M. Simon, H. Arkowitz, & L. Beutler (Eds.), *Handbook of cognitive therapy* (pp. 267–282). New York: Plenum Press.

Chapter 11

Cognitive Therapy with Depressed Elderly Inpatients

David A. Casey, M.D., and
Robert W. Grant, Ph.D.

TREATING DEPRESSION IN THE ELDERLY

America is an aging society. In 1900, one in every 25 persons in the United States exceeded the age of 65. Today, this figure is about one in every eight. Persons over age 65 represent the fastest-growing segment of the population, and the population of elders is expected to double from the current figure of approximately 25 million to more than 50 million over the next half century (Bureau of the Census, 1986; Jenike, 1985). This profound demographic change will create significant challenges for those who provide care for the elderly.

Depression is a common disorder among older persons. Estimates of prevalence have varied widely (Gurland, 1976). Early studies reported frequencies of around 10% but newer research, using more rigorous diagnostic criteria, has yielded prevalence figures in the range of 2% (Blazer, Hughes, & George, 1987; Klerman et al., 1986). However, recent research has also revealed that approximately 27% of elders experience significant depressive symptoms that do not necessarily fit DSM-III-R diagnostic categories (Blazer et al., 1987). Depression is particularly common among institutionalized elders, such as those in nursing homes and hospitals.

Depression is often overlooked in elderly persons. Currently, most older patients with major depression do not receive treatment (German, Shapiro, & Skinner, 1985). A variety of factors contribute to this problem. First, many older patients view any type of mental health treatment as a stigma or as a sign of personal weakness. They rarely seek out psychiatric care for themselves and may resist referral by their physicians or family members.

Second, physicians often fail to recognize depression in the elderly because, in this age group, patients often present with atypical features (e.g., higher incidence of somatic complaints than are usually seen in other age groups) and denial of depressed mood. Physicians, psychologists, nurses, and other health care workers should be attentive to the various ways in which a depression (or other functional disorders) may covary with underlying medical conditions. Although many other groups of patients may also deny feelings of depression and distress or find it more acceptable to ascribe symptoms to a reaction to a physical disorder, such responses appear to be more pronounced in the elderly (Raskin & Rae, 1981; Raskin & Sathonanthan, 1979).

Many elderly persons suffer from cognitive deficits that can be worsened by depression. Psychomotor retardation, poor concentration, impaired attention, and lack of interest in usual activities—all common symptoms of depression—can occasionally result in a condition referred to as "pseudodementia." In these situations, depression mimics the cognitive deficits seen in true dementia (Reifler, Larson, & Hanley, 1982; Wells, 1979). The elderly also have the highest suicide rate of any population group, and the rate has risen further in recent years (Casey, 1991). The reasons for this troubling finding are complex and not fully understood, but lack of recognition and appropriate treatment of depression probably play an important role.

Treatment of depression in the elderly frequently involves the prescription of antidepressant medication. Antidepressants often can be very effective, especially in cases of severe depression. A combined approach in which biological treatments are integrated with social and psychological interventions may prove to be the most effective strategy (Wright, 1987; Wright & Schrodt, 1989). However, the use of medication in this age group is complicated by physical illnesses and the general frailty that often exists. Antidepressant medication can produce anticholinergic and cardiovascular side effects as well as sedation. These reactions are difficult for elderly patients to tolerate. Side effects may include confusion, urinary retention, dry mouth, blurred vision, constipation, and tachycardia. Orthostatic hypotension, a common problem, can contribute to ataxia or impaired gait. Ataxia may lead to falls with severe consequences such as hip fractures (Salzman, 1984). Electroconvulsive therapy (ECT) may be useful in many cases of geriatric depression, but patients are often reluctant to accept this treatment.

Clearly, depression in the elderly is a major public health problem that will become even more critical in the future. Innovative strategies will be required to address this problem. The intolerance to medication and reluctance to undergo ECT displayed by many elderly patients make psychotherapy a highly desirable alternative form of treatment. Traditionally, however, the elderly have not been considered good candidates for psychotherapy.

Older individuals have been viewed as being too inflexible, having too much life experience to explore, and lacking sufficient remaining life span to justify their participation in long-term psychoanalytic psychotherapy. This pessimistic view originated with Freud, who believed that patients over age 50 did not have the necessary "elasticity of mental processes" for psychoanalysis (Freud, 1904/1950). Others have challenged this view (e.g., Lazarus, 1980), and interest in using psychotherapy with elderly patients has grown. Unfortunately, the scientific literature in this area is very sparse. Elderly patients are usually excluded from psychotherapy research. Reasons for this include the possibility of cognitive dysfunction or physical illness as confounding factors. The elderly are an extremely heterogeneous group, making independent variables harder to control. Thus, systematic study has been difficult.

Ageism can play a role in the avoidance of outcome research with elderly patients. Therapists may possess common prejudices about aging and the elderly. Aged patients also may activate the therapist's own anxieties in regard to eventual old age and death. In addition, the discrepancy in age between therapist and patient often hinders the development of a therapeutic relationship. Young therapists may have difficulty seeing elderly patients as individuals, tending to view them instead as members of a group with certain stereotyped characteristics.

There are a small number of studies that support the view that psychotherapy is a useful treatment for depression in the elderly. Lazarus and associates (1984) reported that brief, psychodynamic, individual psychotherapy was useful in the treatment of depressed outpatient elders and that patients responded best to supportive rather than insight-oriented interventions. Studies of cognitive therapy (CT) with depressed elders have generally reported favorable results. Several investigations by Gallagher and Thompson (1982, 1983), Thompson, Davies, Gallagher, and Krantz (1986), and Thompson, Gallagher, and Breckinridge (1987) support the use of psychotherapy in the outpatient treatment of elderly depressives. They found that patients with fewer endogenous features responded more favorably to psychotherapy and that improvement tended to be maintained better with cognitive or behavioral therapies than with psychodynamic therapy. Dobson (1989) performed a meta-analysis of 28 studies that evaluated the efficacy of CT in the treatment of depression. He found that greater improvement was positively related to younger patient age. However, significant symptom relief was found in all age groups examined, including the elderly. Dobson considered his conclusions to be equivocal because various age groups were not adequately represented in the meta-analysis.

Beutler et al. (1987) reported that group CT was effective in the treatment of elderly depressives. Also, Steuer et al. (1984) found that group cognitive–behavioral therapy was effective in the outpatient treatment of elderly depressives and was superior to psychodynamic group therapy on some measures. In a study of bibliotherapy, both cognitive and behavioral techniques using structured reading materials were found to be useful (Scogin, Jamison, & Gochmaur, 1989). All of the above cited research studies were conducted in outpatient settings. Controlled studies of inpatient cognitive therapy for geriatric depression have not yet been undertaken.

GEROPSYCHIATRY INPATIENT UNITS

In recent years, the field of geriatric psychiatry has grown to be recognized as a subspecialty area, and in some hospitals separate geropsychiatry inpatient units have been organized. Patients on such units can display a full range of psychopathology such as dementia, delirium, delusional disorders, and mixed medical and psychiatric problems. However, depression is the predominant reason for hospitalization on most geropsychiatry inpatient services (Spar, Ford, & Liston, 1980).

The Edward E. Landis Geriatric Psychiatry Center at Norton Hospital in Louisville, Kentucky, is a geropsychiatry teaching unit affiliated with the University of Louisville School of Medicine. The treatment program of the Landis Center will be briefly described to provide an overview of a geropsychiatry unit. The 10-bed unit is located in a general hospital and serves patients referred from the community, emergency room, and medical/surgical wards. The average length of stay is approximately 17 days. Many patients have significant medical problems and thus are followed concomitantly by medical specialists. The unit is equipped to treat patients with a high degree of medical illness.

Treatment involves a wide array of modalities including pharmacotherapy, electroconvulsive therapy, family therapy, behavioral therapy, structured social activities, and group therapy as well as individual psychotherapy. Patients are encouraged to participate in these activities and groups in order to overcome isolation, rebuild self-esteem, counter hopelessness and helplessness, and recover social skills. Cognitive therapy principles and methods are an integral part of most activities and group treatments. The Landis Center, like other cognitive therapy units

(CTUs) at the University of Louisville, has made steps toward the implementation of a comprehensive treatment model (see Chapter 3). Nurses and other staff members, such as occupational and activity therapists, have received training in cognitive therapy principles and techniques. The chief barrier to the implementation of a comprehensive CTU is the necessity to provide care for psychotic and organically impaired patients. Our location in a general hospital means that patients of all psychiatric categories must be admitted.

Geropsychiatry units usually have a high degree of structure. Many depressed elders are unable to effectively manage a daily schedule. Indeed, inability to attend properly to basic needs such as cooking, cleaning, and paying bills may have precipitated the hospitalization. The structured routine of the Landis Center helps patients resume an organized and constructive life style. A sample daily schedule and a listing of weekly therapeutic activities and groups are displayed in Tables 11.1 and 11.2. The schedule for the day is presented and reviewed at the daily unit-community meeting.

The treatment program at the Landis Center also includes an assessment of functional capacity. Whereas accurate diagnosis is essential for appropriate application of somatic therapies, patients with the same diagnosis may have widely divergent functional abilities. The treatment program utilizes a rehabilitation approach based on this functional assessment. The patient is encouraged and assisted to address specific functional deficits and maximize areas of strength. For instance, the treatment program might include such things as gait training,

TABLE 11.1. Sample Daily Schedule: Edward E. Landis Geriatric Psychiatric Center, Louisville, Kentucky

8:00–9:00	Breakfast
9:00–9:30	Personal care
9:30–10:00	Therapy session with doctor or nurse
10:00–10:30	Exercise group
10:30–11:00	Unit-community meeting
11:00–12:00	Recreational therapy
12:00–1:00	Lunch
1:00–2:00	Occupational therapy group
2:00–3:00	Free for rest or individualized activities
3:00–4:00	Leisure skills group
4:00–5:00	Community outing
5:00–6:00	Dinner
6:00–7:00	Current events group
7:00–9:00	Unit activities (e.g., TV, games, discussion groups)
9:00	Bedtime

TABLE 11.2. Therapeutic Activities: Edward E. Landis Geriatric Psychiatry Center, Louisville, Kentucky

Art therapy (once weekly)
Community outing (once weekly)
Cooking group (once weekly)
Current events group (five times weekly)
Exercise group (daily)
Family therapy (variable)
Individual sessions with nurse (variable)
Individual therapy and/or physician rounds (daily)
Leisure group (weekly)
Occupational therapy group (three times weekly)
Recreational therapy (daily)
Reminiscence group (two times weekly)
Sing-along (two times weekly)
Unit community meeting (daily)

audiology evaluation, speech therapy, and a nutritional assessment in addition to medical and psychological procedures. This approach requires a variety of staff members to work together in a true multidisciplinary effort. Team members provide verbal updates during daily staff meetings as well as written progress reports on the patient's chart.

COGNITIVE THERAPY IN GEROPSYCHIATRY UNITS

Although somatic, group, and activity therapies have usually been the major types of treatment on geropsychiatry units, CT has been adopted as the primary psychotherapeutic intervention at the Landis Center. Elderly patients generally respond well to CT. The emphasis on learning skills to cope better with depression fits well into the overall emphasis on rehabilitation of function. Cognitive therapy may be acceptable to patients who are biased against traditional psychodynamic psychotherapy, which they see as endless and difficult to understand. The collaborative nature of the therapeutic relationship helps limit regression and excessive dependency. Also, the "here-and-now" problem-solving focus circumvents potential problems related to the large volume of life material typically processed in more traditional psychotherapy.

Because of the short length of stay on the Landis Center, CT has a distinct advantage over traditional psychotherapy. Meaningful therapeutic work can often be accomplished during a brief hospital stay.

Cognitive therapy meshes well with the structured approach used on the geropsychiatry unit. In fact, behavioral assignments can usually be incorporated into the unit's daily schedule.

The simplicity, usefulness, and accessibility of the basic concepts of cognitive therapy appeal readily to staff who are already steeped in a rehabilitation model that stresses problem solving and adaptation. In addition, geropsychiatric staff members are rarely committed to traditional psychoanalytic concepts of psychotherapy and are often open to cognitive approaches. Cognitive therapy can provide a unifying treatment philosophy for staff from a variety of disciplines on the geropsychiatry unit.

Cognitive Therapy Techniques with the Elderly

Although all of the general principles of CT described in earlier chapters are applicable to work with elderly inpatients, certain changes in technique may be necessary. The following modifications are presented as a general guide for cognitive therapy with elderly inpatients.

1. *Prepare the patient for therapy*. Special attention to orienting the patient for therapy is needed. It is common for elderly patients to have very negative views, common to their generation, about psychiatric treatment. Much of the early work in cognitive therapy with older individuals may be directed at dispelling such negative attitudes and expectations regarding treatment. The goals of CT should (at least initially) be modest and be presented in a simple and jargon-free manner. This will help the patient to think of therapy as a practical and common-sense way of learning to cope with the stresses of aging.

2. *Adjust the framework of therapy to the patient's capabilities*. Short and frequent therapy sessions (15 to 25 minutes, five or more times weekly) are indicated because of the greater severity of disorders on an inpatient ward, the frequent cognitive or physical impairments of the aged, as well as the short treatment period during an inpatient stay. Therapy sessions are paced slowly, with much repetition of key ideas to insure patient understanding. As the patient progresses and displays improved mood and greater self-efficacy, longer and more intensive sessions may be possible.

3. *Use the structure of the unit*. The high degree of structure on the inpatient unit provides a haven from stresses and responsibilities that have often been viewed by the patient as overwhelming. The hospital program provides support and allows the patient to concentrate his or her energies on the specific factors or assumptions contributing to the

depressed mood. In addition, much of the CT homework can be integrated with the unit's structured activities (such as groups, activities, and out-trips).

4. *Use a variety of techniques and resources in treatment.* Cognitive therapy is usually combined with other treatments, such as pharmacotherapy or occupational therapy. Elderly patients, because of physical illness and declining self-care skills, often require treatment that embodies biological and social components in addition to psychological techniques. Examples include medical interventions, physical therapy, referral to the Visiting Nurses Association, and contracting for live-in help after discharge.

5. *Involve the family in treatment.* Inclusion of the family in the treatment program is often a crucial part of therapy. Long-standing family conflicts frequently reemerge as members confront the increasing dependency of a depressed elder. Family therapy, based on CT principles, can be used to alter some of the harmful assumptions and attributions family members hold regarding each other and the family as a unit. Using CT techniques to examine beliefs about aging and depression that are held by the elder's family and significant others helps them develop new, less hopeless points of view. This is especially important in those situations in which the patient will be living with the family after discharge. The rudiments of CT can usually be taught to the family, after which their aid can be enlisted in the task of countering the patient's negative thoughts and behaviors.

6. *Adopt a flexible treatment approach.* It may be necessary to modify the traditional rigid schedule of therapy hours and allow the patient to request assistance as needed. For instance, this may be done on an inpatient basis by using a nurse or aide as cotherapist, thus allowing the patient a resource for CT that can be applied on a more frequent and timely basis. Similarly, the increased dependency manifested by many elderly patients can often be used to advantage. The experienced therapist can use this dependency to form a therapeutic alliance more easily and to insure compliance with behavioral assignments. Cognitive therapy techniques, such as Socratic questioning or examining the evidence, may have to be expressed in a more concrete or literal form in cases where the patient is poorly educated or displays cognitive deficits.

7. *Plan the transition between inpatient and outpatient treatment.* Cognitive therapy techniques should be used prior to discharge to explore and counteract negative expectations that the patient may have regarding discharge or the home situation. The timing of the initial outpatient follow-up should be based on the patient's diagnosis, functional capacity, and home situation. To reduce the possibility of decompensation after discharge, the termination process should be a gradual one. The

patient should be expressly given the freedom to request additional sessions or to resume therapy when needed.

Simplification of Cognitive Techniques

In many ways, work with depressed elderly inpatients represents cognitive therapy stripped to its basic elements. The therapist attacks hopelessness and helplessness as directly as possible while attempting to maximize a patient's sense of mastery and pleasure. Collaborative empiricism, such as experienced with younger patients, often must evolve over time. Very withdrawn or despondent patients may be unable to participate fully as partners in the therapy and, especially at the beginning, must depend on the therapist to provide most of the "energy" for therapy. A few negative beliefs closely related to feelings of hopelessness or helplessness can be selected by the therapist for modification by techniques such as Socratic questioning or examining the evidence. Looking at false conclusions, rather than logical errors in the thinking process itself, is usually helpful in getting a regressed elder started in therapy. Such patients often find it difficult to identify automatic thoughts or logical errors, but they may be able to recognize the erroneous beliefs that are the outcome of these thought processes.

During an early therapy session, Mrs. A., a 78-year-old woman, was able to grasp the concept that thoughts are an important determinant of feelings. However, she was unable to spot any of her own automatic thoughts without considerable assistance from the therapist. These thoughts were characterized by an exaggerated sense of hopelessness and helplessness about her poor relationship with her husband. Rather than persisting in the attempt to help the patient recognize these automatic thoughts and the logical errors involved, the therapist shifted strategies.

THERAPIST: Let's put aside our work on your automatic thoughts for today and just look at some of the conclusions you have drawn about your situation. You seem to believe there's nothing you can do to change your marriage.

MRS. A.: I've tried everything, and nothing works. He'll never change.

THERAPIST: Is it possible there could be approaches you haven't considered? Maybe your children could convince your husband to start marital therapy.

MRS. A.: I don't think they would try to stand up to their father.

THERAPIST: Have you discussed this with them?

MRS. A.: No. What's the use? I know what they'll say.

THERAPIST: It seems to me that you don't have much to lose by trying. Can we call them today?

MRS. A.: You can go ahead. It couldn't get any worse than it is now.

In this example, the therapist focuses directly on a specific belief, namely that the patient's marital conflict is hopeless and nothing she can do could ever bring her husband into marital therapy. For the moment, the automatic thoughts and logical errors associated with the belief are not considered in depth. Instead, the therapist simply explores a dysfunctional belief with the patient and attempts to generate alternatives. This example also illustrates that, early in treatment, the energy for change often must come primarily from the therapist.

Homework assignments are usually simple ones, such as keeping a journal of some type. Occasionally a two-column thought-recording technique is useful. Many elders feel overwhelmed by complex homework assignments such as the standard Daily Record of Dysfunctional Thoughts (DRDT) (see Chapter 1). A case example illustrates this point:

Mrs. B., an 80-year-old widow, became extremely depressed following a minor physical illness. During an early session, she stated, "I suddenly realized how old I am; an 80-year-old cannot do very many things anymore." Her illness had brought out a number of negative beliefs about aging and old people that she had not previously applied to herself. Therapy was initiated by teaching the patient the basics of the cognitive model. The chalkboard was used to illustrate schematically the relationship among external events such as her illness, her own beliefs about the illness, related beliefs about the aging process, and finally her depressed mood. These concrete, visual illustrations made it easier for her to see the linkages between these concepts.

Although Mrs. B. had many negative thoughts about herself, it was decided to concentrate on one central idea of the relationship between her age and her abilities. She was given a homework assignment involving the DRDT, but Mrs. B. found this task to be overwhelming and interpreted this as a further sign of her declining abilities. After the therapist challenged this conclusion, Mrs. B. was given a simpler homework assignment that involved keeping a list of her beliefs about aging. During therapy sessions, she was encouraged to reconsider her dogmatic beliefs about negative consequences of "being 80." The evidence for and against her conclusions was explored. The patient acknowledged that just a few months before she had been quite vigorous and content, despite her advanced age. Mrs. B. was helped by the therapist to see that many of her friends were still happy and active at age 80 and beyond. She began to see her depression as a consequence of her negative beliefs about aging. As she improved, further work was done to explore her illogical thought processes, such as dichotomous thinking and selective abstraction. Eventually, she was able to articulate a more realistic view of the aging process.

Behavioral Techniques with Elders

Depression in the elderly often presents with demoralization, apathy, inertia, and excessive self-absorption. Behavioral techniques are frequently useful in addressing these problems. At the Landis Center, the patient's individual activities schedule is used to promote a gradual increase in physical and social activity. Staff are quite persistent in encouraging adherence to the behavioral program. The schedules are presented to patients and families as a central part of treatment. Whenever possible, an acceptable schedule is achieved through negotiation between staff and the patient. Families are often recruited to help the patient follow the activities schedule. Behavioral techniques used in CT sessions are often integrated with the individual activities schedule. This information is communicated to nursing staff who are responsible for implementing the behavioral plan, and the patient's behavioral progress is reviewed daily in staff meetings.

Mrs. C., an 85-year-old married woman, was transferred from the medical service for treatment of depression and profound apathy. She had grown increasingly dependent on her family for daily care. Eventually, this evolved into dressing and feeding her. No physical cause for this disability could be found. The patient had little formal education and distrusted psychiatrists. She told her doctor "I'm weak, and weak people need rest and care, not talk." Underlying this behavior, there appeared to be severe depression as well as a variety of complex beliefs about herself, aging, and her family. Attempts to engage her in "talking" cognitive therapy were unsuccessful.

A conference was held among the therapist, the patient, and her family. The difficulties with the patient's belief that rest and caretaking were the only solutions to her problems were discussed. Her family readily agreed to the need for increased physical activity and eventually prevailed on the patient to accept a new approach. The idea that "weak people can improve by gradually building up strength" was suggested as a substitute for her dysfunctional belief. The physical therapist, occupational therapist, and nursing staff collaborated with the individual therapist to set up a behavioral program incorporating the concept of graded-task assignments. As the patient gradually became more physically active and resumed self-care, she also became more open to talking about her problems. However, this was limited largely to a discussion of her beliefs about illness, aging, and the benefits of physical activity.

Coping with Realistic Loss

Probably the major theme expressed by elderly patients in psychotherapy is that of loss. The elderly experience myriad types of loss: vigor, health, cognitive skills, status, income and occupation, as well as loss of loved ones. Some elderly patients become overwhelmed by negative events that accumulate more rapidly than can be tolerated. Therapists commonly encounter helplessness and hopelessness in such instances. Often patients also are preoccupied with physical symptoms that may be influenced by depression. The struggle with physical pain may be an important aspect of therapy with medically ill patients. Those with terminal illness usually anticipate death and try to come to terms with it, but many elderly patients in psychotherapy do not volunteer any thoughts or feelings about death.

For elderly patients who have developed depression as a reaction to realistic loss, the therapist's task is to maximize the patient's ability to cope with these adverse events. In these situations, there may be no cognitive distortions about the events themselves. Rather, patients may have exaggerated negative beliefs about themselves and their ability to cope with problems. The therapist helps the patient develop a realistic plan to cope with the event taking into account the patient's past abilities to meet such challenges successfully. Many cognitive techniques can be applied, such as Socratic questioning, examining options, and listing advantages and disadvantages. The cognitive therapist's own beliefs and attitudes about aging may influence his or her ability to separate the patient's realistic concerns from distorted depressive cognitions. Considerable experience may be necessary before therapists can fully recognize and understand their attitudes about growing old.

Treatment of patients who have experienced real, negative life events is illustrated by the case of Mrs. D., a 67-year-old widowed female, who became depressed following the death of her husband. They had been married for over 40 years. Mr. D suffered from an inoperable brain tumor, and his behavior over the last 15 months of his life had been bizarre and unpredictable. Despite these problems, Mrs. D. insisted on caring for her husband at home. After Mr. D's death, Mrs. D. became increasingly despondent, lost interest in many former activities, and began to isolate herself from family and friends.

The therapist did not deny the extent of Mrs. D.'s loss—indeed she had lost the person who was closest and most important to her. Mrs. D.'s feelings of loss and abandonment were acknowledged by the therapist, and an empathic and supportive approach was maintained throughout. Also, cognitions regarding the consequences of her husband's death were carefully examined in a sensitive manner. Depressogenic thoughts regarding her inability to cope with life's demands, the impossibility of enjoying activities ever again, and her perceived lack of self-worth were elicited. Through the use of techniques such as examining the evidence, the patient was able to start to recapture some of her previous vitality. Homework assignments, designed to counter maladaptive beliefs, required her to enlarge her circle of social contacts and activities. These exercises concretely disproved her assertions regarding the futility of trying to carve out an existence as a single person. Mrs. D. continued to grieve but was able to start focusing more on the demands and opportunities of her current circumstances.

Existentially Oriented Cognitive Therapy with the Elderly

The attempt to come to terms with the meaning of one's personal existence is an important theme in psychotherapy with elderly patients. This process has been viewed as the final developmental task of the life cycle (Erikson, 1963, 1968; Peck, 1968). Depressed patients often cannot realistically evaluate their lives because of the systematic errors in thinking that characterize depressive disorders. Cognitive therapy for such patients may take on an existential tone as CT techniques are used to help the patient develop a more balanced, less negative life appraisal. The usual "here-and-now" focus of CT may require modification in such therapies. Life review or reminiscence, using a cognitive approach, focuses on the patient's valuable and enduring accomplishments. An equally important aspect of existentially oriented cognitive therapy involves assisting the patient in regaining a sense of control, purpose, and self-efficacy in the present. Two case illustrations examine these points.

A 76-year-old woman suffered from major depression superimposed on chronic dysthymia. She was an extremely energetic, intelligent woman with a variety of talents. As a young adult, she had developed lofty goals as she struggled to free herself from an impoverished background. Although she had significant accomplishments, she had not been able to meet many of her original goals. A series of losses precipitated her depression, and she developed a pervasive view that her whole life had been a failure.

The patient received extensive supportive and psychodynamically oriented psychotherapy as well as antidepressant medication, with only mild improvement. However, CT proved to be a much more useful treatment for her. Early in the therapy process, traditional "here-and-now" approaches were used to help her regain the ability to participate in her many activities. As the treatment progressed, more time was spent reviewing her life, with an emphasis on dispelling negative, dichotomous beliefs about her children, her career, and, ultimately, herself.

Mr. E. was a 76-year-old man who had been recently widowed. Not only had his wife's death devastated him, but he had depended on her to actively maintain their social ties with friends and relatives. In addition to his feeling of loss regarding his wife, Mr. E. found himself socially isolated because of his lack of interpersonal skills. When initially seen in therapy, Mr. E. verbalized feelings of his life not having been worthwhile because "no ever comes to visit me" and "my kids never write or call." Mr. E.'s beliefs were compared to the reality of the situation; and he admitted that his friends and children *did* sometimes initiate visits, telephone contact, and letters.

Social skills training and behavioral homework that required Mr. E. to originate social interaction became an integral part of therapy at this time. For instance, he was given assignments to invite friends to accompany him to the theater and to begin writing letters to his children who lived out of town. Mr. E. became much less socially isolated and acquired some skill in recognizing his negative thoughts. As his mood improved, Mr. E. started to put his whole life in perspective rather than merely focus on his wife's death. He acquired a sense of pride as his social skills and assertiveness increased. Mr. E. was able to view his children and grandchildren as a part of his heritage to the world, and he verbalized feelings of satisfaction regarding his life's effects and accomplishments.

Cognitive Therapy with Anxiety Disorders

Although the literature focuses on cognitive therapy as a treatment for depression in the elderly, this form of treatment can be used for other disorders, such as anxiety and panic (Clark, 1986; Wright & Borden, 1991; Alford, Freeman, Beck, & Wright, 1990; Barlow, Cohen, & Waddell, 1984).

The use of CT for anxiety in elderly persons is illustrated in the case of Mr. F., a 71-year-old man who suffered from a longstanding panic disorder. His panic attacks were triggered whenever he perceived that his heart rate was increasing. His thinking processes were characterized by an obsessional, hypochondriacal style. Medications were unacceptable to him, because previous courses of tricyclic antidepressants had caused tachycardia. The patient had a rigid belief that a rapid heart beat would ultimately lead to a heart attack, and he spent much of his psychological energy in an effort to prevent this from happening. An extensive cardiac evaluation found no evidence of significant heart disease.

Cognitive therapy involved recording Mr. F.'s beliefs, illustrating how these cognitions precipitated panic attacks, and challenging the inherent logical errors. A systematic desensitization program was designed involving a very gradual increase in activities while monitoring heart rate, thoughts, and anxiety level. Biofeedback and relaxation techniques were used as adjunctive forms of therapy. The patient responded with a marked reduction in frequency and severity of panic attacks.

Supportive Cognitive Therapy

Much of the daily work in the care of geropsychiatric patients (medical management, discussion of medical problems, and so on) is not conducted in standard therapy sessions but during "rounds." Indeed, formal sessions may not be viewed as a central part of the care of many geropsychiatric patients. However, it is useful to consider all interactions with the patient as a form of psychotherapy and to incorporate CT techniques into rounds on a regular basis. In so doing, one may create a cognitive milieu in which patients are regularly encouraged to recognize dysfunctional thoughts and to counter them. Patients who are seen as poor candidates for standard CT may still be treated with supportive psychotherapy based on cognitive–behavioral, rather than psychodynamic principles. This type of psychotherapy is suitable for patients who have depression along with mild dementia or depressive pseudodementia. Supportive CT focuses on the day-to-day interactions on an inpatient unit. Discussions of medical tests, medications, unit activities, privilege levels, and passes are conducted with an emphasis on dispelling hopelessness and helplessness. Every opportunity is taken to encourage patients to reexamine negative beliefs about themselves, their environment, and the treatment itself.

For example, a 75-year-old man with depression and mild dementia was being treated with antidepressant medication. He always tried to "look his best" when seen on morning rounds. However, the nursing staff reported that he would sometimes be tearful after the physicians left his room. When asked about this, he first denied being upset but later acknowledged that he always felt sad after his medicine was discussed. "When you change my medication, I know you doctors must think it's not working. I must really be sick. I don't think you can help me." Although his cognitive impairment precluded extensive psychotherapy, he was able to accept alternate views about changes in his medication regimen. His beliefs about his medicines were discussed with him daily and reviewed with his family as well.

A major aspect of supportive CT is the use of the empirical "try it and see" idea toward activities such as groups, exercise, and outings. Predictions about the patient's progress are elicited in therapy sessions, and then the patient's true experiences are compared with these predictions in subsequent sessions. Positive experiences obviously tend to rebuild hope and improve mood. Negative experiences provide the therapist with the opportunity to encourage persistence and to reframe the negative experience as a problem to be addressed, rather than a personal failure.

In this type of therapy, the burden is on the therapist to teach the cognitive model and provide the impetus to further the therapeutic process. Sessions are brief, informal, and frequent. A review of the patient's progress for that day suggests one or two items for further discussion as therapeutic issues. The agenda is kept very short, and there is no effort to be overly inclusive within any given session. An attempt is made to keep jargon to a minimum. The patient may not even label these discussions as "psychotherapy." Homework is often based on participation in some particular ward activity. Self-rating instruments such as thought records or activity rating scales are simplified as much as possible and may be customized for the needs and cognitive abilities of each patient.

Case Example

Many of the important elements of CT on a geropsychiatric unit can be illustrated by a more in-depth case example. Mrs. F., a 68-year-old widow, was admitted to the geropsychiatry unit because of an overwhelming depression that had not responded to outpatient supportive psychotherapy. She gave a history of depression for approximately 1 year, during which her 90-year-old mother had come to live with her. Her initial enthusiasm for this move gradually gave way to increasing hopelessness, helplessness, anger, and self-blame, as her perception of her mother changed. She came to view her mother as controlling, intrusive, and suspicious. The patient felt powerless to change the situation because of her belief that to challenge her mother would mean that she was a disloyal, unworthy daughter. Her frustration and anger at her mother contributed to intense guilt and self-deprecation. She withdrew from her usual activities such as church, and isolated herself at home, where the negative interaction with her mother continued.

The patient began individual CT and started on antidepressant medication. Although her concentration and attention were poor, she was not found to suffer from an actual dementia. Initially, her ideas regarding her mother were so rigid that little progress could be made in altering them. Therapy focused on teaching the cognitive model, openly discussing her thoughts of hopelessness and helplessness, and beginning an activities program involving many social interactions. As she started to form attachments to staff and other patients and her mood improved slightly, she was given homework assignments that involved a progressive increase of activities and a notation of the effects of these activities on her mood. Reviewing the homework allowed the patient to see that her pessimistic beliefs about her ability to enjoy herself with others were inaccurate.

At this point, Mrs F. was able to recognize negative automatic thoughts flowing from her relationship with her mother. One example was, "I am an evil person because I have angry thoughts about my mother." Examination of automatic thoughts of this type presented a number of opportunities to work with the patient's tendency toward rigid, dichotomous thinking. She was able to see ample evidence that she was not an "evil person" in other aspects of her life. She was also able to acknowledge that even the most loving person would eventually have some negative reaction to her mother's behavior. The CT sessions that had initially been brief and integrated with daily rounds, became longer and more intensive as her concentration improved. The therapist also focused on automatic thoughts related to Mrs. F.'s belief that she was powerless to change her problems. Finally, Mrs. F. was able to examine her belief that she was obligated to have her mother live with her. Her guilty thoughts regarding her desire to have her mother leave were countered. At this juncture, the patient's children were involved in family therapy sessions. They supported her and made arrangements for a retirement home for the patient's mother. Much to Mrs. F.'s surprise, her mother welcomed the move. Mrs. F. continued to improve and was discharged after an 18-day hospital stay.

SUMMARY

Depression in the elderly is a problem that will increase in magnitude as our society ages. Unfortunately, depression is often overlooked in this age group. Although antidepressant medications can be beneficial, there are many problems associated with their use in this population. Therefore, psychotherapy is an attractive alternative.

Although the elderly have often been viewed as poor candidates for psychotherapy, research supports the use of cognitive therapy for elderly depressives. Cognitive therapy procedures can be adapted for use with depressed geriatric inpatients, including those with mild dementia. Modifications include a simplification of therapy techniques, using short, frequent sessions, and combining cognitive therapy with other interventions. "Real-life" losses are frequently experienced by elderly patients, and treating depression in such instances is a challenge for the therapist. However, the cognitive therapist can help patients recapture past means of coping and rediscover remaining strengths.

This chapter introduces the concept of supportive cognitive therapy. Strategies derived from standard CT are applied in repetitive informal contacts in the inpatient setting. In this manner, the benefits of the CT approach can be offered to a wide variety of individuals who would not ordinarily be considered to be good candidates for psychotherapy. We conclude that cognitive therapy offers pragmatic and effective tools for treating elderly psychiatric inpatients.

REFERENCES

Alford, B. A., Freeman, A., Beck, A. T., & Wright, F. D. (1990). Brief focused cognitive therapy of panic disorders. *Psychotherapy, 27,* 230–234.

Barlow, D. H., Cohen, A. S., & Waddell, M. T. (1984). Panic and generalized anxiety disorders: Nature and treatment. *Behavior Therapy, 15,* 431–449.

Beutler, L. E., Scogin, F., Kinkish, P., Schretlen, D., Corbishley, A., Hamblin, D., Meredith, K., Potter, R., Bamford, C., & Levenson, A. (1987). Group cognitive therapy and alprazolam in the treatment of depression in older adults. *Journal of Consulting and Clinical Psychology, 55,* 550–556.

Blazer, D., Hughes, D. C., & George, L. K. (1987). The epidemiology of depression in an elderly community population. *Gerontologist, 27,* 281–287.

Bureau of the Census. (1986). *Age structure of the United States population in the 21st century* (D.C. statistical brief SB-1-86). Washington, DC: U.S. Government Printing Office.

Casey, D. A. (1991). Suicide in the elderly: A two-year study of death certificate data. *Southern Medical Journal, 84*(10), 1185–1187.

Clark, D. M. (1986). A cognitive approach to panic. *Behaviour Research and Therapy, 24,* 461–470

Dobson, K. S. (1989). A meta-analysis of the efficacy of cognitive therapy for depression. *Journal of Consulting and Clinical Psychology, 57,* 414–419.

Erikson, E. (1963). *Childhood and society* (2nd ed.). New York: W. W. Norton.

Erikson, E. (1968). The human life cycle. In D. Sills (Ed.), *International encyclopedia of the social sciences* (pp. 286–292). New York: Macmillan.

Freud, S. (1950). On psychotherapy. *Collected papers,* Vol. 1 (pp. 249–263). London: Hogarth Press. (Original work published 1904.)

Gallagher, D. E., & Thompson, L. W. (1982). Differential effectiveness of psychotherapies for the treatment of major depressive disorders in older adult patients. *Psychotherapy: Theory, Research, and Practice, 27,* 482–490.

Gallagher, D. E., & Thompson, L. W. (1983). Effectiveness of psychotherapy for both endogenous and non-endogenous depression in older adult outpatients. *Journal of Gerontology, 38*, 707–712.

German, P. S., Shapiro, S., & Skinner, E. A. (1985). Mental health of the elderly: Use of health and mental health services. *Journal of American Geriatric Society, 33*, 246–252.

Gurland, B. J. (1976). The comparative frequency depression in various adult age groups. *Journal of Gerontology, 31*, 283–292.

Jenike, M. A. (1985). *Handbook of geriatric psychopharmacology*. Littleton, MA: PSG Publishing.

Klerman, G. L., Lavori, P. W., Rice, J., Reich, T., Endicott, J., Andreasen, N. C., Keller, M. B., & Hirschfield, R. M. A. (1986). Birth-cohort trends in rates of major depressive disorder among relatives of patients with affective disorder. *Archives of General Psychiatry, 47*, 689–693.

Lazarus, L. W. (1980). Self-psychology and psychotherapy with the elderly: Theory and practice. *Journal of Geriatric Psychiatry, 13*, 69–88.

Lazarus, L. W., Groves, L., Newton, N., Gutmann, D., Ripeckyj, A., Frankl, R., Grunes, J., & Havasy-Galloway, S. (1984). Brief psychotherapy with the elderly: A review and preliminary study and outcome. In L. Lazarus (Ed.), *Psychotherapy with the elderly* (pp. 15–35). Washington, DC: American Psychiatric Press.

Peck, R. C. (1968). Psychological developments in the second half of life. In B. L. Neugarten (Ed.), *Middle age and aging*. Chicago: University of Chicago Press.

Raskin, A., & Rae, D. S. (1981). Psychiatric symptoms in the elderly. *Psychopharmacology Bulletin, 16*, 23–25.

Raskin, A., & Sathonanthan, G. (1979). Depression in the elderly. *Psychopharmacology Bulletin, 15*(2), 14–16.

Reifler, B., Larson, E., & Hanley, R. (1982). Co-existence of cognitive impairment and depression in geriatric outpatients. *American Journal of Psychiatry, 139*, 623–626.

Salzman, C. (1984). *Clinical geriatric psychopharmacology*. New York: McGraw–Hill.

Scogin, F., Jamison, C., & Gochmaur, K (1989). Comparative efficacy of cognitive and behavioral bibliotherapy for mildly and moderately depressed older adults. *Journal of Consulting and Clinical Psychology, 57*, 403–407.

Spar, J., Ford, C., & Liston, E. (1980). Hospital treatment of elderly neuropsychiatric patients. II: Statistical profile of the first one-hundred twenty-two patients in a new teaching ward. *Journal of American Geriatric Society, 28*, 529–543.

Steuer, J., Mintz, J., Hammen, C., Hill, M., Jarvik, L., McCarley, T., Motoike, P., & Rosen, R. (1984). Cognitive behavioral and psychodynamic group psychotherapy in treatment of geriatric depression. *Journal of Consulting and Clinical Psychology, 52*, 180–189.

Thompson, L. W., Davies, R., Gallagher, D., & Krantz, S. E. (1986). Cognitive therapy with older adults. In T. L. Bring (Ed.), *Clinical gerontology: A guide to assessment and intervention* (pp. 245–279). New York: Haworth Press.

Thompson, L. W., Gallagher, D., & Breckinridge, J. S. (1987). Comparative effectiveness of psychotherapies for depressed elders. *Journal of Consulting and Clinical Psychology, 55*, 385–390.

Wells, C. F. (1979). Pseudodementia. *American Journal of Psychiatry, 136*, 895–900.

Wright, J. H. (1987). Cognitive therapy and medication as a combined treatment. In A. Freeman & V. B. Greenwood (Eds.), *Cognitive therapy: Applications in medical and psychiatric settings* (pp. 36–51). New York: Human Services Press.

Wright, J. H., & Borden, J. (1991). Cognitive therapy of depression and anxiety. *Psychiatric Annals, 21*, 424–428.

Wright, J. H., & Schrodt, G. R., Jr. (1989). Combined cognitive therapy and pharmacotherapy. In A. Freeman, M. K. Simon, H. Arkowitz, & L. Beutler (Eds.), *Handbook of cognitive therapy* (pp. 267–282). New York: Plenum Press.

Chapter 12

Cognitive Therapy of Alcoholism

Curtis L. Barrett, Ph.D.,
and Robert G. Meyer, Ph.D.

"Stinkin' thinkin' leads to drinkin'."
—AA saying

". . . the main problem of the alcoholic centers in his mind, rather than in his body."
—The "Big Book" (AA, 1976)

The condition or disease that we call alcoholism has existed for all of humanity's recorded history. If we were to follow tradition and name the disease for an individual who described its course in great detail, alcoholism might be called "Jellinek disease" after the pioneering work of E. M. Jellinek (1960). However, cognitive therapy theorists and practitioners might find it more comfortable to name the disease for the first victim who was documented as showing the major cognitive symptoms of alcoholism. In this case, we would recommend using "Noah disease."

The ninth chapter of the *Book of Genesis* describes Noah's drunkenness and loss of control to the extent of falling asleep naked before rolling down the sides of his tent. His son Ham saw what his father had done and sought help from Noah's other two sons, Shem and Japeth. Shem and Japeth literally "covered up" Noah's nakedness by putting a garment between their shoulders and *backing* up to their father so as to avoid having direct knowledge of his drunkenness and nakedness. Thus, Shem and Japeth also can qualify as the first documented enablers. They protected Noah from the full consequences of his drunken behavior.

When he awoke, Noah apparently realized what had happened but, exhibiting distortions that are familiar to those recognized in the cognitive model of psychopathology, "knew what his younger son had done *unto* him" [italics added]. That is, he interpreted Ham's actions as done to him rather than for him. He discounted, or denied, the facts of his own drunken behavior. As we might expect, the enablers Shem and Japeth were rewarded by Noah. Then Noah cursed Ham's son, Canaan, and declared: "a servant of servants shall he be unto his brethren." Once more, we see a feature of the coping styles used by alcoholics: *indirectness*. To punish Ham, Noah cursed Ham's son.

We will not settle here the issue of naming the condition commonly called alcoholism. These historical perspectives are noted simply as a vehicle for explaining why we are choosing to avoid any attempt to deal with the myriad of scientific and clinical controversies about alcoholism and its treatment. We acknowledge from the outset that some will debate whether addiction of any sort exists, whether alcoholism is best thought of as a disease or habit, whether genetic loading is a factor in developing alcoholism, whether an abstinence-based approach to therapy is essential, whether nonalcoholic therapists can treat the disorder, and hundreds of other important issues. At the present time, controversies about alcohol abuse rage around us, and, all too frequently, these controversies find their way into economic and political arenas. There need be no satisfactory resolution of these issues for us to describe some things that we think help patients who suffer from alcoholism, however these individuals are diagnosed or labeled.

It is not our purpose here to provide an extensive review of the literature on applications of cognitive therapy to the treatment of substance abuse or addictions. However, we would be remiss in not inviting attention to that literature. One of the earliest contributions was by Beck and Emery (1977), who provided a general guidebook for applying cognitive therapy (CT) to problems of substance abuse. This work was continued by Emery and Fox (1981). More recently, Beck, Wright, and Newman (in press) extended this line of inquiry to treatment of cocaine abuse. In a series of papers, the "Philadelphia group" (e.g., Woody et al., 1983) explored use of psychotherapy with opiate addicts. Marlatt and Gordon (1985) provided a comprehensive volume describing use of CT in preventing relapse, on which Gorski and Miller (1986) have anchored a full program for relapse prevention. Schlesinger and Horberg (1988) developed a systematic CT-based approach to therapy for families of addicts. We suggest that any application of CT, for a total program in treating the addicted, be based in this literature. Finally, we note that Walsh et al. (1991) have demonstrated the value of inpatient experience to initiate therapy over referral to self-help groups or outpatient therapy.

The focus of this chapter is limited. Our interest is the use of cognitive therapy with alcoholics, not addicts in general, and with alcoholics who are admitted to an inpatient treatment setting. In our view, the cognitive therapist who deals with hospitalized alcoholic patients has several advantages. The hospitalized patient can be observed 24 hours per day in a wide variety of situations (e.g., group therapy, milieu activities, unit-community meetings, and following return from therapeutic passes). Confrontation about whether the patient is "using" is simple: the hospital laboratory arbitrates this with accurate and rapid test results.

Unfortunately, inpatient treatment of alcoholics has drawbacks also. The era of 28- to 90-day inpatient treatment programs, as a norm, is gone. Today, inpatient therapists usually see precious time spent in detoxification of very ill patients. Thus, when detoxification is complete, the patient may have little time left in the hospital. Further, the patient's ability to deal with abstract concepts may be severely impaired for days. Drugs necessary for good medical practice (e.g., to protect the patient from undue distress or seizures) also may impair cognitive processes. For these reasons, the cognitive therapist must develop very specific goals for each patient and must meet them efficiently if long-term therapy is to succeed. The therapist may even have to advocate for limited use of scarce inpatient resources in order to leave the patient a reserve "account" of insurable days for the future in the fairly likely event of relapse.

In our approach to treating alcoholics on an inpatient psychiatric ward of a general hospital, it has proved useful to take, as given, the following propositions.

1. Alcoholism is a progressive disease that can be fatal if unchecked.
2. Alcoholism has four aspects that must be treated. These may be called the biological, the psychological, the sociological, and the spiritual.
3. Once alcoholism has developed, the human body seems to require some 9 to 15 months to adjust to an alcohol-free life style. The vast majority of relapses and outright treatment failures occur in the first 15 months after the onset of abstinence.
4. Even though recovery from alcoholism is a lifelong proposition, most successful alcoholics have achieved a relapse-resistant program of recovery within 2 to 3 years.

These propositions amount to underlying schemas that govern the behavior of cognitive therapists who work with inpatient alcoholics. Progress in therapy, in large measure, may be judged by the degree to which the patient comes to share the therapist's schema and begins to behave in ways that are consistent with this philosophy of treatment. Therapeutic activity aims at identifying other schemas that govern the alcoholic's behavior and modifying or extinguishing these schemas. Thus, there is very little that distinguishes the therapeutic *strategy* associated with treating alcoholism by cognitive therapy from the therapeutic strategies used in treating depression, anxiety, or personality disorders. However, there *are* major differences in tactics as well as in the content of automatic thoughts that are manifest as a result of underlying schemas. Perhaps the best illustration of these differences lies in the way the patient's verbalizations of helplessness or powerlessness are viewed.

HELPLESSNESS AND POWERLESSNESS

Persons who suffer from depression often perceive themselves as helpless and powerless. The negative cognitive triad is reliably observed. That is, depressed patients view themselves, their present experience, and their future in a negative perspective. Cognitive therapy aims at changing these perceptions.

Very soon after admission to an alcoholism treatment unit, alcoholics typically demonstrate almost the opposite cognitive pattern. Despite overwhelmingly negative input from the biological and sociological aspects of their lives, alcoholics paint a positive picture of their health and circumstances; optimism reigns. For example, liver function tests that are not indicative of imminently terminal illness are taken as evidence that the disease of alcoholism has "not yet" taken hold of the patient's body. Psychological testing that shows significant, though probably not permanent, brain dysfunction is received by the patient almost with elation. Implications of these effects of chronic intoxication for coping with the stressful events of returning to family and work are similarly discounted. The alcoholic often expects the therapist to accept that the patient's spouse is overjoyed at the patient's being so quickly "cured" and that the employer is imploring the patient to return to work at once. Of course, the therapist's moves to obtain first-hand contact with spouse or employer may be rebuffed or frankly forbidden. The idea that the alcoholic patient may be seeking discharge in order to regain access to alcohol is, of course, vigorously refuted by the patient.

What of the perception of personal power in the recently admitted alcoholic? Again, unlike the depressed individual, the alcoholic patient on an inpatient ward is soon to be found on the phone trying to take charge of his or her life. Indeed, an experienced therapist often can pick out the alcoholics on an inpatient ward by observing who spends the most time on the telephone. Typically, the alcoholic patient soon appears outwardly self-assured and positive that he or she knows exactly what to do and how to do it. With great confidence, the alcoholic patient takes a few days of hospital-based abstinence as incontrovertible evidence that the disease has not really affected him or her. Far from presenting as powerless or helpless, the recently abstinent alcoholic shows an unrealistic sense of power to deal with the disease even when he or she is able to admit that it is present.

Often the staff of a psychiatric ward will appear to agree with the patient. Compared with psychotic patients and some others found on a general psychiatric ward, the alcoholic patient can appear to be rather sound. This is particularly so if the alcoholic patient is successful in avoiding situations on the ward that require clear thinking rather than socializing. Thus, one of the first tasks of the therapist is to establish with staff that the patient is more impaired than is readily apparent. Also, the therapist has to engage the patient's collaboration in order to *induce* perceptions of powerlessness and helplessness (rather than to counter them as would be necessary with depressed patients).

Therapists who have worked with alcoholics, utilizing more conventional treatment methods, may respond to the foregoing by labeling the patient's behavior as "denial." They may also view the process of resistance as "old hat" and say, simply, that the patient has not yet reached a useful "bottom." It follows in such models that about the only alternative is to wait until the patient is "ready." We have worked in settings where such models were dominant. To us it seemed that the model might be perfectly appropriate for a self-help program that claims to work with "those who want to recover and not those who need to recover." However, such models are not at all satisfying to professional therapists. These therapists view the alcoholic, on admission, as little different from the trauma patient admitted to an emergency room. A life-threatening condition is presented, and it does not matter that the patient cannot understand the threat to his or her life. It is the expertise of the professional that is on the line, and time is of the essence. If the first window of opportunity to treat the alcoholic is not used successfully, there may not be another one. Nearly every therapist who works with alcoholism has learned of a relapsed patient who committed suicide or died in an accident before successful treatment could be accomplished. There is little comfort in lamenting that the patient was "not ready." It is equally true that the therapy was "not ready" to deal with the state of illness with which the patient presented.

How may we use cognitive therapy to induce powerlessness and helplessness in alcoholic inpatients and, thereby, reach both those who are "ready" and those who are not? It is best to start with the relatively simple strategy of providing information to the patient without lecturing, cajoling, or otherwise precipitating pathological resistance in the patient. By *direct questioning*, the therapist may learn what the patient believes to be the nature of alcoholism in others and need not insist that the patient apply that to his or her own case. Usually the patient presents rather stereotyped views such as: "Alcohol is just a crutch. . . . alcoholics are skid-row bums. . . . I'm not that bad yet. . . . I know a lot of people who drink more than I do, and they aren't alcoholics. . . . I might have let it get out of hand, but now I know to cut back or just quit using it altogether."

Once the therapist knows how the patient views alcoholism and alcoholics, the next (and, perhaps, the most crucial) step is to establish that *collaborative empiricism* will be used in developing a factual base that the therapist and the patient will come to share. The reason that this step is so critical is that an alternative approach is so tempting. For example, it may appear that the therapist should attempt to batter through the patient's denial system by use of authority or threat. Such techniques are well known to stiffen resistance to therapy or to induce outwardly compliant passive–aggressive behavior. It is very common at this stage of treatment for the patient to decide to adopt a strategy of compliance for the duration of the hospitalization, which is known to be short, and to begin thinking of resumed drinking as a "reward" on discharge for such compliant behavior. It is absolutely necessary, in our experience, to establish that the therapist will not degrade the patient and will preserve the patient's dignity. It also is highly useful in the beginning of therapy, especially for the therapist who is not recovering from a substance abuse-problem, to attribute any socially noxious or criminal behaviors of the patient to the disease process. The therapist should suspend any judgment of the patient's character until the patient has been abstinent for a year or more.[1]

[1]It should be apparent that the cognitive therapist who works with alcoholics must examine, rather closely, his or her own automatic thoughts and schemas concerning alcoholism. We have observed therapists who, while insisting that alcoholism is a chronic disease like any other chronic disease, will hold the alcoholic patient responsible for socially noxious or illegal behaviors, e.g., nonpayment of child support, loss of bowel or bladder control, drug seeking, or manipulative behaviors. They probably would not respond similarly to a stroke victim even if that person had neglected treatment for hypertension or otherwise "brought it on himself."

Generally, we ask the patient to accept, as a starting point for therapy, the idea that "properly diagnosed" alcoholism is a progressive, usually fatal, disease. We sidestep initial resistance by using the term "properly diagnosed" and allow the patient to keep his or her own diagnosis an open issue. Rarely do we find patients who will not take this step. We then explain that progressive means that the disease, once established, continues to worsen throughout the course of life. One does not become abstinent for a time and then get to start all over again. If relapsed, the alcoholic picks up where he or she would have been if the drinking had continued. The term "usually fatal" is not elaborated at this point. We simply ask the patient to recognize that properly diagnosed but unsuccessfully treated alcoholics have a very high rate of suicide, traffic accidents, and medical disorders related to alcohol abuse.

We place our emphasis on the concept of "disease." We ask the patient to tell us about some diseases that he or she believes might be like alcoholism. As much as possible we use *guided discovery* to move the patient toward diseases that have some rather clear physical cause, such as diabetes or malaria. We may also, at this point, suggest that injuries such as those from burns are comparable conditions in that they may be caused by toxic chemicals or fire.

Once the patient is willing to examine the nature of disease, including that of alcoholism, we raise the question of pitting one's "will power" against the disease. We may ask the patient directly to suggest some common diseases that he would treat using will power. Following the principles of *guided discovery* and *collaborative empiricism*, we start with whatever the patient may give us. Our goal is to set up a parallel between dealing with, say, malaria, through will power and dealing with alcoholism through will power.

Sooner or later, we introduce the idea that alcohol itself is a chemical and, therefore, has similarities to other chemicals or substances. At this point we are ready to suggest that both diseases and chemicals present forces that we, as human beings, cannot oppose without help. We may ask what the patient would think of a person who poured gasoline on his arm and proposed to set it aflame and prevent injury to his arm by force of will. We have also found it useful to use *hyperbole*, gently, by asking the patient to imagine having to oppose the effects of an enema or laxative by using will power. Generally, by this time, the patient has become willing to accept that "properly diagnosed" alcoholism is no more treatable by "will power" than is any other such disease. At a later time, this realization may be related to the first step toward

[2]We are aware, of course, that this is a point of debate in the literature. For purposes of therapy, we accept it as at least a useful theory and possibly as scientifically reliable.

recovery, as it is defined by Alcoholics Anonymous. That step says: "We admitted we were powerless over alcohol—that our lives had become unmanageable." However, we carefully suggest that the patient does not have to admit powerlessness over *all* alcohol. It is only necessary to admit powerlessness over alcohol that has been introduced into the diseased body of an alcoholic.

We depict "alcohol" as a neutral substance that will behave reliably according to basic rules of chemistry, thereby attempting to remove the emotional association with the substance. It is made clear that without a decision to introduce the alcohol into his or her body, the alcoholic is no more harmed by alcohol than is anyone else. It is often surprising to see how much this face-saving device can mean to a recently admitted, ambivalent alcoholic patient. Much of the defensiveness (denial) that is encountered in other models seems to be circumvented by this cognitive therapy technique. Yet it also establishes effectively that the patient is, if alcoholic, "powerless over alcohol."

Continuing along this line, with guided discovery, we test the patient's progress in taking what amounts to the "first step" suggested by Alcoholics Anonymous. Because the patient is usually more cognitively impaired at such times than is readily apparent, we are rather concrete in what we ask of the patient. For example, we may ask: "If alcoholism is a disease, and if it is automatically triggered by taking alcohol into the body of a person who has that disease, does it make any sense at all for a person who is alcoholic to use alcohol?" When the almost inevitable answer is given, we may move on to the next logical question. That is of the sort: "What would you say is the mental condition of a person who takes into his or her body a chemical that is poison for that person?" We may use the examples of allergic reactions to penicillin, bee stings, and other substances before setting up the question about alcohol. The hoped-for result is that the patient will suggest that it is, in some way, "crazy" or "insane" for a person to act in this way. If the patient gives us this point, and usually the patient will do so, we are ready to suggest the second step of Alcoholics Anonymous. That is, active alcoholism (using alcohol when properly diagnosed as "allergic to alcohol") is a form of "insanity." The second step of AA suggests, at the same time, a reaching out for help in some form: "Came to believe that a Power greater than ourselves could restore us to sanity." Thus, the therapist has taken the patient, by guided discovery, through a reversal of ideas of personal power to the point of acknowledging helplessness in the face of an overwhelming chemical force. The patient has not been demeaned or humiliated by the therapist. The patient has not been defined as weak or lacking moral courage. Further, the idea of reaching out for help when faced with something beyond one's control, has been made logical and, we hope, acceptable.

Why such meticulous attention to these parallels to AA's first and second steps? As we explain to the patients, using examples, we know of no tasks that can be completed successfully without taking the first step. Somehow, every successful treatment for properly diagnosed alcoholism seems to have been based on a period of sustained abstinence. That period of abstinence typically is based on the belief that one will be powerless over alcohol if it is ingested. When these steps, or their equivalent, have not been taken, we have observed that the failure to maintain sobriety is just a matter of time. We do not argue here whether tapering or controlled drinking may work for some alcoholics. We simply assert that these have not proved to be viable strategies for hospitalized alcoholic patients.

FROM BIOLOGICAL TO PSYCHOLOGICAL

As indicated above, we hold that there are four aspects to the disease of alcoholism: biological, psychological, sociological, and spiritual. The first two steps of Alcoholics Anonymous, as described above, facilitate acceptance that alcoholism is a biological phenomenon, a disease. Yet, they do not give an understanding of "alcoholic thinking." Nevertheless, the "Big Book" of Alcoholics Anonymous makes clear that the psychological processes related to relapses are baffling.

> . . . the main problem of the alcoholic centers in his mind, rather than his body. If you ask him why he started on that last bender, chances are he will offer you any one of a hundred alibis. . . . If you draw this fallacious reasoning to the attention of an alcoholic, he will laugh it off, or become irritable and refuse to talk. Once in a while, he may tell the truth. And the truth, strange to say, is usually that he has no more idea why he took that first drink than you have. Some drinkers have excuses with which they are satisfied part of the time. But in their hearts they really do not know why they do it. Once this malady has a real hold, they are a baffled lot. (AA, 1976, p. 23)

We postulate that there is a biological basis for relapse in the first 9 to 15 months of abstinence that probably is not present later in the recovery process. Using guided discovery again, we suggest to the patient a very simple exercise to illustrate how biological processes may dictate psychological (thought) processes. We ask the patient to hold his or her breath and, after a deep breath has been taken, we indicate that the task is to hold the breath for about 3 minutes. Often the patient exhales at once and gives us a puzzled look! We assure the patient that what we ask is possible, and usually they start again. Naturally, well before 3 minutes, the patient takes a breath. The next step is to debrief the patient on the thoughts that he or she had while holding the breath. With some adroit questioning the patient usually can identify thoughts that are similar to those commonly occurring in other patients. The patient may start out with optimistic or competitive thoughts. Next, they may think of reasons to discontinue but save face, such as an outside noise to blame for distraction. At some point, the patient usually starts to have angry or hostile thoughts toward the task and, perhaps, toward the therapist. These thoughts are used to illustrate the manner in which the biological process seemed to create the thought pattern that was necessary in order to justify taking a breath. There were even thoughts of the sort needed to justify violating a social situation such as a promise to try hard. Whenever possible, the patient is asked to write down the thoughts that occurred while holding a breath. This exercise may even be done usefully in a group setting to illustrate that the thoughts that come are similar across individuals. If there is a relapsed person in the group, that person may volunteer that the thoughts are similar to those he or she had at relapse, such as resentments, anger, or "what the hell."

This exercise may have to be repeated several times in the course of therapy in order to reinforce the important point that is being made. That is, the biological need (e.g., for alcohol or oxygen) seems to elicit *whatever thoughts may be necessary* in order to justify satisfying that biological need. Further, the thoughts are most likely to be indirect rather than direct. Patients will not think "breathe, you need oxygen" any more than they will think "drink, you need alcohol." The thoughts that come will serve to *justify* breathing or drinking, for example, "That man is crazy to ask me to hold my breath that long" or "With a wife like mine griping day in and day out, anyone would have to have some relief." Even if these self-statements are true, the final response is to the actual body message—breathe, drink.

In our experience, patients accept the *reattribution* that their behavior, in relapsing, has been driven by a biological process that was out of their awareness. There is often a sense of profound relief that they show physically and can report. It is important for the therapist to pick up on this emotional shift and to explore the automatic thoughts that accompany it. When all goes well, the patient takes the next step in therapy and asks what to do about this process in order to stay abstinent. If the patient does not ask, the therapist primes this process with the suggestion that the time has come to deal with that question.

FROM TRUSTING ONESELF TO TRUSTING ONE'S TREATMENT PROGRAM

Earlier, we indicated that alcoholics voice unrealistic positive views of themselves and their capabilities. When the techniques of cognitive therapy have brought the patient to accept powerlessness over alcohol once it is taken into his or her body, as well as the idea that a biological process can dictate thinking that may justify a relapse ("stinking thinking"), the patient often expresses uncharacteristic hopelessness. This may be taken as a sign of progress in the treatment of alcoholism. The patient may ask for help in a more genuine, authentic way. When this happens, the therapist may introduce the idea of "ganging up on the disease." A visualization exercise that has proved useful for this purpose is as follows. The patient first visualizes trying to hold back a huge boulder all by himself and then visualizes the same situation equipped with various tools and with other individuals available. The analogy is usually persuasive. "Ganging up on the disease" is interpreted to mean using various components of an overall therapy plan. The plan is articulated to include professional therapy (including group treatment), any prescribed medication, and self-help or twelve-step organizations. This is often the moment to use a time-honored phrase from the "Big Book" of Alcoholics Anonymous: "Remember that we deal with alcohol—cunning, baffling, powerful! Without help it is too much for us" (AA, 1976, p. 58).

We may contrast the cognitive therapy approach with the more common, directive style of some twelve-step-based programs. With the guided discovery technique, the *patient* discovers a need to attend group therapy, AA meetings, and other helpful activities. The *patient* takes ownership of the therapy process and can be reinforced by the therapist for taking a step toward coping with his or her disease. Many twelve-step programs give succinct instructions that, although helpful to those who accept and follow them, do not offer much new learning for the patient. Worse, such instructions may precipitate even more resistance in the patient. Typical of these is the instruction: "Don't drink, read the 'Big Book,' get a sponsor, and go to meetings." Sometimes specific goals are set: "Make ninety meetings in ninety days." It is true, no doubt, that one who follows these instructions will come to have a sense of "owning" the program that is being followed. However, too much is left to chance. The cognitive therapist, by contrast, assesses in an early session from ample receipt of feedback whether the patient is progressing toward owning a program of recovery. If the patient is at that point, there is no reason not to use suggestions just like those used in traditional programs. On the other hand, such therapeutic shortcuts may cost dearly later in the process. The best strategy assures that the patient owns and trusts the treatment program.

COGNITIVE THERAPY AND THE SOCIOLOGICAL ASPECTS OF ALCOHOLISM

It is very seldom that one treats an individual in an inpatient setting who has no family, occupational, or other social entity affected by his or her disease. Even the most serious, frequently relapsed cases are likely to be in a problematic relationship with the courts or social welfare organizations. In our experience, it is useful (and perhaps even imperative) to involve in the therapy process some representative of every social entity still important to the patient. This includes not only family members and the employer but also the patient's priest or minister, neighbors who care, drinking buddies, extended family, social welfare agencies, and so forth. Often these individuals are not identified by the patient but become known when they visit the patient on the ward.

In our view, the patient's consent should be routinely obtained so that every visitor understands why the patient is in the hospital and what role he or she may play in the patient's recovery. Generally, it is fruitful to have the patient show the visitor a movie or video on alcoholism such as that made by Father Joseph Martin: *Chalk Talk* (Ashley, 1975). In this way, the patient not only reviews the points made in the movie but benefits from the changed attitude or understanding that the visitor may develop. Very destructive "enabling" behavior can be reduced in many cases by this technique. We recall one instance in which a visitor initially took issue with the patient's diagnosis, since the visitor said he "spilled more whiskey than [the patient] drank." In the process of viewing the videotape, the visitor decided that he too should stop drinking! This had an obvious effect on the patient.

Whenever possible, a meeting of the "members of the problem" is arranged, and standard group process techniques are used to elicit data in order to clarify the diagnosis and its dimensions. Nearly always there is diversity of opinion in the group and evidence that secret-keeping, conspiracies of silence, jockeying for family position, and other processes abound. In one case, we found that the family's opinion leader, who seemed at first blush to have little family power, believed that her brother could quit drinking anytime that he desired to do so. To her, it was simply a matter of will power, and she knew, from living with him, that he had plenty of will power. In another case we learned to our great surprise that the most leverage over the patient's behavior was held by his adult mentally retarded child. The patient was able to resist all attempts to bring him into the hospital for treatment of alcoholism until the child said: "I don't like you any more. You scare me when you are drunk." Hearing that, the patient began to cry and consented to come in for treatment. Later we learned of the guilt he carried at having conceived a child late in life, while drunk, and learning subsequently that the child's Down syndrome was associated with late-life conception.

Almost always in these sessions some family member postulates that "will power" is the answer to the problem of alcoholism. Usually this comes up despite our best efforts at teaching the family and others that alcoholism, as a disease, is not defined as a deficiency of will power. Cognitive techniques, usually of the guided discovery variety, are very helpful when the "will power solution" surfaces. Generally, when this occurs, we shift from group process techniques to one-on-one in a group. We persist until the "will power advocate" concedes that his or her position is that biochemical processes are subject to voluntary control. Since "will power advocates" usually do not suffer from alcoholism, they are likely to accept that what applies to the patient applies to them as well. Continuing with the technique of guided discovery, we suggest that they should demonstrate the point so that it can be understood by all. We suggest, more specifically, that they demonstrate their proficiency in controlling biochemical processes through will power. Using mild hyperbole, we ask them to consider eating several bars of a special kind of candy bar, which is actually a powerful over-the-counter laxative, and then returning to the group to demonstrate their control over this chemical. Properly done, this usually precipitates a good-humored laugh from all present, and the point is made. Naturally, clinical sensitivity is necessary to avoid embarrassing the "will power advocate" and to avoid any suggestion that individuals coming to the group meeting will be humiliated or demeaned.

Once there is agreement among the patient's sociological network that a program of treatment is needed and that the members have a role to play, attention can be directed at bringing out the group's memories of the patient's drinking behavior. At first, the "members of the problem" are only asked to recall general events. However, when the group is comfortable with talking about the past events, the therapist asks that they recall instances in which they acted as "enablers." Emphasis is kept on the instances in which the person covered up for the patient or, in other ways, participated in the deceptive strategy adopted by the patient.

Faced with the fact of past enabling behavior, the "member of the problem" is asked to suggest alternative actions or statements that he or she could have used in the situations. The participants can take turns in presenting situations, including the old responses and the new responses that have been generated. The timing is almost always appropriate then to develop a *contract* stating that members of the patient's sociological network will use the new, nonenabling strategies in the future.

A prominent problem among the members may be referred to as a "secrecy pact." In time, it is usually revealed that the patient has made agreements with each member of the problem on the condition that the agreement not be revealed to others in the group. When the secret pacts are discovered, the therapist acknowledges that such arrangements usually have some logical basis in the minds of those who make the pacts. The therapist then elicits automatic thoughts associated with the making of a secret pact and proceeds to examine them in the usual way. In one case, the secret pact was with a sister whose automatic thoughts centered around her being the only one who had the sort of relationship with the patient that would lead him to sobriety. She thought of herself as "always special" in his life and "the one he really counts on for help." The patient seemed to agree with her, she thought, but also seemed not to want others to know of their special relationship. To her surprise, she discovered that her parents (individually), her siblings, and others in the family had the same thoughts. Indeed, it was discovered that the patient, in times of crisis, had confided these "facts" to nearly every member of the family. Thus, it was revealed that nearly every member of the problem had alternated from "savior" to excluded person to villain as the patient extracted what was needed to keep on drinking. The therapist, of course, took pains to explain that this reflected the priority that alcohol had come to have in the patient's life. The behavior was not explicated to the group as evidence of character disorder but, rather, was interpreted as the result of the state of the disease at the time. After all, the patient was in desperate straits trying to maintain the addiction.

In situations such as this, the therapist can find it useful to suggest that the members of the problem attend self-help, twelve-step groups such as Alcoholics Anonymous, Alanon, or Alateen. The opportunity to discover that other alcoholics and their families have had much the same experience reinforces the idea that alcoholism is a disease rather than a weakness in the patient's moral make-up. The therapist capitalizes on the well-known concept of "learning readiness" in determining when to recommend attendance at other helpful meetings.

INTERNAL DIAGNOSIS OF ALCOHOLISM

Several times in the foregoing we have used the phrase "properly diagnosed" before the term "alcoholism." From the professional, clinical, and scientific perspective we are referring to such diagnostic systems as those found in the *Diagnostic and Statistical Manual of Mental Disorders* (DSM-III-R) published by the American Psychiatric Association (APA, 1987). Such diagnoses are, in our thinking, "external diagnoses." They reflect observations and data available from outside of the patient, including self-report. However, the more important diagnosis in the treatment of alcoholism is that made, at an intensely personal level, by the patient. It is significant that Alcoholics Anonymous does not provide a formal definition of alcoholism. In the famous twelve steps the word alcoholism is not mentioned at all. It is to be found in the "three pertinent ideas":

1. That we were alcoholic and could not manage our own lives.
2. That probably no human power could have relieved our alcoholism.
3. That God could and would if He were sought. (AA, 1976, p. 60)

The "system" of self-diagnosis that is used in AA is simple. One reads stories describing alcoholism as it occurred in real persons and one hears the stories of real individuals claiming to be alcoholic at AA meetings. If there is a match, the diagnosis may be made by the individual. In time, the identity is accepted and endorsed, and the individual begins to announce himself or herself, at least at AA meetings, as alcoholic.

Obviously, cognitive therapy of alcoholism will be helpful sooner if the patient accepts that a proper diagnosis has been made. Therefore, efforts in this direction are made just as soon as the patient seems to accept that alcoholism is a disease that has biological and psychological aspects.

The first step in assisting with self-diagnosis is to elicit the automatic thoughts that the patient has when thinking of the term "alcoholic." In most cases, given the familial nature of the disease, the automatic thoughts will center around one or more family members. Also, there probably will be events around which concepts of alcoholic behavior are organized. It is unlikely that the patient will refer to himself or herself in this phase. From what the patient produces, the therapist may infer the patient's "assumptive world" (Frank, 1963) that has been constructed with regard to alcoholism and alcoholics. It is likely that cognitive distortions, such as absolutistic or global thinking, will become apparent. If this happens, the patient may be asked to state the evidence that alcoholics and alcoholism fit the description that has been given. It may be useful to use the *double-column technique* to examine the strengths and weaknesses of each bit of evidence that the patient offers (e.g., that only "bums" become alcoholic, that saying he or she is alcoholic means that he or she is like the town drunk, or that being alcoholic signals character pathology). With the double-column technique, alternative formulations emerge, and the patient should come to a realistic and accurate perception of what alcoholism and alcoholics are like.

Once this step is completed, the patient may go on to using the double-column technique to list evidence, both pro and con, for the proposition: "My proper diagnosis is alcoholism." The patient is asked to list all possible evidence *for* the proposition and all possible evidence *against* the proposition. The therapist ensures that the evidence is written and, to facilitate this, makes sure that paper and pen are available for both the patient and the therapist. Once all of the evidence has been listed, the therapist suggests that each item be weighted in terms of its importance. Finally, the patient is asked to make a tentative diagnosis and to defend it. Regardless of what the patient decides, the therapist reviews the evidence and then gives the patient the opportunity to request the therapist's diagnosis. Usually, although the diagnosis is self-evident, it is important for the therapist to be prepared for a strong emotional response from the patient. There may be an unexpected breakthrough of emotion. Supportive therapy techniques, of empathy and genuineness, are used to help the patient handle such traumatic self-acceptance.

If the patient is stable enough and otherwise able, the peak emotional response situation is *the* opportune time for the patient to develop a program of recovery and to write it down. The act of surrender (James, 1923) combined with a commitment to recovery make very powerful therapeutic forces.

Regardless of whether surrender and commitment are apparent, it is important that the patient accept the veracity of the personal diagnosis and the program of recovery that follows from it. This is what we refer to as "ownership." The therapist should take the role of guide and facilitator of the program that will be developed in collaboration with the patient. Thus, the therapist should not appear to "own" the recovery program.

PROGRAM OF RECOVERY

Restraints on the length of hospital stay almost always require that the patient be discharged well before the plan of recovery is fully tested. This fact of life makes it imperative that the aftercare treatment plan be intensive and broadly based. If at all possible, a formal relapse-prevention group, preferably based on cognitive therapy, should be provided for patients. We have found Gorski and Miller's (1986) program to fit cognitive therapy well. Attendance at self-help or twelve-step groups also should be made part of the program of recovery except in the most extraordinary circumstances. For example, one of our patients absolutely refused to attend AA meetings because, he said, of an especially humiliating experience that he had had. We did not challenge his story early in his recovery. Eventually, he associated with AA members in our therapy group and was able to be desensitized sufficiently to attend AA. We cite this as an example of being cautious in labeling avoidance of AA as inherently pathological and of being patient with recovering persons.

It is necessary to reinforce frequently the belief that 9 to 15 months are required for the human body to return to normal after prolonged use of alcohol. Just as cognitive therapy calls for recognizing thoughts and addressing maladaptive information processing, it also calls for reinforcing cognitions that may enhance the probability of recovery. The idea of using 2 to 5 years to develop a resilient program of recovery (i.e., one that can be resistant to life's stresses without succumbing to alcohol use) also should be reinforced at every opportunity.

Following discharge, patients are urged to use cognitive therapy techniques in daily living. These techniques do not conflict in any way with the steps and traditions of Alcoholics Anonymous. In fact, one can find clear parallels between the conventional wisdom of AA and the technical requirements of cognitive therapy. Such skills include conflict resolution, collecting evidence, rational decision making, seeking outside opinion, enhancing assertiveness, cognitive rehearsal, avoiding projecting (an AA term) and catastrophizing, and developing more appropriate dependence on others.

COGNITIVE–BEHAVIORAL THERAPY AND USE OF DISULFIRAM

For patients who have had previous relapses and for patients whose work or legal situation makes relapse extremely risky, the use of disulfiram (Antabuse®) may also be considered. This substance has been termed a "chemical fence" that the alcoholic can choose to place between himself or herself and alcohol. Unfortunately, disulfiram treatment has not been shown to have a very high success rate. As Barrett (1985) has discussed, this is mostly because of the failure of clinicians to apply known technology to enhance compliance. All too often, the medication ends up in the medicine cabinet rather than in the patient for whom it was prescribed. Then, of course, the medicine cabinet remains abstinent, and the patient's relapse is just a matter of time.

We have found it best to use cognitive techniques to establish disulfiram as "a chemical to fight a chemical." Once the patient has accepted the biological aspect of alcoholism (using methods described above in considerable detail) and has assessed the risks of relapse, the use of a chemical to fight a chemical can make some sense. If the patient doesn't initiate a request for help, the therapist can suggest it.

We recommend that the procedures developed by Barrett (1985) be followed. The patient is required to come to the clinic daily for the medicine, and there is ongoing cognitive therapy each time the patient appears. At the very least, the patient is reinforced for program compliance that day. Reluctance to coming in daily can be countered with usual cognitive techniques used to deal with "resistance." One technique that has been helpful is to let the patient conclude, through guided discovery, that he or she was always able to make it to the source of alcohol (e.g., liquor store) whether broke, walking, hot, cold, or wet.

The value of supervised ingestion of the prescribed drug has been shown in several of our cases. These patients came to the clinic faithfully, for months, but held the medicine in the mouth rather than swallowing it ("cheeking"). Until we caught on, their relapse the day after taking disulfiram was very surprising. A patient who avoids supervision is very likely to be relapsing.

Disulfiram therapy, combined with cognitive therapy, can be useful for "members of the problem" also. Frequently, the patient's behavior has taken those who care for him or her to the limit of tolerance. Suspicious that the patient has started to use alcohol secretly again, the members of the problem may begin to "play detective." Such checking on the patient, particularly just after discharge from treatment, may combine with usual resentments to justify relapse in the mind of the patient. When members of the problem are assured that the patient is on disulfiram, they are more likely to focus on the reality of the patient's behavior. Day by day, week by week, month by month, they know the patient is recovering. Focus can be on the positive aspects of what the patient is doing, and, when negative behavior has to be confronted, accurate attributions are possible. That is, the patient's behavior and not his or her disease may now be the focus.

In addition to moving patients and "members of the problem" toward the idea of disulfiram as "a chemical to fight a chemical," the therapist may want to use other analogies. For example, we have found it useful in some cases to liken disulfiram to a cast for a broken bone. As we put it, "disulfiram acts as a cast to support the alcoholic while the healing goes on inside." Another view that we have found to be useful is that disulfiram reduces the number of daily decisions that the patient must make about alcohol to *one*. This contrasts with the countless decisions that have to be made when the "chemical fence" is not in place but the environment is full of drinking opportunities.

We are careful to point out that disulfiram does not, in itself, "cure" or "heal." It is just a tool, though an important tool, that promotes the recovery process. This is an important counterattribution. All too often the patient, or others, will perceive disulfiram as another chemical on which to depend and therefore will consider it to be a pathological crutch. For example, at an AA meeting we heard a speaker, sober for 20 years, report that he had been on disulfiram for the first 18 months of this sobriety. One might have expected him to be grateful that he had made it through the first 18 months with the assistance of disulfiram. Instead, he said authoritatively that in his opinion disulfiram was "just a damned crutch." We have wondered how many newcomers took that as a mandate to refuse prescribed disulfiram.

COGNITIVE THERAPY AND THE SPIRITUAL ASPECT OF ALCOHOLISM

Beck and Emery (1977, p. 3), in their treatment manual for cognitive therapy of substance abuse, include biological, social, and behavioral concomitants of addictions but do not deal directly with the "spiritual" aspect of these disorders. However, they observe that cognitive therapy addresses the problems, including personal relationships, that give meaning to life. Our use of the term "spiritual" differs somewhat from the way that it is commonly used in twelve-step self-help groups. If there are significant "spiritual" problems, we ask a pastoral counselor who has special training in cognitive therapy to see the patient. A description of pastoral counseling in a cognitive milieu is contained in Chapter 3.

Our approach is to determine the automatic thoughts and schemas that the patient associates with spirituality and to work at modifying only those that impair recovery (e.g., pathological guilt, blaming God). In the early phases of treatment, including most of the hospitalization stage, we are therefore likely to accept whatever the patient brings to us. Later, in outpatient treatment, we explore the "spiritual" aspect in more detail. Often, for those who do not have well-developed religious orientations or who are frankly agnostic, we substitute "morale" for "spiritual." That is, we foster the idea that humans are social beings and that they are most effective when attacking problems through a shared group effort that respects basic values.

SUMMARY

For purposes of this chapter we have avoided dealing with the myriad of controversies concerning alcoholism and its treatment. We have proposed a working definition of alcoholism as a progressive, often fatal, disease that has four aspects: biological, psychological, sociological, and spiritual. Also, we have focused on ways that cognitive therapy may be used as a component of a program of treatment for alcoholics who have been hospitalized. This hospitalization, in the 1990s, is conceptualized as brief and, in some settings, may rarely exceed 15 days. Alcoholics treated in such settings are likely to be chronically ill and to have relapsed three or more times. Moreover, they are likely to be involved in some problematic relationship with family, employer, courts, or social agencies.

We have outlined cognitive therapy strategies and techniques that have proved useful in overcoming the alcoholic's resistance to treatment, usually termed "pathological denial." In our practice, this approach minimizes the rate of discharges against medical advice. For the most part these strategies and techniques appear little different from those applied in the treatment of depression. However, there are some important exceptions. Notably, alcoholics present with unrealistic self-assessments as being powerful, competent, and optimistic about the future. Techniques used with depressed individuals should be modified, in ways indicated here, to accommodate the specific cognitive psychopathology of alcoholism. Alcoholics must move to an act of surrender and then recognize (reattribute) that they suffer from a disease more powerful than they alone may manage and that strength can come from "ganging up" on the disease.

As far as we can discern, there is nothing in our adaptation of cognitive therapy to the treatment of alcoholism that runs counter to the principles of Alcoholics Anonymous. Nevertheless, there is a difference between the cognitive set of the professional and the helping member of AA. The social role taken by concerned volunteers in AA includes caring but accepting limitations on what can be accomplished. Indeed, the main motivation is defined as "selfish," that is enhancing or maintaining one's own sobriety. Volunteers are helped, in the face of frequent failures to convince alcoholics to seek assistance, by the phrase: "AA is for those who want it, not for those who need it." Professionals, by contrast, have the obligation to respond to the patient's need and to develop technology (e.g., medication or attitude-changing procedures) that will benefit the addicted person even when he or she is not receptive.

In our experience, cognitive therapy is an especially useful approach to treating the alcoholic. Many of the pitfalls of more directive and confrontive techniques, such as those used in "breaking down" denial, are avoided by the collaborative nature of cognitive therapy. The patient and therapist are allies in the process of recovery. However, as treatment proceeds, ownership of the therapy and the responsibility for preserving what has been learned fall increasingly on the recovering person.

We close with one last appeal for those who have the opportunity to work with a suffering alcoholic. Treat the situation as an emergency, analogous to a patient with severe arterial bleeding or the like. In his book *The Cup of Fury*, Upton Sinclair (1956, p. 12) commented on Jack London's writing in *John Barleycorn*.

In this slim volume he described what he called "the Long Sickness" and "the White Logic"—respectively, the pessimism and the skepticism produced by alcoholism—and when he came to the end, he summoned up his conclusions with these words.

> Mine is not a tale of a reformed drunkard. I was never a drunkard and I have not reformed. . . . No . . . I shall take my drink on occasion. With all the books on my shelves, with all the thoughts of the thinkers shaded by my particular temperament, I have decided coolly and deliberately that I should continue to do what I have been trained to want to do. I will drink—but oh, more skillfully, more discretely than ever before. Never again will I be a peripatetic conflagration.

Thus, proudly, Jack London (1913) concluded his story. He went on with his drinking, "more skillfully, more discretely," for 2 or 3 more years. And then, at the age of 40, he gave his last word on the subject by taking his own life. Nearly every alcoholic meets a helping professional on his road to the "bottom" or to death. It is our hope that, in the 1990s, these alcoholics will encounter a therapist who knows and utilizes the new strategies and methods of cognitive therapy.

REFERENCES

AA World Services, Inc. (1976). *Alcoholics Anonymous: The story of how many thousands of men and women have recovered from alcoholism* (3rd ed.). New York: Author.

American Psychiatric Association. (1987). *Diagnostic and statistical manual of mental disorders*, (3rd ed. revised). Washington, DC: Author.

Ashley (1975). *Father Martin's Chalk Talk: The Original*, videotape. Havre De Grace, MD.

Barrett, C. L. (1985). Use of disulfiram in psychological treatment of multiply hospitalized alcoholics. *Bulletin: Society of Psychologists in Addictive Behaviors, 4,* 4.

Beck, A. T., & Emery, G. D. (1977). *Cognitive therapy of substance abuse*. Philadelphia: Center for Cognitive Therapy.

Beck, A. T., Wright, G. D., & Newman, C. F. (in press). Taking the kick out of the habit: Cognitive therapy of cocaine abuse. In A. Freeman & F. Datillio (Eds.), *Casebook of cognitive behavioral therapy*. New York: Plenum Press.

Emery, G. D., & Fox, S. (1981). Cognitive therapy of alcohol dependency. In G. Emery, S. D. Hollon, & R. C. Bedrosian (Eds.), *New directions in cognitive therapy: A casebook* (pp. 181–200). New York: Guilford Press.

Frank, J. (1963). *Persuasion and healing*. Baltimore: Johns Hopkins Press.

Gorski, T., & Miller, M. (1986). *Staying sober: A guide for relapse prevention*. Independence, MO: Independence Press.

James, W. (1923). *Varieties of religious experience*. New York: Longmans, Green.

Jellinek, E. M. (1960). *The disease concept of alcoholism*. New Haven: Hillhouse Press.

London, J. (1913). *John Barleycorn*. New York: Grosset & Dunlap.

Marlatt, G. A. & Gordon, J. R. (Eds.). (1985). *Relapse prevention*. New York: Guilford Press.

Schlesinger, S. E. & Horberg, L. K. (1988). *Taking charge: How families can climb out of the chaos of addiction*. New York: Simon & Schuster (Fireside).

Sinclair, U. (1956). *The cup of fury*. Great Neck, NY: Channel Press.

Walsh, D. C., Hingson, R. W., Merrigan, D. M., Levenson, S. M., Cuddles, A., Heeren, T., Coffman, G. A., Becker, C. A., Barker, T. A., Hamilton, S. K., McGuire, T. G., & Kelly, C. A. (1991). A randomized trial of treatment options for alcohol-abusing workers. *New England Journal of Medicine, 235*(11), 775–782.

Woody, G. E., Luborsky, L., McLellan, A. T., O'Brien, C. P., Beck, A. T., Blaine, J., Herman, I., & Hole, A. (1983). Psychotherapy for opiate addicts: Does it help? *Archives of General Psychiatry, 40,* 639–645.

Chapter 13

Cognitive Therapy for Eating Disorders

Wayne A. Bowers, Ph.D.

The use of cognitive therapy (Beck, Rush, Shaw, & Emery, 1979) and related cognitive–behavioral therapies has grown over the past 10 years because it has consistently been shown to be an effective treatment for depression (Hollon & Beck, 1986). In more recent years, reports have begun to appear on the treatment of anxiety disorders (Barlow, 1988; Beck, Emery, & Greenberg, 1985), adolescents (Schrodt & Wright, 1987), alcoholics (Glantz, 1987), chronic psychiatric disorders (Greenwood, 1987), and personality disorders (Freeman & Leaf, 1989).

Cognitive therapy (CT) has also been applied to the treatment of eating disorders (i.e., anorexia nervosa and bulimia nervosa). Bruch (1962, 1985) noted that cognitive factors influence the development and maintenance of anorexia. Pathological cognitions have also been described in patients with bulimia (Fairburn, 1985). Cognitive therapy for eating disorders is directed at the persistence of underlying dysfunctional beliefs and values concerning food, body shape, and weight (Cooper & Fairburn, 1984; Fairburn, 1985; Garner & Bemis, 1982, 1985).

Using principles of CT described by Beck and co-workers (Beck, 1976; Beck et al., 1979), Garner and Bemis (1982, 1985) integrated cognitive strategies into a "multidimensional" treatment of anorexia nervosa. Following the model of treating depression, they adapted cognitive and behavioral interventions to deal with the specific types of thinking patterns often seen with anorexia nervosa. In a similar fashion, Fairburn (1985) developed a treatment approach for bulimia using cognitive–behavioral interventions. He observed that many of the features of bulimia nervosa can be viewed from a cognitive perspective rather than simply as symptoms of the disorder. For this reason, Fairburn and others (e.g., Agras, Schneider, Arnow, Raeburn, & Telch, 1989) designed treatment programs to produce cognitive change. These authors consider changes in attitudes, beliefs, and automatic negative thoughts to be prerequisites to full recovery.

Central to the cognitive model for treatment for eating disorders is what Beck (1976) calls "systematic errors in thinking" or faulty information processing. Garner and Bemis (1982) have focused on cognitive errors as contributors to the disorder. These errors include arbitrary inference, selective abstraction, overgeneralization, magnification and minimization, personalization, and absolutistic or dichotomous thinking (see Chapter 1 for a full explanation). These disturbances in information processing provide ongoing support for relentless dieting, extreme ideas about food or body size, and overall negative self-perceptions. As in the treatment of depression, the therapist's ability to teach the patient to challenge and reframe these faulty assumptions becomes a focal point for cognitive therapy of eating disorders.

Several studies have found CT to be an effective treatment for outpatients with eating disorders, particularly bulimia nervosa (Agras et al., 1989; Connors, Johnson, & Stuckey, 1984; Lacey, 1983; Lee & Rush, 1986; Wolchik, Weiss, & Katzman, 1986). Much less has been reported on the use of cognitive interventions for eating disorders in hospital settings. Inpatient treatment programs for eating disorders have traditionally used a behavioral approach that emphasizes contingency management techniques (Andersen, Morse, & Santmyer, 1985; Andersen, 1986; Halmi, 1985; Levendusky & Dooley, 1985). However, within many behavioral programs, the use of cognitive therapy techniques has become an integral part of the hospital treatment (Andersen et al., 1985; Garfinkel, Garner, & Kennedy, 1985). This chapter describes how CT can be effectively utilized in treating anorexia nervosa and bulimia nervosa during hospitalization.

INDICATIONS FOR HOSPITALIZATION

The decision to hospitalize an individual with an eating disorder is usually made when outpatient treatment fails to restore the patient's weight to a healthy level or there has been a failure to stop chaotic eating behavior. Indications for hospitalization have been described by several authors (Andersen, 1986; Garfinkel & Garner, 1982). Common reasons for hospital admission include the following: (1) weight loss has reached such significant proportions that intervention is required to curtail starvation; (2) it is necessary to break an unending cycle of binging–purging in nonemaciated patients; and (3) the patient is profoundly depressed, suicidal, or psychotic.

Brief hospital admissions may be indicated occasionally for diagnostic observation, treating complications or crises, confronting the patient's denial, or initiation of individual and family psychotherapy. Health concerns are by far the most frequent reasons for admission to a hospital.

CONTINGENCY MANAGEMENT

Inpatient treatment programs for eating disorders commonly employ contingency management techniques to restore weight and "normalize" eating habits. Descriptions of such programs have been set forth in several different books (Andersen, 1986; Andersen et al., 1985; Garfinkel & Garner, 1982; Halmi, 1985) and are not repeated in detail here. However, a brief overview of contingency management procedures is provided as a background for understanding CT interventions for inpatients with eating disorders. Cognitive therapy programs are usually developed in concert with a contingency management treatment system.

Patients who have anorexia nervosa are often admitted after they have reached a danger zone of low body weight, electrolyte imbalance, cardiovascular dysfunction, or other serious physical pathology. The behavioral pattern of food restriction, excessive exercise, emesis, and/or laxative abuse must be broken to avoid significant morbidity or even mortality. Also, starvation can impair learning and memory functioning to the point that the patient is unable to think effectively or participate actively in psychotherapy. Refeeding and weight gain thus become essential targets for treatment.

Contingency management protocols may appear to be heavy-handed to the cognitive therapist who is most familiar with highly collaborative therapeutic relationships. Rather strict rules and obvious reinforcers are used because the destructive behavioral patterns are unlikely to change unless definitive measures are taken. Ideally, the patient and his or her family agree that behavioral interventions are required; they then contract with the treatment team to institute a contingency management program. However, in some life-threatening cases, a court order must be obtained in order to initiate behavioral measures.

The general format for a contingency management program involves setting clear weight-gain objectives, rewarding the patient for attaining goals, and using restrictive measures when goals are not met.

Reinforcers are designed for the short term (e.g., going on a daily activity with the patient group) and the long term (e.g., an opportunity to go off the ward unescorted). Great care is taken to weigh the patient under controlled conditions in order to avoid possible manipulations of the behavioral system. Usually, patients are weighed three times a week, before the first meal of the day (after voiding). After the dietician consults with the patient to plan a reasonable diet, a firm expectation is made that the entire amount of each meal will be eaten. Usually a staff member sits with the patient during meals to be a supportive coach. The patient's room may be locked for an hour or longer after the meal.

The level of physical and social activity is one of the main reinforcers. If weight goals are not achieved, the patient may not be allowed to attend desired activities such as a craft shop experience, a group walk, or a family visit. However, as progress is made, the patient is gradually rewarded with an increasing sphere of activities. Physical exercise is a particularly important element of the program. At the beginning of treatment, exercise may be severely limited. In some instances, bed rest may be required. As the patient gains weight and begins to restore her or his health, a reintroduction to reasonable levels of exercise may be considered.

Patients with bulimia nervosa are less likely to be admitted to the hospital than those with anorexia nervosa because they do not commonly have problems with malnutrition. However, medical sequelae of bulimia (such as electrolyte imbalance or gastrointestinal disorders) or severe depression may lead to hospitalization. If weight is in the normal range, as it frequently is, the behavioral goals become weight maintenance and disruption of the binge–purge cycle. Careful monitoring of intake during meals and prevention of emesis by keeping the patient out of his or her room until the meal is fully digested are the main behavioral interventions. Reinforcers are used to shape responses as in cases of anorexia nervosa.

INDIVIDUAL COGNITIVE THERAPY FOR EATING DISORDERS

When the patient has severe malnutrition or cognitive impairment, the aforementioned contingency measures must be used before initiating cognitive therapy. However, many patients can be treated simultaneously with contingency management and CT. It must be emphasized that cognitive therapy, to be effective, should be introduced at a level that can be assimilated by the patient.

It is important to begin therapy by helping the patient to understand the rationale for treatment (Kornblith, Rehm, O'Hara, & Lamparksi, 1983). Describing the cognitive model of psychopathology is a good starting point for patients who have intact learning and memory functioning. This process includes such things as explaining the cognitive triad, automatic thoughts, and the interaction of thoughts, feelings, and behavior. Also, giving details about the different phases of therapy (e.g., behavioral interventions early in the therapy and cognitive procedures later) can facilitate a collaborative atmosphere for treatment.

Generally, the degree of emphasis on behavioral techniques depends on the severity of the disorder. For most inpatients, symptoms are so extreme that the initial sessions are primarily behavioral in nature. Behavioral procedures set the stage for subsequent cognitive interventions by establishing situations that generate thoughts and feelings regarding food, weight, body size, and control over the environment.

Behavioral Interventions

It is extremely important that the patient understands the rationale for the various behavioral procedures. Thus, emphasis should be placed on increasing the individual's level of knowledge about her or his disorder and methods of treatment. Interventions are action-oriented so that the patient has the opportunity to practice specific methods for dealing with concrete problems. Successful experiences on behavioral tasks can help break the cycle of demoralization, avoidance, and self-disparagement (Beck et al., 1979). When describing these interventions, the therapist should avoid generalizations that may imply that the completion of one task will make the patient immediately feel better or have a rapid change in his or her fears over food, weight, and body image.

Behavioral assignments are graded to the patient's level of understanding or motivation. The therapist needs to keep in mind that some individuals with an eating disorder may have difficulty in working with complex ideas or procedures. It is also important not to assign behavioral tasks for completion outside the therapy session until the therapist is certain that the patient understands their rationale and method of implementation. A similar exercise should usually have been completed within a therapy session before a homework assignment is made.

Activity Scheduling

Daily activity scheduling and mood monitoring are useful early in the course of treatment. Since an inpatient program often contains planned activities, the therapist can have the patient monitor mood (e.g., anxiety or depression) during the day. An hour-by-hour collection of an individual's moods can point to those situations that are uncomfortable for the patient. It is especially important to monitor the level of affect that surrounds mealtime (immediately before, during, and just after eating) and when the individual is weighed. These are times that anxiety or feelings of dysphoria may be most intense. Such monitoring may also reveal what mechanisms a patient uses to decrease anxious thoughts and feelings. The activity schedule provides an additional benefit by utilizing structure to help counteract hopelessness, helplessness, and loss of motivation.

Mastery and Pleasure

The activity schedule is also used to monitor the mastery and pleasure associated with the patient's experiences in the treatment setting. To do this, the patient rates each completed activity for both mastery and pleasure on a scale from 0 to 10. These ratings give patient and therapist immediate feedback on responses to the therapy milieu. Often, simple interactions with other patients or staff can elicit thoughts of being fat or out of control or concerns about one's competency. Fluctuations in mastery and pleasure ratings will accompany these dysfunctional cognitions. By monitoring the types of tasks in which the individual engages while having these thoughts, the therapist can begin to focus individual or group sessions on those situations that can benefit from cognitive interventions. For example, activities rated as low in mastery or pleasure may lead to identification of events that trigger specific problematic behaviors, such as dietary restriction or increased exercise. Mastery and pleasure ratings also may be used to generate homework assignments that challenge the patient's hypotheses of being fat or out of control.

Graded-Task Assignments

Graded-task assignments are used to assist the individual to complete a series of actions successfully. This is accomplished by working with the patient to break down an apparently overwhelming task into subtasks, ranging from the simplest to the most complex. Subsequent completion of the graded subtasks may provide immediate and unambiguous proof that the patient can successfully manage challenging or difficult situations. Key features of a graded-task assignment are (1) problem definition (for example, assisting the patient to believe that eating a full meal is important), (2) formulation of a project (method of step-wise assignment of tasks is taught—see Table 13.1 for an example), (3) im-

TABLE 13.1. Graded-Task Assignment

Problem: Eating a full meal.

Steps:

1. Assess negative or fearful concerns about the meal.
2. Go into the dining room and get meal tray.
3. Sit down at the table.
4. Assess the degree of difficulty of eating each of the foods on the tray.
5. Start with the food that causes the least anxiety.
   a. Take one bite at a time
   b. Do not put down utensils between bites
6. Take a bite of the next easiest food and go up the hierarchy of foods from easiest to most difficult. Repeat step 5a with each new food.
7. When meal is completed, assess physical status and negative or fearful concerns.
8. Leave dining room and focus on what it has been like to eat.
9. Identify negative concerns.
10. Affirm to yourself that you can eat a full meal even though it creates discomfort.

mediate, direct observation by the patient that there has been success in reaching a specific goal, (4) recognition and ventilation of the patient's doubts, cynical reactions, and belittling of the achievement, (5) encouragement of a more realistic evaluation by the patient of the actual performance of the task, (6) emphasis on the fact that the patient has reached the desired goal, and (7) devising new, more complex assignments that can build on previous successful experiences.

Graded-task assignments and daily mood ratings are particularly important in the early stages of treatment. These procedures help the therapist establish a base line for further work and also offer the patient short-term results that encourage hopefulness and further involvement in therapy. The assignments should be designed so that there is a high probability of success. A poorly arranged graded-task assignment may result in a failure, which is likely to increase the patient's sense of demoralization.

Rehearsal

This procedure, based on a graded task paradigm, encourages the patient to *imagine* each successive step in a sequence leading to a desired outcome. Rehearsing the steps often uncovers a sequence of behaviors the patient can use during the assignment. Rehearsal can also be used to identify potential "roadblocks" that might impede successful completion of the assignment. One such use of behavioral rehearsal is at mealtime. Using imagery, the therapist helps the patient to "walk" through a hospital meal. Helping an individual to visualize the food, identify and work with thoughts and fears, and successfully "eat" a meal in imagination can increase confidence in the patient's ability to overcome his or her disorder.

Another related behavioral intervention is practicing with tasks *in vivo*. For example, a patient with bulimia nervosa is first shown where "junk food" can be purchased within the hospital setting. Next the patient and therapist go to the vending machines, purchase food (non-diet), and eat the food together. As with rehearsal in imagery, the therapist can use this type of learning experience as a springboard to working with the patient's thoughts and concerns about impulse control.

Cognitive Interventions

Adaptations of Beck's model (Beck et al., 1979) are necessary when working with an individual with an eating disorder. Garner and Bemis (1985) recommend that specific features of eating disorders should be addressed. These include (1) the relative intractability of the disorder (including reluctance to enter treatment); (2) interaction between physical and psychological elements; (3) prominence of deficits in self-concept related to the patient's lack of self-esteem and awareness of (and confidence in) internal states; (4) idiosyncratic beliefs related to food and weight; and (5) the patient's perception of the desirability of retaining certain focal symptoms (e.g., low body weight, control over others). It is suggested that the level of motivation for treatment can be improved by the gradual evolution of a trusting therapeutic relationship (Garner, 1986; Garner & Bemis, 1985).

Basic characteristics of the cognitive structure of individuals with eating disorders have been detailed by several authors (Agras et al., 1989; Fairburn, 1985; Garner & Bemis, 1982). Patients with eating disorders often perceive that body weight or shape can serve as the sole criterion for self-worth and complete self-control and regimentation are desirable. Eating disorders are also associated with a profound fear of becoming fat and or an intense desire to be thin. Perfectionistic tendencies frequently pervade most aspects of the lives of these patients.

A comprehensive review of the use of all types of cognitive–behavioral therapies in the treatment of eating disorders is beyond the scope of this chapter. Interested readers are encouraged to consult Agras et al. (1989), Fairburn (1985), Garfinkel and Garner (1982), Garner and Bemis (1982, 1985), and Wilson, (1986). In general, these authors suggest that several of the interventions described by Beck (1976) be utilized. These include (1) monitoring thoughts and feelings and/or increasing the individual's awareness of thoughts, (2) becoming aware of and understanding the interaction among thoughts, feelings, and dysfunctional behaviors, (3) identifying negative automatic thoughts and challenging these cognitions, (4) increasing the ability to accept more realistic and appropriate interpretations, and (5) identifying and modifying underlying schemas that maintain the disorder.

Eliciting Automatic Thoughts

Cognitions intervene between the perception of an external event and the patient's emotional response to this event. These "automatic thoughts" often are not within the awareness of the patient because they occur in such a habitual fashion. Automatic thoughts are usually spontaneous, on the edge of awareness, and evaluative in nature (positive or negative). Also, there is a tendency for them to be global or general. These types of thoughts tend to be repetitive, plausible to the patient, and idiosyncratic. Examples of typical automatic thoughts of eating disorder patients are contained in Table 13.2. The therapist works to make the patient aware of when these thoughts occur and how they influence his or her behavior. To accomplish this the therapist can employ several interventions, including Socratic questioning, imagery, and thought recording. These basic CT procedures have been described earlier in the volume (Chapters 1 and 4). Several other cognitive techniques are illustrated here with brief case vignettes.

TABLE 13.2. Common Automatic Thoughts of Patients with Eating Disorders

If I eat this food, no one will like me.
Without my 1 hour of exercise, I'll blow up like a balloon.
If I eat one cookie, I'll never be able to stop.
Walking through the dayroom makes me feel like a cow.
If my weight goes over 100 pounds, I'll never be able to lose it again.
Eating this food will mean I'm out of control.
If I eat in front of other patients, they'll think I'm a fat pig.
Seeing my weight go up each morning means I'm a weak person.
If I'm not thin, then I'm nobody.
When my weight goes up, I feel bad, and when it goes down, I feel good.
If I eat more than others at dinner, I feel guilty.
The staff wants me to get fat.

Role Playing

Role playing is a useful tool to elicit automatic thoughts, especially when the problem is an interpersonal one. The therapist plays the role of the other person involved in an upsetting situation while the patient plays himself or herself. The roles may then be reversed. The role play often elicits automatic thoughts as it is being carried out.

PATIENT: I'm having a hard time talking to the dietitian about my menus.

THERAPIST: What sort of things seem to get in the way?

PATIENT: I'm not quite sure!

THERAPIST: Let's role play the situation to see what is happening.

PATIENT: Okay! I think I'm getting too many calories on my tray at lunch time.

THERAPIST: *(as Dietitian)* You need to eat at least a minimum amount of calories to be healthy.

PATIENT: I know, but there seems to be too much food for one meal. Are you sure that you haven't made a mistake in your calorie counts?

THERAPIST: No, there hasn't been a mistake; we have all agreed on this level of caloric intake.

PATIENT: All right, I'm sorry that I bothered you.

THERAPIST: You look angry now. What was going through your mind during the role play?

PATIENT: I was thinking that I can't ask any questions and that everybody else is trying to control what I do. I should be able to handle my diet by myself.

Examining the Evidence

Hypotheses are set forth, and the patient is engaged in exercises to test the validity of cognitions. The inpatient milieu provides many opportunities to gather evidence that can be used to modify dysfunctional thoughts.

PATIENT: My thighs are bigger today than yesterday. I'm so fat!

THERAPIST: How does that affect you?

PATIENT: No one will want to be with me after I've gained so much weight.

THERAPIST: How will others be aware that your thighs are bigger then the day before?

PATIENT: They will just know! They can see the difference.

THERAPIST: What would happen if you tested out your hypothesis during group today? And what would you do if no one in group could tell that your thighs were bigger.

PATIENT: I guess my ideas of how others see me might change. Maybe my view isn't always shared by others, but I'll bet they'll notice.

Decatastrophizing

This technique, originally developed by Ellis (1962), attempts to transform extreme predications about problems into more realistic expectations. Inpatients who suffer from eating disorders frequently visualize their reactions to situations in a catastrophic manner. This is illustrated by a patient who described what might happen after she was discharged.

PATIENT: If I go out to eat with friends, they'll see how out of control I am with food.

THERAPIST: How will that be a problem?

PATIENT: Once they know that I'm out of control they won't want to do things with me ever!

THERAPIST: What do you mean by being out of control?

PATIENT: It could be anything . . . eating too much, not being able to eat, or just getting nervous at a meal.

THERAPIST: How often have these things happened when you're with your friends?

PATIENT: Well, I get nervous most of the time, but I usually can eat something. I can't remember really losing it.

THERAPIST: And how often have people refused to be with you because of this?

PATIENT: I don't know. They hardly ever say anything about it. I suppose I think they're watching me a lot more than they really are.

THERAPIST: You've used the words "out of control." How well do these terms fit the actual situation as you've described it?

PATIENT: I guess I tend to exaggerate. I'm learning how to eat more normally here in the hospital, and I hope I'll be able to do better when I leave.

Challenging "Should" Statements

This intervention attempts to change overly demanding self-constructs and driven behavior. Patients with eating disorders are highly prone to having problems with perfectionistic standards.

THERAPIST: How are you doing with the eating disorder program?

PATIENT: Not as well as I would like.

THERAPIST: What seems to be giving you difficulty?

PATIENT: Well, this program is designed to help me feel more comfortable with eating three meals a day. I've been here 10 days, and I'm still afraid I am going to binge.

THERAPIST: How does that create a problem?

PATIENT: I should be more comfortable with food and eating. But, I'm just as scared as the day I came into the hospital. I feel awful . . . like I'm letting myself and my parents down. I should be working harder!

THERAPIST: I noticed a few "shoulds" in your statements. What effect do you think they have on how you feel?

PATIENT: I'm not really sure what you mean about "shoulds."

THERAPIST: Often a "should statement" implies that the individual is not meeting certain expectations or demands. It's also likely that a feeling of guilt occurs when you have a "should statement." I wonder if that could be true of how you have described your progress in the program?

PATIENT: Well, I do feel bad about how things have been going.

THERAPIST: What might happen if you could alter the "should" part of one of your statements. For example, "I *should* be more comfortable with eating three meals a day" could be changed to "I *want* to be comfortable with three meals a day?"

PATIENT: It does make it sound different.

THERAPIST: If you change your perception of the situation how does that affect the way you feel?

PATIENT: Well, I do feel a little better now. It doesn't seem like I'm letting people down as much.

Articulation of Beliefs

An attempt is made to organize or consolidate the distorted perceptions and assumptions. This may be as simple as identifying a specific, repetitive cognitive distortion (i.e., by "mind reading" while eating, the patient's automatic thought is that those around her think she is a "pig"). However, this procedure can be more complex when the therapist assists in identifying maladaptive schemas. These assumptions, or "rules for living," guide the way a patient reacts to many situations. Schemas provide templates for judging oneself, other people, or the future. In order to identify these assumptions, the therapist listens closely for themes that cut across several different situations or problem areas. Often the schemas are stimulated by experiences in the hospital setting, as illustrated by the following vignette.

PATIENT: When I walk through the dayroom, people think I'm fat.

THERAPIST: What leads you to that conclusion?

PATIENT: I just know that is what they are thinking.

THERAPIST: Do you have direct evidence of what others are thinking?

PATIENT: No! But if I think I'm fat then surely others must see me that way also.

THERAPIST: What might be another way of explaining the situation you just described?

PATIENT: Well, I guess I could be jumping to conclusions by believing that they see me in exactly the way that I see myself.

THERAPIST: So then, what is the basic belief that you have about yourself?

PATIENT: I'm fat . . . no matter what I do about it or what anyone else says.

Challenging Beliefs Through Behavioral Exercises

This is often a part of homework. Such assignments help the individual to test specific behaviors in order to understand better the interaction among thoughts, feelings, and behavior. They also permit the patient to gather evidence about his or her own perceptions. Behavioral exercises are set up in a variety of milieu activities. For example, mealtimes on the unit can be engineered to challenge and modify pathological cognitions.

PATIENT: If I eat three meals a day I will gain tons of weight.

THERAPIST: What information do you have to support this idea?

PATIENT: In the past my weight has gone up whenever I eat like other people.

THERAPIST: How could we test out your belief that you will gain "tons of weight" by eating three meals a day?

PATIENT: By not eating three meals we could see if my weight is stable or goes down.

THERAPIST: How about a different approach? What if you ate three meals and each day we look at how much, if any, your weight goes up?

PATIENT: I can try, but what if it does go up?

THERAPIST: First, we need to learn exactly what happens when you eat regular meals, including how you think and feel about doing this.

Prospective Hypothesis Testing

Garner and Bemis (1985) describe hypothesis testing as the translation of specific predictions and conclusions into formal hypotheses that may be evaluated by collecting information from planned experiments. For the eating-disorder patient, this often means moving from very global or diffuse concepts to specific hypotheses that can be tested in the hospital milieu.

THERAPIST: As part of the inpatient program you will be eating more food than you usually do.

PATIENT: I'm afraid that if I eat any more than I do now, my weight will get out of control, and I'll never stop eating.

THERAPIST: Are there any other fears that you have about eating?

PATIENT: My stomach will stick out and people around me will think I'm fat.

THERAPIST: Is it possible that your concerns could be tested while you are in the hospital?

PATIENT: I don't know how that would be done. If I eat anything I'll get fat.

THERAPIST: Lets look at your fears and try to place them into an experimental framework, something that can be tested in a concrete fashion.

PATIENT: How would you do that?

THERAPIST: Let's look at the idea that your weight will be "out of control." How could we set up an experiment to test this hypothesis?

PATIENT: I get weighed three times a week; that would be a good test. I'll bet that by tomorrow I've gained 10 pounds.

THERAPIST: That's a start. But I'd like to add something. How about a definition of what out of control weight would be?

PATIENT: All right. Any day my weight gain is more than one pound would be out of control. Does that sound about right?

THERAPIST: I think you came up with a reasonable definition for now. I would like for us to be able to refine it as we go along. Do you agree?

PATIENT: It's okay with me.

Reattribution Techniques

This strategy assists patients to alter maladaptive perceptions of the significance of environmental events. Patients learn that attributions may be inaccurate and that the validity of subjective experience must be questioned.

THERAPIST: I think you've made good progress while in the hospital.

PATIENT: Maybe, but the staff looks at me funny . . . like there was something wrong with me.

THERAPIST: What's happened to make you think that they look at you funny?

PATIENT: They don't spend much time with me anymore. They seem to have more time for others and less for me.

THERAPIST: So the amount of time that they spend with you influences how you think they see you?

PATIENT: Yes. If they cared as much as before, they would spend the same amount of time.

THERAPIST: Do you have other evidence that they do not care as much?

PATIENT: Not really.

THERAPIST: If you don't have any direct evidence, what might be another way of looking at the situation?

PATIENT: Well the other patients are pretty demanding. There have been lots of new admissions. That could explain the staff having less time for me.

THERAPIST: If that were part of what was going on, how would you see the staff's reactions to you?

PATIENT: I guess I would have to rethink how much they care.

THERAPIST: Maybe we could brainstorm to come up with ways to test out your current beliefs.

GROUP THERAPY

Group psychotherapy has gained recent support as a primary intervention in the treatment of eating disorders (Hall, 1985; Schneider & Agras, 1985). Research suggests that the group provides an opportunity to incorporate a wide array of therapeutic techniques within one format. For example, experiential and social learning methods can help alleviate symptoms of bulimia and result in changes in self-acceptance, social presence, self-control, and body image. Fairburn (1981) documented the impact of group therapy on symptom reduction and adaptive changes in attitudes toward food, body shape, and weight.

A Structural Format for Group Therapy

Treating inpatients poses several challenges. Group size and composition, for example, can change noticeably from week to week. Inconsistent attendance makes it difficult to pursue individual issues or topics in depth, and it hinders group members from effective interaction with each other. Thus, standard procedures for group building as described by Yalom (1985) can be quite difficult in the hospital setting.

Several factors deserve consideration when one is running an inpatient group for eating disorders. As noted above, therapists should be aware that a group's membership may change dramatically from week to week. Careful selection and preparation of members are therefore very important to the success of this type of group. Screening is necessary to avoid inclusion of psychotic, organic, or excessively hostile persons. Such individuals will either be unable to grasp the content of group sessions or will disrupt the work of the other patients. Preparation for participation in the group can be formal and structured (Gauron, Steinmark, & Gersh, 1977; Yalom, 1985) or can be informal (for example, asking existing members to describe the purpose and procedures of the group to each new member).

One approach that works well in an inpatient setting is to consider a format in which the entire life of the group process is viewed in terms of a single session. This method, suggested by Yalom (1983), is discussed in detail in Chapter 5 of this volume. In practical terms, this means that the therapist plans a structured session for each group meeting. The therapist maintains a high level of activity throughout and guides the process so that closure on homework or other follow-up therapy issues can be reached by the end of the session. The frequency of group meetings depends on the nature of the inpatient setting. However, it is recommended that the eating disorder group meet for 90 minutes at least twice each week. This allows sufficient time for a meaningful discussion of topics of shared interest and development of homework assignments.

The structural framework for group cognitive therapy suggested here consists of three parts. The first component of the session, lasting for about the first 10 or 15 minutes, is devoted to setting an agenda. This may consist of asking whether there is a desire to discuss some aspect of the previous session or a new topic. Homework is consistently placed on the agenda. If several suggestions for agenda items are made during this time, they are noted and rank-ordered by the group. Also, this early part of the session can be used to introduce new patients to the cognitive model. A brief explanation of cognitive therapy is often included, and handout material can be distributed at this time and developed into the new member's first homework assignment.

The middle part of the session takes the largest share of time, usually about 50 to 60 minutes. The focus is on the specific agenda items developed by the group. Topics might include preoccupation with weight and body image, anxiety about attaining social approval, or issues of self-esteem. During this time the therapists assist members in developing an understanding of which automatic thoughts, cognitive errors, and schemas are involved in their disorder. Challenging these beliefs within the group can help others see how their own thoughts affect their emotions. The support and sharing of other members enhances the patient's understanding of what can be done to effect change.

The last part of the session (10 to 15 minutes) is devoted to a synthesis of the group process, homework assignments, and closing statements. Members are encouraged to discuss how they were affected personally by the group session. They can give direct feedback to another group member or to the therapists. The homework for the next session is clearly specified, after which the session concludes with the therapist(s) making comments about the overall progress of the group.

CONCLUSION

Successful inpatient treatment of eating disorders using contingency management to restore weight and reestablish controlled eating has been well documented. Also, cognitive–behavioral methods have been shown to be useful with patients suffering from eating disorders. This chapter describes the use of cognitive therapy and related behavioral procedures for the treatment of eating disorders when one is working within a comprehensive inpatient program. In the future, research is needed to identify the specific aspects of treatment that are successful and to discover how to incorporate them into a maximally effective treatment plan.

REFERENCES

Agras, W. S., Schnieder, J. A., Arnow, B., Raeburn, S. D., & Telch, C. F. (1989). Cognitive–behavioral and response prevention treatments for bulimia nervosa. *Journal of Consulting and Clinical Psychology*, *57*, 215–221.

Andersen, A. E. (1986). Inpatient and outpatient treatment for anorexia nervosa. In K. D. Brownell & J. P. Foreyt (Eds.), *Handbook of eating disorders: Physiology, psychology, and treatment of obesity, anorexia and bulimia* (pp. 333–350). New York: Basic Books.

Andersen, A. E., Morse, C. L., & Santmyer, K. S. (1985). Inpatient treatment of anorexia nervosa. In D. M. Garner & P. E. Garfinkel (Eds.), *Handbook of psychotherapy for anorexia nervosa and bulimia* (pp. 311–343). New York: Guilford Press.

Barlow, D. H. (1988). *Anxiety and its disorders: The nature and treatment of anxiety and panic*. New York: Guilford Press.

Beck, A. T. (1976). *Cognitive therapy and the emotional disorders*. New York: International Universities Press.

Beck, A. T., Emery, G., & Greenberg, R. L. (1985). *Anxiety disorders and phobias: A cognitive perspective*. New York: Basic Books.

Beck, A. T., Rush, A. J., Shaw, B. F., & Emery, G. (1979). *Cognitive therapy of depression*. New York: Guilford Press.

Bruch, H. (1962). Perceptual and conceptual disturbances in anorexia nervosa. *Psychosomatic Medicine*, *24*, 187–194.

Bruch, H. (1985). Four decades of eating disorders. In D. M. Garner & P. E. Garfinkel (Eds.), *Handbook of psychotherapy for anorexia nervosa and bulimia* (pp. 7–18). New York: Guilford Press.

Connors, M. E., Johnson, D. L., & Stuckey, M. K. (1984). Treatment of bulimia with brief psychoeducational group therapy. *American Journal of Psychiatry*, *141*, 1512–1516.

Cooper, P. J., & Fairburn, C. G. (1984). Cognitive behavior therapy for anorexia nervosa: Some preliminary findings. *Journal of Psychosomatic Research*, *28*, 493–499.

Ellis, A. (1962). *Reason and emotion in psychotherapy*. New York: Lyle Stuart.

Fairburn, C. G. (1981). A cognitive behavioral approach to the treatment of bulimia. *Psychological Medicine*, *11*, 707–711.

Fairburn, C. G. (1985). Cognitive–behavioral treatment for bulimia. In D. M. Garner & P. E. Garfinkel (Eds.), *Handbook of psychotherapy for anorexia nervosa and bulimia* (pp. 160–191). New York: Guilford Press.

Freeman, A., & Leaf, R. C. (1989). Cognitive therapy applied to personality disorders. In A. Freeman, K. M. Simon, L. E. Beutler, & H. Arkowitz (Eds.), *Comprehensive handbook of cognitive therapy* (pp. 403–434). New York: Plenum Press.

Garfinkel, P. E., & Garner, D. M. (1982). *Anorexia nervosa: A multidimensional perspective*. New York: Brunner/Mazel.

Garfinkel, P. E., Garner, D. M., & Kennedy, S. (1985). Special problems of inpatient management. In D. M. Garner & P. E. Garfinkel (Eds.), *Handbook of psychotherapy for anorexia nervosa and bulimia* (pp. 344–359). New York: Guilford Press.

Garner, D. M. (1986). Cognitive therapy for bulimia nervosa. *Adolescent Psychiatry, 13,* 358–390.

Garner, D. M., & Bemis, K. M. (1982). A cognitive–behavioral approach to anorexia nervosa. *Cognitive Therapy and Research, 6*, 123–150.

Garner, D. M., & Bemis, K. M. (1985). Cognitive therapy for anorexia nervosa. In D. M. Garner & P. E. Garfinkel (Eds.), *Handbook of psychotherapy for anorexia nervosa and bulimia* (pp. 107–146). New York: Guilford Press.

Gauron, E. F., Steinmark, S. W., & Gersh, F. S. (1977). The orientation group in pre-therapy training. *Perspectives in Psychiatric Care, 15*, 32–37.

Glantz, M. D. (1987). Day hospital treatment of alcoholics. In A. Freeman & V. Greenwood (Eds.), *Cognitive therapy: Applications in psychiatric and medical settings* (pp. 51–68). New York: Human Sciences Press.

Greenwood, V. B. (1987). Cognitive therapy with the young adult chronic patient. In A. Freeman & V. Greenwood (Eds.), *Cognitive therapy: Applications in psychiatric and medical settings* (pp. 103–106). New York: Human Sciences Press.

Hall, A. (1985). Group psychotherapy for anorexia nervosa. In D. M. Garner & P. E. Garfinkel (Eds.), *Handbook of psychotherapy for anorexia and bulimia* (pp. 213–239). New York: Guilford Press.

Halmi, K. A. (1985). Behavioral management for anorexia nervosa. In D. M. Garner & P. E. Garfinkel (Eds.), *Handbook of psychotherapy for anorexia nervosa and bulimia* (pp. 147–159). New York: Guilford Press.

Hollon, S. D., & Beck, A. T. (1986). Cognitive and cognitive–behavioral therapies. In S. L. Garfield & A. E. Bergin (Eds.), *Handbook of psychotherapy and behavior change* (pp. 443–482). New York: John Wiley & Sons.

Kornblith, S. J., Rehm, L. P., O'Hara, M. W., & Lamparksi, D. M. (1983). The contribution of self-reinforcement training and behavioral assignments to the efficacy of self-control therapy for depression. *Cognitive Therapy and Research*, 7, 499–528.

Lacey, J. H. (1983). Bulimia nervosa, binge eating and psychogenic vomiting: A controlled treatment study and long-term outcome. *British Journal of Psychiatry, 286*, 1609–1612.

Lee, N. L., & Rush, A. J. (1986). Cognitive–behavioral group therapy for bulimia. *International Journal of Eating Disorders, 5*, 599–615.

Levendusky, P. G., & Dooley, C. P. (1985). An inpatient model for the treatment of anorexia nervosa. In S. W. Emmett (Ed.), *Theory and treatment of anorexia nervosa and bulimia: Biomedical, sociocultural, and psychological perspectives* (pp. 211–233). New York: Brunner/Mazel.

Schneider, J. A., & Agras, W. S. (1985). A cognitive behavioral group treatment for bulimia. *British Journal of Psychiatry, 146*, 66–69.

Schrodt, G. R., & Wright, J. H. (1987). Inpatient treatment of adolescents. In

A. Freeman & V. Greenwood (Eds.), *Cognitive therapy: Applications in psychiatric and medical settings* (pp. 69–82). New York: Human Sciences Press.

Wilson, C. P. (1986). The psychoanalytic psychotherapy of bulimic anorexia. *Adolescent Psychiatry, 13*, 274–314.

Wolchik, S. A., Weiss, L., & Katzman, M. A. (1986). An empirically validated, short-term psychoeducational group-treatment program for bulimia. *International Journal of Eating Disorders, 5*, 21–34.

Yalom, I. D. (1983). *Inpatient group psychotherapy*. New York: Basic Books.

Yalom, I. D. (1985). *The theory and practice of group psychotherapy* (3rd ed.). New York: Basic Books.

Chapter 14

The Chronic Patient

Jan Scott, M.B., B.S., M.R.C.Psych.,
Susan Byers, Ph.D., and
Douglas Turkington, M.B., B.S., M.R.C. Psych.

The use of cognitive therapy (CT) in patients with long-term and severe mental health problems has been a relatively recent development. There are no controlled trials available, but open studies have provided encouraging results (Kingdon & Turkington, 1991; Scott, 1992). We begin with a brief overview of the shared characteristics of chronic patient populations and the reasons why CT might be a helpful therapeutic approach. Cognitive therapy interventions are then described for three specific subpopulations: chronic depression, chronic personality disorders, and chronic schizophrenic disorders. The concluding section of the chapter reviews similarities in the treatment of these conditions.

COGNITIVE THERAPY AND THE CHRONIC PATIENT

Patients with long-term difficulties often have failed to respond to standard therapeutic interventions. Therapists find these patients a challenge to both their clinical skills and their professional self-esteem. Not only does the primary disorder lead to great suffering on the part of the patients, but sequelae such as family or marital disharmony, social isolation, and loss of function contribute to a further erosion of quality of life. In the past, many chronic patients resided permanently in institutions. With the advent of community-based services and the shift away from long-term hospitalization, such individuals are increasingly seen in an outpatient setting. Admissions are usually the result of a severe clinical exacerbation, a major life crisis, or failure to cope on a day-to-day basis.

Admission of the chronic patient to the hospital does not usually yield a substantial benefit in itself. The patient and his or her family may obtain some relief from the respite, but a systematic approach to inpatient care is needed to reverse the symptoms that led to hospitalization. There are several components of inpatient CT that make it a useful treatment for patients with chronic disorders.

1. *Structured problem-solving approach.* An inpatient unit provides a safe and structured environment in which to offer treatment. The focus on problem solving is valuable because a wide range of difficulties experienced by the patient are addressed, and practical coping strategies are learned.
2. *Collaboration.* Staff often find themselves in challenging relationships with these patients. The style of CT encourages patient and therapist to explore data together in a collaborative rather than confrontational way.
3. *Empirical approach.* The patient with chronic difficulties may have experienced previous treatment failures or may find it difficult to identify particular gains that may lead to discharge from the hospital. The patient's skepticism or apprehension about both the treatment and the durability of improvement can be tackled through hypothesis testing.
4. *Accessibility and acceptability to staff.* Chronic patients may make staff members feel pessimistic or even inadequate as therapists. The structured goal-directed approach of CT helps to combat ineffective use of therapeutic contact time with the patient. Staff also may find the cognitive model of treatment to be more accessible and acceptable for use with chronically ill patients (Scott, 1988b).
5. *Adaptability of the model.* Cognitive therapy utilizes a flexible approach, and the format and content of therapy sessions can be modified to suit the needs of a broad spectrum of patients (Beck, 1976; Wright & Schrodt, 1989; Freeman, Simon, Arkowitz, & Beutler, 1989).

Cognitive therapy with the chronic patient can be provided through a comprehensive milieu therapy model or an "add on" model (see Chapter 3). The length and intensity of the program can be adapted to individual requirements, and therapy can be continued after discharge. Also, CT can be used as part of a combined treatment approach with psychopharmacology (see Chapter 7). Biological treatments are an important component of therapy for many chronic patients. The next three sections describe the use of CT with specific types of patients with chronic psychiatric disorders.

COGNITIVE THERAPY WITH CHRONICALLY DEPRESSED INPATIENTS

Chronic depressive disorders are defined by the persistence of symptoms for two years or more (Scott, 1988a). Severe chronic major depressions may require extended periods of inpatient care. Earlier work at the University of Newcastle Upon Tyne has identified several individual and family characteristics of chronically depressed patients that may dilute the efficacy of the standard inpatient CT approach (Barker, Scott, & Eccleston, 1987; Scott, 1988b).

Individual Factors

These patients have high scores on measures such as the Global Chronicity/Severity Index (Fennell & Teasdale, 1982) that may predict poor treatment response to either drugs or CT (Rush, Beck, Kovacs, & Hollon, 1977). Moreover, when compared to acute depressives, chronic depressives have a significantly higher prevalence of unipolar depression in first-degree relatives, higher neuroticism scores, and a greater number of adverse life events both before and after the onset of the depressive episode (Scott, Barker, & Eccleston, 1988). Chronic depressives also appear to show specific cognitive vulnerabilities such as low self-esteem, generalized hopelessness, persistently biased recall of personal memories, poor subjective awareness, and failure to generalize learning (Scott, 1992).

Family Factors

Both chronic depressives and their families have a high prevalence of interpersonal problems. The spouse of a chronic depressive is rarely "neutral" and may openly express anger or frustration toward the patient. Each member of the family may harbor automatic negative thoughts regarding the patient, and the behavior of the family unit may not change despite improvement on the part of the depressed individual. Patients must be helped to renegotiate their role in the family or to deal with the family's negative expectations and beliefs.

Cognitive Milieu Therapy

Taking the above factors into account, a CT milieu approach was developed for chronic depression that produced significant improvements in 70% of the patients admitted to our unit for treatment-resistant patients (Scott, 1992). The program tackles chronic depression through an extended and a more intensive treatment package than used with acute patients. Although the basic techniques of CT are not changed, the style of delivery is significantly modified. There is a prolonged initial emphasis on engaging the patient in CT and "action-oriented" behavioral techniques. The initial CT sessions are often shortened (20 minutes) but are held frequently. Much of the CT is carried out in the ward setting by the nursing staff (Scott, 1988b). These interventions serve the purpose of helping patients to overcome their inertia about engaging in activities and also provide objective "second opinions." Another component of this model is an evening debriefing session—typically conducted by a nurse.

Family CT sessions are educational (e.g., explaining depression and CT) and also look at specific issues (e.g., examining the family members' automatic thoughts regarding the patient's depression). Coping strategies for all family members are discussed. Most families require at least two or three sessions (see Chapter 6).

Work relating to changing or modifying the individual's underlying schemas is usually delayed till the later phases of hospitalization and continues after discharge. In our opinion, outpatient CT sessions should be held for at least 6 months. The value of continued outpatient CT has been confirmed by several recent studies (Miller, Norman, & Keitner, 1989; Thase, Bowler, & Harden, 1991). In order to demonstrate some of the components of an inpatient therapy program for chronic depression, a case example is described.

Case Illustration

Elizabeth was a 36-year-old married woman who lived with her husband and two children. She had suffered from chronic major depression that had remained unresponsive to a number of antidepressant medications over a period of 4 years. Elizabeth had a history of two previous episodes of major depression, including a postpartum episode 12 years previously, following the birth of her first child a daughter. She had always felt insecure in her relationship with this child, and was increasingly threatened as her daughter took over domestic roles within the home.

The current episode of depression was partially ameliorated by antidepressant medication, but about 2 years into the episode her mother had a stroke. Elizabeth persuaded her husband and children that they should move their home to be nearer to her mother. However, shortly after the move, her mother died. Elizabeth's husband was angry at "being made to move," losing his social network, and having to change jobs. The marriage, already under strain, deteriorated further. Her depression became worse, and her distress was difficult for the family to manage.

A local physician prescribed diazepam, which Elizabeth took excessively. Eventually, she took an overdose of this medication. Admission was arranged at a local psychiatric hospital, where a variety of medications and psychotherapies proved ineffective over a period of 6 months. Elizabeth had become self-obsessed and talked at length about every aspect of her depression. She refused to take part in bereavement work or other forms of counseling, stating that these issues were "too painful" to discuss. However, if staff stopped talking to her about such matters, she expressed the view that they were rejecting her. Relationships with the staff on the unit became increasingly tense, and weekend passes were distressing to all the family. Problems came to a head when, as a last resort, her doctor suggested ECT. Elizabeth refused, and the unit staff concluded that they "had nothing left to offer." She was therefore transferred to the Newcastle Chronic Depression unit.

Sessions 1–3

The initial interview was not an easy affair. Elizabeth felt angry with her therapists at the previous unit and saw transfer to Newcastle as a punishment. Thoughts such as "the other unit gave up on me" and "my family wants to get rid of me" were very near to the surface. Despite her reticence about talking to the cognitive therapist, she was able to generate alternative beliefs such as "perhaps my family wants me to come here for a specialist's help because they care about me and want me to recover." The interview appeared to progress slowly, and it was agreed to continue the assessment over two more (daily) sessions. Unit staff were asked to have brief conversations with Elizabeth to help her settle into the unit and to encourage her engagement in therapy.

By the end of this initial phase of treatment, Elizabeth and her therapist were able to generate a list of problems in three general areas: (1) self-esteem (e.g., feeling inferior and unlikable, guilt about her mother's death); (2) relationship problems (e.g., her husband's resentment about moving and leaving his friends, her fear that "he will leave me, and I will not cope," tension about her older daughter taking on a surrogate mother role with the younger child, thoughts about being a "bad mother," and social isolation); and (3) problems in day-to-day functioning (e.g., poor self-care, difficulty occupying her time, loss of pleasure in activities, taking diazepam to escape, and inability to manage basic tasks).

The introductory sessions also revealed important background information that allowed the therapist to develop hypotheses about underlying depressogenic assumptions and the patient's potential for acceptance or rejection of treatment. There was a family history of affective disorder in her grandfather and her mother. Elizabeth had vivid memories of feeling rejected by both individuals. She had always believed that her mother preferred her older brother to her. This raised the possibility of underlying schemas such as "I am an inferior person" or "I am unlovable." When her mother was not well, Elizabeth was expected to remain at home and look after the family. Frequent absences from school kept her rather isolated from her peers.

Her mother often took to her bed, and the children were expected to be quiet and not "cause any distress." Elizabeth was frequently punished for being noisy or having "bad behavior." These infractions usually appeared to be of a minor nature. However, she recalled being told that her mother's continued ill health was her fault. It was hypothesized that, with this background, Elizabeth had derived schemas such as "unless I am perfect, I will be harmful to others." Her family members were highly critical and suspicious of the doctors who were looking after her mother. Furthermore, the night Elizabeth's mother died there was a delay in the arrival of the local doctor. Given these circumstances and her own recent experiences, it was suspected that Elizabeth might have a negative view of the medical profession and might reject any treatment program offered. She admitted to a "lack of faith in therapy," and, with her agreement, this item was added to the problem list.

Sessions 4–5

This phase of therapy focused on the patient's ambivalence about the treatment program and the third category of identified problems (difficulties in day-to-day functioning). One of Elizabeth's most distressing current problems was the marital difficulties she was experiencing. However, the therapist believed it would be countertherapeutic to start with this issue because of the complexity of the problem and because of Elizabeth's low level of ability to manage simple daily activities. A failure with a major problem early in therapy can seem disastrous to a chronically depressed person, perhaps even leading the patient to reject the therapy outright (Scott, 1988b; Thase & Wright, 1991). Thus, two easier tasks were set up in parallel: (1) during the treatment sessions, Elizabeth and the cognitive therapist examined her thoughts relating to CT; and (2) outside the sessions, Elizabeth began to work with her primary nurse on specific behavioral goals. It was agreed that, for the next 3 days, the primary nurse would meet with Elizabeth and that they would jointly complete an activity schedule that she would use to keep track of what she had done during the day.

Automatic thoughts identified at this stage of treatment related specifically to the patient's views of CT:

THERAPIST: You were telling me you didn't have much faith that cognitive therapy would work?

ELIZABETH: Well, nothing else has been helpful so far.

THERAPIST: Can I ask you how much you believe the thought that cognitive therapy won't work.

ELIZABETH: Probably 100%.

THERAPIST: So you believe the statement "cognitive therapy won't work" probably 100%. Does "probably" allow any room for doubt?

ELIZABETH: I suppose it might. . . . No, not really when I think about it. . . . All the treatments are the same.

THERAPIST: Can I ask you if there's anything about cognitive therapy that might help you try it for a while? Is it different in any way from the treatments you had before?

ELIZABETH: *(Pause)* No . . . well actually that's probably not fair. If nothing else, this is the first time people seem to have tried to understand what's going on from my point of view. At least you ask me questions and check if you understand what I'm saying. It's different from that point of view.

As a homework assignment, the patient agreed to examine in more detail the idea that "cognitive therapy won't work." Elizabeth spoke to the staff, who gave her a handout on cognitive therapy, and she talked about the treatment program with staff members who reinforced the therapist's statement regarding a 70% improvement rate. She also talked with current inpatients and got their views on the treatment. At the next session the therapist again questioned Elizabeth about her perceptions of CT.

THERAPIST: What did you learn from the homework assignment?

ELIZABETH: Well, the staff said it works, but you'd expect that—wouldn't you?

THERAPIST: They don't strike me as a group who'd just agree for the sake of it, but I understand your point. Did they say it always worked?

ELIZABETH: Well no, they admitted that a lot of people don't improve.

THERAPIST: Can you remember how many "a lot" is? Is it more than half?

ELIZABETH: No, I think it's less.

THERAPIST: Yes, our current figures suggest that 70% of the patients we admit show a marked improvement. . . . Can I ask what you thought of the handout?

ELIZABETH: Actually, I didn't read it. There didn't seem much point, and I can't really concentrate.

THERAPIST: Okay. Can we come back to that in a moment? I'd like to find out about your discussions with the other patients. Did you ask any of them about the therapy?

ELIZABETH: I don't like anyone here much, but there were two women talking about it in the lounge, so I did have a few words.

THERAPIST: And what did you learn from what they said?

ELIZABETH: Well, one of them said she wasn't sure if it had done much good, but the other one was quite enthusiastic. However, she did say that in the beginning it felt like people pushed her pretty hard . . . just like you do with me. *(At this point Elizabeth smiled broadly.)*

THERAPIST: *(Smiling back)* Well, I promise not to push you too much, but I wonder if we could spend a bit of time going through the handout you didn't get a chance to read?

Elizabeth agreed, and together she and the therapist discussed the material in the handout. The therapist then proceeded with further questions about the patient's view of CT.

THERAPIST: Can I ask you again about the idea that cognitive therapy doesn't work for depression? Can you give me a rating on that?

ELIZABETH: Well, I guess I have to accept the information you and the others have told me. So I suppose I believe the idea about 50%.

Although not particularly convinced by the data presented, Elizabeth was now able to acknowledge that CT might work for some chronic depressions. There was a great deal of negativity in Elizabeth's comments, but the therapist remained task-oriented throughout. Further exploration of the types of difficulties successfully treated at the unit eventually led Elizabeth to rate her belief in the efficacy of cognitive therapy at about 75%.

THERAPIST: I regard this as good news.

ELIZABETH: Why?

THERAPIST: Well, I would have been concerned if you'd said you'd totally changed your mind. A rating of 75% suggests some room for doubt. I'm more than happy to work with "healthy skepticism" about the therapy, and we can continue to check out your beliefs about the treatment on a regular basis.

Further change in the belief that "cognitive therapy will not work for me" now needed to be challenged by experience with the therapy.

Sessions 6–9

The first targets for behavioral change were problems in performing basic tasks such as grooming, keeping her room clean, and attending scheduled activities. The primary nurse developed a daily schedule with Elizabeth that allocated a specified period of time to self-care tasks. Other staff were designated as "motivators" and "reinforcers" to help her engage in these activities. The goal was for her to get as far as she could with a list of self-care tasks in the allocated time, then to move on to the other activities on the schedule (e.g., recreational therapy, occupational therapy, educational groups). This tactic seemed to work. Elizabeth began to complete more tasks within the time period allocated. Furthermore, she spontaneously commented on feeling "a little better."

The occasions when Elizabeth withdrew to her room were used to carry out work on automatic thoughts. It became clear that she characteristically tried to escape from situations where she perceived she might be judged or rejected or might be asked to do something that she feared could not be achieved. The nursing staff turned their attention to these situations in her daily activity schedule. Together, Elizabeth and nursing staff were able to carry out immediate *in vivo* tests of the automatic thoughts. Also, a regimen of phenelzine and lithium (Barker et al., 1987) had been substituted for her previous antidepressants. This permitted an opportunity to explore carefully, in individual therapy, the rationale of the combined treatment with pharmacotherapy and CT (see Chapter 7). Individual CT was also directed, in part, at Elizabeth's desire to escape. The automatic thoughts generated in the sessions with the nurse were examined in more detail and were used as examples of how dysfunctional thinking can lead to dysphoric emotion and ineffective behavior. The patient and therapist continued to build rapport throughout this phase of treatment.

Sessions 10–12

Elizabeth's difficulties in occupying her time were, to a certain extent, overcome by the structuring of the daily activity schedule. The unit had a general routine for all patients that was supplemented with individualized activities scheduled by the primary nurse and the patient. The lack of pleasure in day-to-day activities was addressed with a standard CT approach. Elizabeth was asked to make mastery and pleasure ratings on her daily schedule (see Chapter 1). The primary nurse then negotiated with her about incorporating several potentially enjoyable activities into the day's activities.

In order to demonstrate the alliance between the primary nurse and the individual cognitive therapist, a joint session was held. Elizabeth indicated that she found no activities enjoyable, so she was asked to identify with her primary nurse over the next few days the three "least unenjoyable" activities. She was also provided a list of activities available to inpatients and asked to incorporate the three that she found most attractive (or the least unattractive) into her schedule. The primary nurse then monitored her activities over the next few days to ensure that the plan was carried through.

At the next session, Elizabeth reported on the activities that had been most enjoyable. Although all activities were scored in the low range, she was asked to choose two that she had rated highest and to include them in her next daily activities schedule. She was also asked to select other activities from the list to try or to suggest alternatives. The therapist may need to be directive and provide much of the energy for early behavioral change with severely depressed, chronic patients. The strategy that "if this does not work we will go for something else on the list" often helps overcome the patient's passivity.

Elizabeth's abuse of benzodiazepines was an important complication of her chronic depression. One of the sessions at this phase of the treatment started with a discussion of the use of diazepam:

THERAPIST: You mentioned that the diazepam was prescribed after your mother died.

ELIZABETH: Yes, I was beside myself. No one knew how to help me, and I felt uptight all the time. I wanted some relief so I asked for the pills. The local doctor gave them to me and told me to take them whenever I felt tense.

THERAPIST: Is that how you came to use them so often?

ELIZABETH: Yes, I found after a while that the pills were the only way to feel calm. They made me feel detached from things, and I also felt in control for the first time in a long time, or at least at first.

THERAPIST: Let me check to see if I understand what you've just said to me. After your mother's death you felt distressed in a way that neither you nor anyone else could control. The distress was particularly characterized by feeling tense, which I presume was in response to your thoughts about the loss of your mother. You then found a means of controlling that tension through using diazepam.

At this point, the therapist had deliberately reframed the behavior as a coping strategy, albeit a maladaptive one. This helped Elizabeth engage in a discussion about alternate coping strategies to deal with the thoughts and feelings surrounding the loss of her mother. Elizabeth acknowledged that the use of benzodiazepines was counterproductive, particularly because she had begun to need to take more medication in order to achieve the same level of relief. Also, the diazepam promoted an avoidance of the source of her tension. She had, for example, expressed resistance to exploring her relationship with her mother, but eventually consented to look at her thoughts about her mother's death. Elizabeth and her cognitive therapist agreed to collaborate on an action plan as described below:

THERAPIST: Let's recap our plan to look at your use of diazepam. . . . In fact, perhaps you could review the plan for us?

ELIZABETH: You want me to tell you the plan?

THERAPIST: Yes. I want to be sure that you understand the agreement.

ELIZABETH: Well, first of all you're going to start to gradually withdraw the diazepam, and you will give me a copy of the reduction program so that I know what dose I will be getting each day. Next, I said you'd have to replace the tablets with something, so we decided that I would get involved with one of the staff who runs a program on relaxation. You also said we could work on the thoughts related to the tension, particularly those that are about my mother.

THERAPIST: That's right. Do you want to go on now to talk about how you were thinking after your mother died?

ELIZABETH: Okay. *(Pause)* I just keep thinking that if I'd been well my mother would never have died.

THERAPIST: You believe you could have prevented it in some way?

ELIZABETH: I'm sure I could. It was my fault she died.

THERAPIST: That sounds like a very strong and important thought. Are there any other ideas about this you can identify at the moment?

ELIZABETH: No. *(Pause)* Well . . .

THERAPIST: Go on.

ELIZABETH: Well, except that I think I take after my mother.

THERAPIST: You're looking more depressed now—like we've brought out beliefs that cause a lot of distress.

ELIZABETH: I think you're right. I feel so guilty, and it seems like I could never get over this or change how I act.

THERAPIST: Let's try to start work on helping you with these beliefs. Is that okay with you?

ELIZABETH: No. Well . . . I suppose so.

THERAPIST: Elizabeth, I hope you don't mind my pointing out that you always respond to my questions by saying "No" and then seem to say "Yes." Do we need to look at that?

ELIZABETH: *(Smiling)* I don't know whether to say no or yes.

(Both smile and laugh.)

THERAPIST: Well, maybe next time we could discuss what your immediate thoughts are to my suggestions so that we can check about how you view the therapy. But, for now I want to get started on your beliefs about your mother's death. You've said "It was my fault my mother died," and then you went on to comment that you take after your mother. Could we start to look at the evidence for and against each of these conclusions?

ELIZABETH: Yes. *(Smiles at therapist.)*

Sessions 13–16

Exploration of thoughts relating to responsibility for her mother's death helped Elizabeth to see that she was not the cause of this event. Also, she was able to complete several assignments in which she listed similarities and differences between herself and her mother. Elizabeth began to recognize that she was quite different from her mother and had positive attributes that could be used to advantage. These therapeutic initiatives were accompanied by a significant improvement in her mood.

The therapy now began to turn to issues relating to the patient's current family situation. The recent change of residence had led to a number of marital tensions that needed to be explored. It was also thought that her spouse could assist in reviewing Elizabeth's idea (now weakened) that she was like her mother. Furthermore, Elizabeth's negative self-image was being reinforced by her older child's taking over some of her mothering role. However, the therapist believed that further individual work was necessary before initiating family therapy. Unless Elizabeth was more positive and secure, it would be difficult to prevent negative family interactions from undermining the fragile improvement in self-esteem.

Reattribution techniques were used to help Elizabeth review her sense of responsibility for the house move. She came to the opinion that whereas she had instigated the move, her husband's reaction to the changed situation was not "all my fault." He had taken at least a portion of the responsibility for the move, and she recalled that initially he had been very positive about his new job and the new friends he had made. Her views about being a "bad mother" were revised by exposing the differences between how she had been before she became depressed as opposed to afterwards. The next sessions began to look at the family situation more specifically.

Sessions 17–24

The next six sessions offered support for the forthcoming family therapy while they continued to deal with the items on Elizabeth's problem list. Issues for the family therapy sessions were discussed in detail. The aim was not just to explore the problems but also to encourage cognitive rehearsal in preparation for the family sessions, thus allowing Elizabeth and the therapist to identify and overcome "roadblocks."

During the first family session, her husband and older daughter expressed reservations about relinquishing household duties that they had assumed after Elizabeth became ill. Thus, for a weekend pass, the family members were encouraged to carry out graded reallocation of tasks, so that Elizabeth could slowly increase her level of responsibility in the household. They were encouraged to note the outcome of this experiment and report back at the next session. This exercise was repeated on a number of consecutive weekends in order to help Elizabeth build up her level of activity and confidence.

The next family session focused on specific aspects of interpersonal functioning and associated cognitions. The couple began to look at good and bad aspects of their marriage and resolved to carry out a number of tasks related to trying to "change the negatives." Attention was given to her interaction with both children, particularly her older daughter. Each individual was given the opportunity to give his or her "analysis" of the positives and negatives in the relationships. Positives were reinforced, and negatives were tackled appropriately. An example was that Elizabeth's children had not been telling her about their problems with school or friends because she had seemed preoccupied or distant, and they feared making her worse. They had been confiding only in their father. It was resolved that Elizabeth would set aside particular times on her passes to have the chance to talk with each child individually. In addition, she would schedule some family activities each day.

Elizabeth then began to work on her problem of social isolation. The first exercise was to write a letter to a previous confidante who lived near her old house. The task of reestablishing contacts was carried out in a graded way accompanied by exploration of automatic thoughts. After the letter was sent, a contact was made in person. Recent experiences (her prolonged absence from social networks through illness and hospitalization) were linked to the insecurity she experienced in the past during her prolonged absences from school (because of her mother's ill health). At this point in the therapy, Elizabeth was able to recognize and change underlying schemas relating to a sense of personal weakness and incapacity.

Sessions 24–28

Elizabeth was now having extended periods of leave at home. She had joined a "personal effectiveness" group held near her home as a way to improve interpersonal skills. She also had made several contacts with church members and neighbors and had found them to be sympathetic and supportive. This had countered her fears of rejection "because I'm mad." She had a brief setback when one individual overtly criticized her, but this provided excellent material to reinforce therapeutic techniques, and to "warn" Elizabeth of potential hurdles that would need to be confronted after discharge. This phase of the therapy was devoted primarily to helping Elizabeth manage the transition between the hospital and home (see Chapter 16).

Postdischarge

Elizabeth was discharged from the unit after an 11-week hospitalization. Two crisis calls were received in the first few days. Events, thoughts, and feelings were processed over the telephone using CT techniques. Both contacts were precipitated by feelings of "panic" associated with a fear of not being able to cope with a forthcoming social event and the catastrophic prediction that this would lead to a relapse. Coping strategies were rehearsed, and Elizabeth was encouraged to call back afterwards to report how it had gone. Therapy postdischarge took the form of weekly outpatient CT. Much of the work focused on assumptions and low self-esteem, but it was still important to pay attention to activity scheduling during the first few weeks out of the hospital.

Elizabeth eventually found a part-time job near her new home. She continued to make steady progress and began to come for CT every 2 weeks. She remained somewhat fragile but was able to cope with her problems. There were setbacks around the time of the anniversary of her mother's death, when her younger child had difficulties with the move to senior school, and intermittently when her husband expressed resentments about the move. She had one further brief episode of major depression that was treated as an outpatient by an increase in medication and more frequent sessions of CT. Nevertheless, 3 years after her hospital admission she was functioning well in the community.

COGNITIVE THERAPY WITH CHRONIC PERSONALITY DISORDERS

Patients with chronic personality disorders (CPD) typically have maladaptive schemas that underlie their patterns of dysfunctional behavior. The strategies they use to interact with the world, develop relationships, or "solve" problems are often ineffectual. Beck, Freeman, and Associates (1990) have suggested that the behavioral pathology of different personality disorders is linked to specific clusters of characteristic schemas. For example, the patient with a schizoid personality may believe "I will always be alone," or "keep away from others," whereas the person with a dependent personality may assume that "I cannot live without a man (woman)" or "if he (she) leaves, I'll die." The reader is referred to Beck and colleagues (1990) for a full description of schema development in various personality disorders.

The standard format for cognitive therapy described in Chapters 1 and 4 must be modified somewhat in work with CPD patients. First, these disorders, by definition, are chronic, and the treatment course is therefore usually extended beyond the short-term range. Therapy may be required for more than a year and may span several hospitalizations and periods of outpatient care. Ideally, the same therapist works with the patient during the hospital and aftercare phases of treatment.

Although the therapeutic relationship is important in all forms of CT, the collaborative process is perhaps most important in treatment of personality disorders. Schemas about significant interpersonal relationships are often recapitulated in the therapeutic relationship. This process, sometimes termed "transference," can provide information about the patient's basic assumptions and habitual modes of behavior with significant others. Overly dependent, narcissistic , or aggressive themes can undercut the collaborative and empirical relationship that is necessary for cognitive therapy.

Generally, the cognitive therapist attempts to maintain a problem-oriented, structured approach that encourages the patient to engage in productive therapeutic activity. Psychoeducational techniques, focused homework assignments, and frequent use of feedback also help to prevent the development of a regressive transference. However, the cognitive therapist needs to be prepared to recognize and modify maladaptive or destructive developments in the therapeutic relationship when they occur (Beck et al., 1990). Techniques used in this regard include identification and change of the patient's dysfunctional schemas, recognition of the therapist's own cognitions, increased emphasis on the structure of therapy, and the engaging in more direct problem-solving activity. Consultation with a colleague is indicated when there is an unresolved, troubled therapeutic relationship with a CPD patient.

With patients who have major depression or anxiety disorders, eliciting and modifying automatic thoughts often is enough to initiate substantial symptomatic change. Schema work is usually delayed till the later phases of therapy. With CPD patients, amelioration of the effect of dysfunctional schemas is almost always the core of the therapeutic experience. Cognitive therapy with CPD patients features both intensive and extensive attempts to change schemas. The treatment process involves frequent and repetitive use of CT procedures, such as examining the evidence, listing advantages and disadvantages, developing alternate schemas, and homework assignments.

Trying out new strategies *in vivo* is an important component of CT with chronic personality disorders. Usually, these patients have developed defective social skills after many years of harboring maladaptive self-constructs. Cognitive therapists use role play, modeling, cognitive–behavioral rehearsal, psychoeducational procedures, and graded-task assignments to promote growth of more adaptive behavior. One of the major differences in treatment of CPD patients, compared to acute psychiatric illnesses, is the need for *multiple* repetition of efforts to modify schemas and alter behavior. The therapist must be able to be patient, tolerate frustration, and remain persistent throughout the course of treatment.

Hospital admission is usually only a relatively brief part of the treatment of a CPD patient. Most admissions of personality disorders are necessitated because of dangerous behavior such as suicide attempts or threats toward others. However, some CPD patients are admitted when they develop symptoms that interfere with their ability to carry out tasks of daily living. Examples might include a passive–dependent personality with an associated chronic pain syndrome, or borderline personality disorder with a brief "minipsychosis." Usually CPD patients are discharged and followed as outpatients after the acute crisis subsides, and they are again able to manage independent living.

The inpatient stay can be a particularly important component of the treatment of CPD. The admission is usually associated with an increase in stress that disrupts the usual pattern of functioning and generates "hot" cognitions and intense emotions. For example, a "rejection" may kindle schemas about self-worth, trust, or attractiveness. The patient may be in a more accessible mode for therapy at these times. The hospital itself may also play a role in bringing underlying schemas to the surface. The close proximity to other patients and staff, the unavoidable restrictions of hospital life, and the increased intensity of the therapeutic relationship (because of more frequent treatment sessions) are several of the features of hospitalization that may provoke the expression of dysfunctional schemas and behavior.

As noted in Chapters 2 and 3, there are multiple opportunities for eliciting and testing out distorted cognitions and learning new skills in the hospital milieu. However, CPD patients can be especially challenging for hospital staff members. The actions of patients with personality disorders can be provocative, manipulative, attention-seeking, or hostile. At times, these patients attempt to "split" staff or entrap them into fulfilling dependency needs or aggressive desires. Staff members can interpret the behavior of the CPD patient as signifying resistance, manipulation, defensiveness, or lack of motivation. However, if a CT conceptualization is utilized, there is an alternate explanation: the patient is using learned strategies that are based on maladaptive cognitions.

Patients whose behavior improves in the hospital setting, but consistently deteriorates after discharge, are particularly troublesome. Such "revolving door" patients often present with exactly the same problems each time they return to the hospital. These individuals usually have difficulty generalizing the gains from the inpatient experience to the world outside the hospital. Their choice of coping strategies after discharge continues to be based on dysfunctional beliefs, thus recreating the scenario that led to the initial hospitalization. Ongoing careful and consistent work is needed to reach the ultimate goals of recovery of function and relapse prevention. The following case illustrates cognitive therapy procedures with a "revolving door" CPD patient.

Case Illustration

Betsy, a 32-year-old single woman who had been diagnosed as having borderline personality disorder, was assigned to cognitive therapy after her fifth hospitalization in 3 years. During previous episodes, she appeared to respond well to medication. However, on release she would begin to deteriorate, even though she continued to take medication (usually low-dose haloperidol—Haldol®). Betsy would become enraged and hopeless and would begin a cycle of self-destructive behavior, including binge eating. She also would become sexually involved with men for whom she had no interest, and then, apparently to punish herself, would begin to burn her stomach or slash her wrists and thighs. This behavior usually culminated in a readmission to the hospital.

The pattern of deterioration was perceived by staff as noncompliance with the follow-up phase of treatment. For example, the hospital staff could be overheard saying: "Here she comes again; no matter what we do, she always screws it up on the outside." Betsy believed this statement herself. Although she wanted to stay out of the hospital, by the fifth hospitalization, she was becoming increasingly hopeless. The psychiatric staff had tried numerous treatments prior to referring Betsy for cognitive therapy. The long list of therapies included multiple antipsychotic, antidepressant, and anxiolytic drugs; several trials of other types of psychotherapy; and a full course of electroconvulsive treatment.

The patient's history included longstanding abuse and neglect, including sexual abuse by her stepfather. She had performed poorly as a student, although she did manage to graduate from high school. Betsy had held a variety of jobs for short periods over the last few years. She lived with her mother; her stepfather had died from complications of alcoholism. Although Betsy had had a series of short but intense heterosexual relationships, she had never been married and had no children.

Betsy was treated at a unit with an "add-on" model for cognitive therapy (see Chapter 3). The cognitive therapist provided a "cognitive therapy track" module for selected patients. Staff members had been oriented to cognitive therapy procedures but did not apply these techniques on a regular basis. The role of the cognitive therapist in this milieu was to provide individual CT and to serve as consultant to staff members in using cognitive therapy as an adjunct to standard treatment.

The therapist developed a dual-level case conceptualization that attempted to explain Betsy's frequent relapses:

1. *Failure to change schemas.* Although Betsy had appeared to respond to previous hospitalizations, it was apparent that her improvement had been short-lived and was probably related to the increased structure and nurturance of the hospital setting. Schemas that were thought to "drive" maladaptive behaviors and coping strategies had not been significantly modified by previous treatment efforts.

Currently, Betsy was very hostile and negativistic. Her behavior was labile and hard to predict. Relationships with staff members were strained. Thus, it was thought that a period of relationship building and behavioral work would probably be required before moving to the deeper schema level in therapy.

2. *Staff attitudes.* The frequent hospitalizations, Betsy's efforts to "split" staff, her failure to improve, and recurrent self-destructive acts had led most of the treatment team to develop a rather hopeless view of the chances for recovery. In many ways, the staff was just "going through the motions" with Betsy. The therapist thought that the staff needed to be reenergized and that a reconceptualization of the case from a cognitive perspective might be helpful.

Sessions 1–3

Betsy was reluctant to begin treatment with a new therapist. She verbalized thoughts such as: "You're abandoning me; everybody's given up; there's no use; I'll just stay in my room." Betsy was so angry and hostile at this time that exploration of these cognitions was not feasible. Instead, the therapist focused on demonstrating a hopeful and kindly attitude toward the patient, despite Betsy's efforts to undermine the beginning of therapy. The first three sessions were spent reviewing the history and attempting to engage Betsy in a collaborative effort to change her behavior on the unit.

Betsy acknowledged that she tended to become more dysphoric during periods when she was aimless and had no clear idea of how to spend her time. In fact, the most recent hospitalization had occurred after she lost a part-time job and began to spend her days either sleeping for long periods or wandering the streets. After admission, she had refused most activities and had been isolating herself in her room whenever possible.

In one of the first attempts at hypothesis testing, the therapist posed the following question: "Would you be willing to check out, here on the unit, the idea that a structured day can make you feel better?" Betsy replied: "You're probably right, but I still don't want to do it. I'm better off if you just let me alone." The therapist responded to this typical "mixed message" by focusing on the positive potential in the patient's attitude: "Part of you seems to think that this is a good idea. Let me think of ways that we can start to encourage that part." A simple contingency contract was then proposed that rewarded (with visits from a friend outside the normal visiting hours) adherence to at least 8 hours of a mutually designed activity schedule.

The first three sessions also were used to introduce Betsy to some of the basic procedures of cognitive therapy. The purposes of collaboration, structure, agenda-setting, feedback, problem orientation, and hypothesis testing were explained. It was emphasized that this new form of therapy would require Betsy's active involvement and that if she invested effort in the treatment, she could start to change the repetitive attitudes and behaviors that were interfering with her functioning.

During the first week of CT, the therapist also met with the treatment team at a planning conference. Considerable frustration and anger at Betsy were verbalized by several of the staff members. The therapist acknowledged the difficulties in working with CPD patients and then outlined the CT component of the treatment plan. Betsy's provocative and self-injurious behavior was explained from a cognitive perspective, and examples of her dysfunctional schemas were given. Particular attention was paid to how schemas such as "I deserve to be punished" or "no one can be trusted" are associated with recreation of patterns of rejection or neglect in interpersonal relationships. The cognitive therapist was supportive of the treatment team and approached negative staff reactions in a nonconfrontational manner. Gentle humor was used to diffuse some of the tensions surrounding Betsy's treatment. By the end of the planning conference, there was a renewed, although somewhat guarded, sense of optimism, and the staff members were prepared to assist with the behavioral components of the therapy.

Sessions 4–6

In the second week of treatment, Betsy began to respond to the structure of the activity schedule. She started to eat regular meals and to participate in most scheduled activities. There also was an improved general attitude on the part of the staff toward Betsy. The CT sessions were devoted primarily to behavioral exercises and to an attempt to engage Betsy in the process of monitoring automatic thoughts. The behavioral treatment consisted of an extension of the activities' scheduling to mastery and pleasure recordings. These data were used in sessions 5 and 6 to reorganize the schedule and make specific assignments that Betsy and the therapist agreed might improve her self-esteem and decrease depressed mood.

Efforts also were made to help Betsy improve her grooming. Staff and other patients had noted that Betsy rarely washed her hair and frequently wore soiled clothes. At times, she even had a strong body odor. This rather delicate situation was approached with caution by the therapist:

THERAPIST: You've told me that you think the other patients don't like to be around you. Part of the problem could be your low self-esteem, but we could also look at the things you might be doing to put them off. Would you be willing to do that?

BETSY: Yes, I suppose. What did you have in mind? Am I a "freak" or something?

THERAPIST: You're certainly not a "freak," but sometimes people that are down on themselves do things that aren't in their best interest. The example that I hear about from the nurses and some of the patients is that you haven't been taking very good care of yourself.

BETSY: *(Looks hurt and angry)* So you want to change me too. It's like I'm never good enough for anybody.

THERAPIST: I can see that my idea stirred up lots of thoughts and feelings.

BETSY: It sure did. All I ever hear is criticism. Why don't people try to help me instead of always dumping on me?

THERAPIST: Let's stop for a minute and take a look at the kinds of thoughts you develop when somebody gives you feedback. It sounds like you immediately jump to the conclusion that the other person finds you unacceptable and just wants to put you down.

BETSY: That's right.

THERAPIST: Could you think of any other reasons why I might bring up this topic?

BETSY: *(Pause)* Well, I suppose you could be trying to help me . . . I guess I have to be careful not to always blame things on everybody else. You've been telling me I have to take some of the responsibility if I am going to change.

THERAPIST: That's right. We'll come back later to learn more about how you interpret feedback, but for now let's try to focus on what you're doing to take care of yourself.

They went on to discuss Betsy's grooming and how it might affect her self-concept and her interpersonal relations. A graded-task assignment was then designed to improve grooming in a step-wise fashion. Nursing staff members were recruited to work with Betsy on this project.

By the end of the second week, Betsy had been introduced to the concept of automatic thoughts and was beginning to recognize that outbursts of sadness or anger were often preceded by negatively oriented thoughts. "Affective shifts" (sudden developments of strong emotion) were used in therapy sessions to identify automatic thoughts. A simplified description of cognitive errors, such as selective abstraction, personalization, and absolutistic thinking, was also given. A homework assignment at the end of session 6 included a three-column thought record (event, automatic thoughts, emotion) with a request to label cognitive errors.

Sessions 7–9

The therapeutic relationship was clearly improving by the third week of treatment. "Transference" issues were handled by keeping the therapy directed at the collaborative problem-solving effort and working through negative reactions to the therapist with Socratic questioning and revision of distorted automatic thoughts. Treatment planning conferences and informal conversations with staff members continued to reinforce the utility of the cognitive approach. Betsy was following the activity schedule and participating in further graded-task assignments designed to improve social skills and develop a more positive self-concept. The therapist thought that Betsy was now ready to begin to explore some of the schemas that were thought to be preventing her from sustaining behavioral change.

Information from Betsy's case history and earlier CT sessions suggested that the following schemas were operative: (1) "I am worthless;" (2) "I am only valuable as a sexual object;" (3) "I am a bad girl;" (4) "I deserve to be punished;" (5) "No one can help me;" (6) "It is all my fault;" and (7) "I am unlovable." These "deep" cognitions made it difficult for her to continue to function when exposed to increased stress after leaving the hospital. Specifically, Betsy would become hopeless when these schemas were activated by some real-life event or memory. After this occurred, she would be unable to maintain her daily schedule or even her personal hygiene.

The therapist believed that fundamental change in these schemas would be a long-term goal that could not be fully realized during the hospitalization. However, one of the objectives of the inpatient phase of treatment was to weaken several of the damaging schemas listed above to the point that the risk for relapse would be significantly diminished.

The therapeutic work on schema modification is illustrated in the following vignette:

BETSY: Whenever something goes wrong I get this powerful urge to hurt myself.

THERAPIST: Can you think of an example?

BETSY: Sure, there are plenty of them. I cut my wrists again before I came to the hospital, and that happened after I got into an argument with my mother.

THERAPIST: What happened?

BETSY: It was really such a silly thing when you think about it. We were trying to decide whose turn it was to go grocery shopping, and I began to think how I never do anything right. I mean, I can't even cooperate around the house.

THERAPIST: Then what did you think?

BETSY: That I'm no good . . . that I deserve what I get. And then I went into the bathroom and starting cutting again.

THERAPIST: There must have been another step in your thinking. Try to put yourself back into the situation. You said "I deserve what I get." What was your next thought?

BETSY: I deserve to be punished.

THERAPIST: You've just given a good example how an underlying belief or schema can control your behavior. The situation started with a minor disagreement, and before long this strong belief that you deserve to be punished came out, and then you cut your wrists.

BETSY: I hadn't really thought of it that way, but I guess you're right.

THERAPIST: Sometimes these schemas are based on false information. Let's try to look for evidence for and against this schema.

They proceeded to generate a list of pros and cons for the schema. Betsy was able to find many circumstances in which she had been abused, neglected, or treated poorly. She had come to believe that she deserved this mistreatment. Betsy then had gone the next step to inflict punishment on herself. Therapeutic work at this juncture also revealed many reasons why she did not deserve to be abused. These included the recollection that she had not encouraged any of the ill treatment when she was a child. It was only as an adult that she began to get into a pattern of recapitulating the punishment. Also, Betsy was able to recognize that she had an inherent self-worth, and she had the right to expect decent treatment from others.

Additional work on this schema included homework exercises in the milieu (e.g., recording automatic thoughts in situations where she came in conflict with others). She was instructed to look for situations in which the schema "I deserve to be punished" was likely to reemerge and to weaken the schema by identifying cognitive errors that supported the belief. A similar assignment was designed for her first pass home, which was scheduled for the end of the third week of hospitalization.

Sessions 10–12

After a successful visit home, and further improvement in self-esteem and behavioral control, plans were made for discharge and a continuation of therapy on an outpatient basis. Prior to discharge, the therapist focused on three major tools for relapse prevention: (1) cognitive–behavioral rehearsal; (2) further schema modification; and (3) extension of activity scheduling to the home setting. Cognitive–behavioral rehearsal was used to recognize "yellow-flags" and potential problem areas that might stimulate primitive schemas and a deterioration in functioning. A number of potentially stressful situations, including arguments with mother, going out on a date, or simply feeling bored or unproductive were identified. Betsy and her therapist then "walked through" these situations to practice adaptive coping methods.

Attempts at modifying schemas also continued through the last week of hospitalization. Several procedures were used such as listing advantages and disadvantages of continuing to hold specific schemas, beginning to write down alternate beliefs, and using homework exercises to try out new schemas. For example, the statement "I deserve to be punished" was reformulated as follows: "I have received lots of punishment; I deserve to be treated better." Finally, an effort was made to continue the structuring of daily activities that had started at the beginning of hospitalization. A weekly schedule was developed that included regular sleeping hours, meals, therapy appointments, exercise, recreational activities, and time to search for a job. Betsy and her therapist agreed that a program of purposeful activity would help to maintain the gains that she had made during the hospitalization.

COGNITIVE THERAPY WITH SCHIZOPHRENIC INPATIENTS

Cognitive therapy was not originally designed for psychotic patients, although Beck considered the cognitive aspects of schizophrenia in one of his early papers (Beck, 1952). Pharmacotherapy is, of course, the mainstay of treatment for schizophrenia. However, recent efforts have been made to develop cognitive therapy procedures that can serve as an adjunct to neuroleptic treatment (Wright & Schrodt, 1989; Fowler & Morley, 1989; Perris, 1989; Kingdon & Turkington, 1991). This section of the chapter will describe methods of using CT with schizophrenic inpatients.

The cognitive perspective for treating schizophrenia starts with trying to understand the situation in which the baffled patient finds himself or herself. If explanations for the illness are conflicting, or are considered to be inadequate by the patient, then catastrophic cognitions may develop around the meaning of this "madness." The patient's mind set may include images of incarceration in an asylum, terrorization by other "lunatics," and rejection by family, friends, and society. If such thoughts or images are not allayed, they will tend to stand in the way of recovery. In some cases, a diagnosis is reached but not given to the patient because of the treatment team's catastrophic thoughts about the diagnosis of schizophrenia. In such a situation, patients often believe the worst and may come to the most appalling conclusions. Intense hopelessness and significant risk for suicide may ensue. A vital role of CT early in the course of hospitalization is to provide a rationale for symptom emergence, justification of the need for neuroleptic treatment, and a hopeful attitude toward treatment.

It has been suggested that a close examination of the antecedents of a psychotic breakdown may be an important component of the CT approach to schizophrenia before any direct attempt is made to modify psychotic symptoms (Beck, 1952). This phase of therapy, beginning with development of a therapeutic alliance, can reduce symptoms in its own right. History taking is directed, in part, at revealing the patient's most pertinent automatic thoughts and underlying schemas. Such information is most often accessed using careful inductive questioning. Often, the patient's "hot" cognitions and schemas can be used to make sense of the specific content of delusions or hallucinations. Some patients can find this work upsetting, and a worsening of symptoms has occasionally been noticed. Should an increase in symptoms occur, it is obviously important to reduce the intensity of the therapy for a period and treat the exacerbation supportively. However, if a good working relationship can be established, and the patient is able to respond to inductive questions, the next phase of the therapy, reality testing, can be initiated.

Reality testing is initiated in a gentle and collaborative way, with patient and therapist examining the information together using the guided discovery mode. Confrontation is to be avoided at all times (Milton, Patwa, & Hafner, 1978). The need for medication is usually one of the important agenda items in CT with schizophrenics. The therapist presents a biopsychosocial model, in which a "chemical imbalance," or underlying biological vulnerability, interacts with maladaptive cognitions and life stress in the development of symptoms. It is also suggested that a multifaceted treatment approach, including medications, cognitive therapy, and social interventions (e.g., family therapy, social skills training, day hospitals, etc.) offers the most comprehensive and potentially useful approach to treatment.

One of the important components of the reality-testing phase of treatment is an examination of the validity of this biopsychosocial treatment philosophy. A psychoeducational orientation is used to explain and demonstrate the utility of medication, CT, and social interventions. Standard CT techniques, such as guided discovery and examining the evidence, also may be used. In the hospital setting, a portion of this work can be accomplished in focused group therapies (see Chapter 5). Nursing and occupational therapy staff need to be aware of the nature of individual and group therapy so that they can help patients with homework assignments. Ideally, the patient is involved in CT procedures throughout the treatment milieu (see Chapter 4). A common goal of CT for schizophrenia is to change the locus of the psychotic symptoms. For example, auditory hallucinations previously believed to have an external origin may come to be seen as unpleasant, internally driven thoughts (essentially like obsessional thoughts in character). Hallucinations and delusions are approached systematically using techniques such as examining the evidence and generating alternative hypotheses. The most accessible symptoms (usually hallucinations) are addressed first.

In the treatment of delusions, the strangeness of the patient's experiences militates toward an acceptance of the value of testing out even the most unlikely hypotheses (e.g., a patient might rate brain dopamine overactivity as a very unlikely cause of his or her symptoms, but he or she might consider hypnosis, witchcraft, or voodoo as credible explanatory constructs). These hypotheses can all be rated for credibility, and, using behavioral homework exercises, gradual testing of these delusional beliefs can take place until more reasonable explanations are accepted. Therapist attributes of patience and determination are particularly valuable in attempting to treat delusions with CT. Sessions may need to be cancelled or terminated prematurely if the patient is unable to proceed. Another meeting can be scheduled at a later time. Although sessions are variable in length (10 minutes to over an hour), the therapist usually does not suggest continuing the treatment beyond 30 to 45 minutes. On occasion, a longer interview may be indicated when a patient is productively exploring a systematized delusion.

A delusion also may be modified by reducing the emotional charge that is associated with it (e.g., a delusion of infidelity is often "protected" from reality testing by the strength of the anger that surrounds it, whereas delusions of persecution may be associated with marked fear).

Dampening these emotions with techniques such as relaxation exercises can succeed in exposing the underlying delusion to reality testing. Some delusions that remain resistant to affectively targeted interventions can be addressed using an inference chain (or "downward arrow") technique to find the underlying schema (see Chapter 1). Although delusions are usually given up gradually by the patient, their plausibility may never be fully rejected, and delusions can remain as lingering doubts. Eventually, some patients are able to laugh at the incredible nature of a delusion that has been "given up."

Relapse prevention is another important component of CT with schizophrenic inpatients. Providing a rationale for therapy to the family and describing how the patient will be working to cope with symptoms can instill hope, decatastrophize the meaning of possible relapses, and reduce guilt. The family and individual formats for therapy can be used to: (1) explain the early symptoms of psychotic relapse; (2) learn to identify and avoid triggering situations, thoughts, or feelings; (3) recognize the need for seeking help; (4) increase compliance with neuroleptic treatment; and (5) identify cognitive strategies to cope with symptom exacerbation. Reducing expressed emotion in the home may also be a goal for family sessions before discharge (see Chapter 6). A case illustration of CT with a schizophrenic inpatient is described below.

A Case of Witchcraft?

Anna was a 20-year-old single woman who was brought by her father and mother to the hospital's emergency service in an acutely disturbed state. She had been diagnosed as having schizophrenia at 16 years of age, but she could not recall ever being told exactly what was wrong with her. Since that time, Anna had never been free of psychotic symptoms, and she had been rehospitalized twice during acute exacerbations. She had persistent auditory hallucinations in association with the paranoid delusion that witchcraft was being used against her. The voices were in the third person and often abusive in nature. Over 4 years of illness, Anna had been treated with extensive courses of neuroleptics. She had become increasingly disturbed during the 48 hours prior to her admission. Her parents reported that she started "talking nonsense" and behaving in a frightened and agitated manner. They did not know why this deterioration had occurred.

Examination at the time of admission revealed Anna to be in a reasonable state of hygiene with appropriate grooming and dress. She was relieved to be in a protected environment away from her neighborhood, because "evil forces are at work there." Anna spoke at a normal rate, but had definite loosening of associations and intermingling of themes that lapsed, at times, into incomprehensibility. She indicated that witchcraft was at the root of her problems, and it was being used to harm her body in various ways. She regularly felt "pins being stuck into my body" and believed that the witchcraft was causing headaches and insomnia. All knives in the house had been hidden because she was terrified that they might be used against her. Anna frequently turned objects around three times in a ritual way. This seemed to offer comfort at her most anxious times.

Anna's parents reported that she had had a normal birth and development. She mixed well with other children, and there were no problematic habits or traits. School performance was excellent until her first breakdown at age 16. Her premorbid personality was described as well balanced, with the ability to make friends easily. There was evidence of perfectionistic and hard-working tendencies during childhood and adolescence. She was an agnostic with no particular interest in the occult.

Over the 4 years of illness, she had been treated mostly with neuroleptic medications. Her outpatient care and home support were managed by a psychiatric nurse. However, repeated attempts to persuade Anna to attend a day hospital, day care, and various support groups had not been successful. At the time of admission, a diagnosis of chronic paranoid schizophrenia was confirmed, and treatment was reinstituted with haloperidol (Haldol®) 2 mg twice daily and 5 mg at bedtime. Cognitive therapy sessions also were prescribed.

Session 1

In this first CT session, Anna indicated that she couldn't understand why she had been hospitalized. She did acknowledge feeling more safe on the ward. Some superficial work was done in therapy to introduce Anna to the cognitive model. For example, initial rational responses to her fearful thoughts and feelings were proposed (e.g., "I haven't been harmed in the past 4 years despite my problems—so why should anything happen now?"). She agreed in a halfhearted way to attempt to use such rational responses to see if they could help. Despite her thought disorder, a reasonable degree of rapport was established, and it was possible to refer Anna back to illogical thought connections and ask for clarification. In this way, three clear themes were identified. The first was that witchcraft was at work and causing problems. The second related to strange feelings in her body. Although these could have been either somatic hallucinations or anxiety symptoms, Anna ascribed these phenomena to the witchcraft. Third, it was noted that the degree of disturbance of thought appeared to fluctuate in relation to the degree of affect attached to the subject matter. Further, Anna's train of thought was better at the end of the interview than it had been at the start.

Session 2

Anna questioned the need for hospitalization. It was decided to give her a clear diagnosis and rationale for treatment. She was told that she had schizophrenia—a type of "nervous breakdown." Anna said that she had expected this because she had seen a film in which someone heard voices all the time and this person had been schizophrenic. She had concluded that schizophrenia is an untreatable illness and therefore had "given up." Anna was told that schizophrenia can be treated and that it is caused in part by overactivity in a region of the brain. It was further suggested that medication could act against this overactivity and thereby help regulate brain function. Evidence of this position was provided in the form of a patient education pamphlet. Anna also was told that schizophrenia can occur under situations of stress. She was able then to relate her recent relapse to repeated arguments at home, lack of sleep, and the death of an elderly relative. When discussing the precipitants for the relapse, her thought processes were much more coherent than at other times. A homework assignment was established that entailed Anna's agreeing to ask three staff members about whether medication helped symptoms of schizophrenia.

Session 3

Homework was reviewed, and Anna had made some notes of staff replies. Most of this session was spent reviewing the purpose and side effects of haloperidol. She agreed to an increase in the dose to 5 mg three times a day. The relationship between sleep deprivation and hallucinations was discussed. Anna's thought disorder appeared to be improving, and the loosening of associations was less dramatic.

Session 4

Guided by inductive questions, Anna discussed the antecedents of the first psychotic breakdown. Initially, Anna could not remember any stresses that might have contributed to the original onset of her illness. However, on close analysis, it could be seen that the family had moved frequently and that she had changed school four times in the 2 years prior to the first episode of illness. When talking about the second change of school, she recalled feeling isolated, sad, and bullied by her new classmates. Depressogenic automatic thoughts were dominant, including: "I'm a failure; this is pointless; and I can't catch up." By the time of the third change in schools, Anna was hyperaroused and displayed somatic anxiety symptoms such as severe tension in her shoulders and neck and unusual abdominal sensations. Anxious automatic thoughts were present: "I must perform better in exams; everything is out of control; I must be a better daughter." The fourth school move only 10 weeks prior to the onset of the first psychotic episode.

By the end of session 4, Anna was able to admit that there was some evidence of a buildup of adverse events prior to symptom onset. This had a normalizing (i.e., decatastrophizing) effect, and she was able to start to see her illness as more understandable.

Sessions 5–9

Anna was more engaged in therapy now and was displaying a greater willingness to discuss thoughts and feelings. Hallucinations were chosen as the next focus for therapy. Heretofore, the reality of the voices had never really been questioned. It was decided to try to find out more about the auditory hallucinations by recording their intensity, frequency, and "triggers." This homework assignment was not done with any great enthusiasm. However, the exercise demonstrated that the voices tended to happen when Anna was alone. Moreover, the hallucinations were noted to be of variable intensity, and, at times, were hardly present at all.

Anna started to show some interest in questioning the validity of her hallucinations. In one homework session she asked several trusted staff members whether they could hear the voices. She returned to the next session to report that all replies had been in the negative. Hypotheses were generated as to what the voices might actually be. She still believed that they were probably "real," but now believed this at only the "70% true" level. This was again tested in a homework assignment in which she attempted to locate the source of the voices. This was a useful maneuver, because her belief in the reality of the voices now dropped below 50%. Possible explanations regarding how the voices might be directed at her alone were discussed, including that she might be a medium hearing the voices of spirits (Anna only believed this at the 30% level), telepathy (20% belief), or a symptom of schizophrenia caused by her "overactivity of a region of the brain" (30% belief). Additional reading material on schizophrenia and continued work in CT allowed her gradually to increase her belief that the voices were a symptom. Anna became less preoccupied and less frightened by the hallucinations after these sessions.

Sessions 10–15

Although Anna's belief in witchcraft was still strong, it had lessened as a result of the work on hallucinations. Anna and her therapist decided to begin to examine the evidence for there being witchcraft in her neighborhood. Much of the evidence that they collected against the witchcraft formulation related to Anna's inability to explain the strangeness of the phenomena she had experienced early in the course of the psychosis. Repeated reframing of this episode as a stress-induced schizophrenic breakdown was useful. The feeling of being stuck by pins was explained as an anxiety symptom associated with hyperventilation. Further, it was demonstrated that the symptoms could be induced by rapid breathing.

Rational responses for negative automatic thoughts also were suggested. Inference chaining of the delusion about witchcraft revealed an underlying schema that demanded total control over life (i.e., "I must be in control at all times"). The activation of this schema in the prepsychotic phase of her illness may have provoked or shaped the specific delusional content. As Anna had lost self-control, she had become convinced that she was being controlled from the outside in a malicious and destructive way. At this phase in the therapy, CT was directed, in part, at modifying the underlying irrational belief about an absolute need for control. By session 15, the delusional beliefs about witchcraft remained as only lingering doubts that did not cause unpleasant emotions or greatly affect behavior.

Sessions 16–20

Reduced motivation in general, and reticence to engage in social interchanges in particular, were approached with relatively slowly paced activity scheduling and mastery and pleasure ratings. By this time, Anna had been transferred to a partial hospitalization program in the same facility (but continued in treatment with the same cognitive therapist). She tended to set goals that were too high and then give up entirely. For example, she would agree to come to the hospital by 9:00 a.m. every morning, but when she realized she couldn't get ready in time, she decided that it would be better not to come at all. This absolutistic thinking was identified, and Anna was told that if she could arrive at the day hospital by lunchtime that it would be okay. Gradually, the starting times were revised, and Anna began to arrive regularly at 9:30 a.m.

Relapse prevention was a major focus of this phase of treatment. Medication compliance continued to be an agenda item. Both cognitive and behavioral procedures were used (e.g., eliciting and changing dysfunctional attitudes about medication, and behavioral interventions to reinforce adherence to the medication regimen). Booster sessions followed completion of session 20 and discharge from the partial hospitalization program. At the time of this manuscript's preparation, Anna was seen by her cognitive therapist every 2 months. She had not relapsed for over 2 years and reported an improved social life and an increased range of interests. She was considering further education. Anna had become very knowledgeable about schizophrenia and appeared to be better equipped to deal with relapse should this occur.

The use of CT with schizophrenic patients, as described above, is still in the early stages of development. Controlled research has not yet been completed to determine whether CT added to pharmacotherapy has an additional benefit over the effects of the drug alone. However, case reports have indicated that CT appears to be well accepted by schizophrenics and is helpful in modifying some of the dysfunctional cognitive and behavioral patterns of this disorder (Wright & Schrodt, 1989; Fowler & Morley, 1989; Perris, 1989; Kingdon & Turkington, 1991). Cognitive therapy may prove to be a useful adjunct to the standard inpatient care for patients with schizophrenia.

CONCLUSION

This chapter describes a cognitive therapy approach to patients with chronic psychiatric disorders. Although specific interventions vary according to diagnosis, severity of symptoms, and characterological structure, there are several general treatment principles that underlie CT strategies for these patients:

1. The treatment program must be realistic. Patients with chronic disorders have many fixed assumptions. Modification of schemas, rather than absolute change, may be the most appropriate initial goal.
2. The treatment program may need to be both intensive and prolonged. Postdischarge continuity of therapy is highly recommended.
3. The involvement of many staff members is required. In order for the program to be maximally effective, the staff needs to be "socialized" to the cognitive model (see Chapters 3 and 9).
4. CT with chronic patients incorporates work on both acute symp-

toms (e.g., hopelessness or delusions) and rehabilitative functions (e.g., reestablishing the individual in the community).

Chronicity is often regarded as being synonymous with poor prognosis. Cognitive therapy offers a new and potentially useful tool in the treatment of this difficult group of patients. The efficacy of CT for chronic patients has not been established in controlled outcome trials, and it is unlikely that this form of treatment will have utility for all individuals with chronic mental illness. Nevertheless, CT may be the psychological treatment of choice (either singly, or in combination with medication) for many individuals in the subgroups described here (Williams, 1992). Galileo once said that if he could see farther than others, it was because he stood on the shoulders of giants. By taking the therapy developed by Beck and adapting it to the chronic patient, we are hopeful that in the future we will be able to see further into the "mist" that surrounds these disorders and reduce the suffering of patients and their families.

REFERENCES

Barker, W., Scott, J., & Eccleston, D. (1987). The Newcastle chronic depression study: The treatment programme. *International Clinical Pharmacology, 2,* 226–232.

Beck, A. T. (1952). Successful outpatient psychotherapy of a chronic schizophrenic with a delusion based on borrowed guilt. *Psychiatry,* 15, 305–312.

Beck, A. T. (1976). *Cognitive therapy and the emotional disorders.* New York: International Universities Press.

Beck, A. T., Freeman, A., & Associates. (1990). *Cognitive therapy of personality disorders.* New York: Guilford Press.

Fennell, M., & Teasdale, J. (1982). Cognitive therapy with chronic drug-refractory depressed outpatients: A note of caution. *Cognitive Therapy and Research, 6,* 455–460.

Fowler, D., & Morley, S. (1989). The cognitive–behavioral treatment of hallucinations and delusions: A preliminary study. *Behavioral Psychotherapy, 17,* 262–282.

Freeman, A., Simon, M. K., Arkowitz, H., & Beutler, L. (1989). *Handbook of cognitive therapy.* New York: Plenum Press.

Kingdon, D., & Turkington, D. (1991). The use of cognitive behavior therapy with a moralizing rationale in schizophrenia. *Journal of Nervous and Mental Diseases, 179,* 207–211.

Miller, I., Norman, W., & Keitner, G. (1989). Cognitive behavioral treatment of depressed inpatients: 6 and 12-month follow-up. *American Journal of Psychiatry, 146,* 1274–1279.

Milton, F., Patwa, V. K., & Hafner, R. J. (1978). Confrontation versus belief modification in persistently deluded patients. *British Journal of Medical Psychology, 51*, 127–130.

Perris, C. (1989). *Cognitive therapy with schizophrenic patients.* New York: Guilford Press.

Rush, A. J., Beck, A. T., Kovacs, M., & Hollon, S. (1977). Comparative efficacy of cognitive therapy and pharmacotherapy in the treatment of depressed outpatients. *Cognitive Therapy and Research, 1*, 17–37.

Scott, J. (1988a). Chronic depression. *British Journal of Psychiatry, 153*, 287–297.

Scott, J. (1988b). Cognitive therapy with depressed inpatients. In W. Dryden & P. Trower (Eds.), *Developments in cognitive psychotherapy* (pp. 177–189). London: Sage.

Scott, J. (1992). Chronic depression: Can cognitive therapy succeed when other treatments fail? *Behavioral Psychotherapy, 20*, 25–36.

Scott, J., Barker, W., & Eccleston, D. (1988). The Newcastle chronic depression study. *British Journal of Psychiatry, 152*, 28–33.

Thase, M. E., Bowler, K., & Harden, T. (1991). Cognitive behavior therapy of endogenous depression: Part 2. Preliminary findings in 16 unmedicated patients. *Behavior Therapy, 22*, 469–477.

Thase, M. E., & Wright, J. H. (1991). Cognitive behavior therapy manual for depressed inpatients: A treatment protocol outline. *Behavior Therapy, 22*, 579–595.

Williams, J. M. G. (1992). *The psychological treatment of depression* (2nd ed.). London: Routledge.

Wright, J. H., & Schrodt G. R., Jr. (1989). Combined cognitive therapy and pharmacotherapy. In A. Freeman, M. K. Simon, H. Arkowitz, & L. Beutler (Eds.), *Handbook of cognitive therapy* (pp. 267–282). New York: Plenum Press.

Part V

EDUCATION AND RELAPSE PREVENTION

Chapter 15

Staff and Patient Education

Christine A. Padesky, Ph.D.

A recent study has shown that mere attendance in a cognitive therapy (CT) group does not guarantee that patients will learn CT skills or experience lower relapse rates (Neimeyer and Feixas, 1990). Patients must be taught cognitive therapy procedures, and they may need repeated practice in order to master skills. Therefore, a key ingredient of a successful inpatient cognitive therapy program is the presence of staff who are able to teach these skills to the patients. This chapter outlines methods for educating staff to help them achieve competency as cognitive therapists and become good teachers of CT skills. Educational programs for admitting physicians and referring therapists also will be discussed. Finally, methods for providing patient education will be detailed.

EDUCATION FOR HOSPITAL STAFF

What Makes a Competent Inpatient Cognitive Therapist?

In cognitive therapy, as in most forms of psychotherapy, the most effective therapists express warmth, empathy, and genuineness (Truax & Carkhuff, 1967; Beck, Rush, Shaw, & Emery, 1979; Persons & Burns, 1985). Beside these "nonspecific" qualities, an inpatient cognitive therapist needs to have a solid grasp of basic CT procedures and experience using these techniques in meeting the special challenges of an inpatient population (e.g., chronic or complex life problems, multiple diagnoses, psychosis, and intense hopelessness with suicidal risk). Most therapists require at least a year of supervised experience doing cognitive therapy before they begin to master this approach. Even more experience is usually necessary to develop the broad variety of skills needed to manage the diversity and severity of problems seen in an inpatient population.

The inpatient therapist should be adept at using fundamental CT procedures, such as Socratic questioning, behavioral techniques, and methods for changing automatic thoughts and underlying assumptions (Beck et al., 1979; Thase & Wright, 1991). Several studies (Jarrett & Nelson, 1987; Teasdale & Fennell, 1982) provide evidence that suggests that depressed patients experience significant improvement in mood following procedures of testing and evaluating their negative cognitions, as compared with simply identifying and exploring thought patterns. Therefore, an effective cognitive therapist needs to learn methods of teaching patients to evaluate and modify negative thoughts. An ability to alter the structure of the therapy to meet the needs of the patient is also important. Many inpatients are disorganized or have significantly impaired learning and memory functioning. These individuals may require a great deal of direction, structure, and learning reinforcement (see Chapters 1 and 4). The degree to which CT is conducted in a structured fashion has been linked to treatment outcome (Shaw, 1988).

The Cognitive Therapy Scale (CTS; Young & Beck, 1980) was devised to measure therapist competency in CT. This scale is used to rate therapist behavior and therapist–patient interactions during therapy sessions. An independent rater reviews an audio or videotape of a therapy session and rates the therapist on both interpersonal factors and the application of CT techniques and procedures. Several studies have found the CTS to be a reliable and valid measure of therapist competency (Dobson, Shaw, & Vallis, 1985; Hollon et al., 1981; Vallis, Shaw, & Dobson, 1986; Young, Shaw, Beck, & Budenz, 1981), and intraclass reliability coefficients for the CTS have ranged from .54 to .96 (Beckham & Watkins, 1989). The CTS can be used by inpatient cognitive therapy programs to: (1) obtain ratings from an outside expert on the competency of staff therapists; (2) give feedback to therapists on strengths and weaknesses; (3) facilitate discussion of CT skills during group or peer supervision meetings; and (4) plan further training.

Who Provides the Education for Primary Therapists?

Cognitive therapy educators can be drawn from several sources. These include: (1) affiliated faculty or hospital professional staff; (2) cognitive therapy consultants; or (3) CT experts who give classes and supervision outside of the hospital. The procedures, advantages, and disadvantages of each of these options are discussed below.

Hospital Staff Members as Educators

Sometimes a hospital will already have a skilled cognitive therapist on staff either as an employee, an affiliated university faculty member, or other member of the treatment team. If so, this person may be able to serve as an educator for those who will provide inpatient CT. The advantages of using an "on-site" professional to educate other staff include convenience, regular availability to answer patient and staff questions, and the possibility of full-time assignment to the CT program to provide consistency and continuity of care. These advantages are great enough for some hospitals (who do not have a cognitive therapist on staff) to decide to invest in either hiring a skilled cognitive therapist or paying for the intensive education of one or more full-time staff members through enrollment in classes and supervision outside the hospital.

The disadvantages of having an on-site staff member teach CT depend on the politics of the hospital, the personal qualities of the individual, and the permanence of the position. Hospital politics are important because even highly skilled employees may be blocked from teaching cognitive therapy for a variety of reasons. For example, some hospitals have a professional "pecking order." Psychiatrists will not attend classes taught by psychologists, psychiatrists and psychologists will not attend classes taught by social workers or nursing staff, and so forth. Moreover, if the staff member is not highly respected, his or her effectiveness as a teacher and supervisor will be jeopardized. An on-site expert will be effective only if supported by other key hospital staff, such as the medical director, chief of nursing, and hospital administrator. Also, an educator may find it difficult to be a strong advocate for the CT program if he or she is involved in other, conflicting political or administrative discussions at the same time.

Employee permanence is another consideration in starting a cognitive therapy program reliant on an on-site professional staff member. It may be desirable to send a staff member to another institution to receive intensive education in CT. In this case, the hospital may want to consider contractual arrangements with the employee so that the hospital will be reimbursed for costs if the individual does not remain at the hospital for a significant period of time after receiving the education. Because of the financial investment needed to start a CT program, it is desirable to try to ensure that employees educated in CT will use these new skills at the hospital that pays for the training.

The Cognitive Therapy Consultant as Educator

If there are no highly skilled cognitive therapists on staff, a hospital may decide to hire a CT consultant for training purposes. The advantages of hiring an outside consultant are: (1) a more experienced or qualified teacher of CT may be available than exists on the on-site staff; (2)

hospital staff may show more interest in learning therapy from an outside expert; (3) the consultant's expertise may extend to program design; and (4) the consultant can provide an "objective" outsider's view of the strengths and weaknesses of a developing program and staff. Some consultants can also provide high-profile visibility in the community for a new cognitive therapy unit (CTU), especially if the consultant is well known and respected as a cognitive therapist either locally or nationally.

Possible disadvantages of an outside consultant may include: (1) problems with long-term availability for follow-up with staff; (2) having relatively little administrative power within the hospital to serve as an advocate for program needs; and (3) not being present to observe day-to-day operations of the program. The first disadvantage usually can be resolved by working out arrangements for use of the consultant's expertise over time. An ongoing arrangement can be developed in which, after an initial period of intensive consultation and education, the consultant remains available to program staff on an hourly basis for supervision, administrative problem-solving, and occasional workshops to update skills and discuss difficult cases. In addition, the consultant may allow videotaping of workshops. If so, these videotapes can be reviewed by staff and also used to orient new staff who are hired after the program begins.

Combining the expertise of an on-site trainer and a consultant can help resolve the disadvantages related to advocacy and daily observation. The professional staff member and consultant can work as a team, suggesting changes in program or resource allocation when necessary. Also, when program needs and problems are identified, the on-site expert and the consultant can pool their efforts to develop potential solutions and share the responsibility for implementing them.

Education through Classes and Supervision Outside the Hospital

Whether or not a consultant is hired, it is often desirable to have one or more members of the staff trained intensively in CT through classes and supervision conducted by experts outside of the hospital. Workshops and conferences on cognitive therapy are held in major cities in the United States at least once a year. Locations for these educational opportunities can be obtained from the various Centers for Cognitive Therapy (see Mooney, 1988, for list). The original Center for Cognitive Therapy at the University of Pennsylvania in Philadelphia can provide information about CT conferences, especially international meetings and those held in the eastern United States. The Center for Cognitive Therapy in Newport Beach, California is a resource for information on

CT workshops in the western United States. Hospitals located near a Center for Cognitive Therapy can usually tap into that Center's programs for supervision. In addition, several Centers for Cognitive Therapy (e.g., Atlanta, Cleveland, New York City, Newport Beach, and Philadelphia in the United States; Santiago, Chile; Stockholm, Sweden) provide intensive training programs and subsequent telephone supervision to therapists throughout their areas.

Participating in these types of educational experiences can help staff members solidify their CT skills. In addition to knowledge of standard CT approaches for depression and anxiety, an inpatient cognitive therapist needs to develop expertise in working with personality disturbances, posttraumatic stress disorder, chemical dependency, and eating disorders, as well as other problems commonly faced during hospitalization. This type of specialty information can be learned through workshops and supervision and then brought back to the hospital and shared with other staff.

METHODS FOR LEARNING COGNITIVE THERAPY

Reading

Most therapists can begin to learn about CT, or to enhance their knowledge, by reading several of the many books written on a variety of clinical topics. The basic text, *Cognitive Therapy of Depression* (Beck et al., 1979), was originally written as a manual to teach therapists CT for depression. It remains an excellent source for learning the essential techniques. Other books and manuscripts provide helpful guides for cognitive therapy of anxiety disorders (Hawton, Salkovskis, Kirk, & Clark, 1989), personality disorders (Beck, Freeman, & Associates, 1990; Freeman, Pretzer, Fleming, & Simon, 1990), eating disorders (Fairburn, 1985; Garner & Bemis, 1985; Garner, 1986), substance abuse (Beck & Emery, 1977; Glantz & McCourt, 1983; Glantz, 1987), couples and family therapy (Beck, 1989; Baucom & Epstein, 1990; Dattilio & Padesky, 1990), and group cognitive therapy (Freeman, 1983; Sank & Shaffer, 1984). More recently, Thase and Wright (1991) have published an abridged manual for individual inpatient CT.

Additional references offer an overview of cognitive therapy for children (Meyers & Craighead, 1984; Kendall & Braswell, 1985; Kendall, 1991), adolescents (Schrodt & Wright, 1987; Wexler, 1991), and a range of other clinical problems (Freeman, Simon, Beutler, & Arkowitz, 1989; Hawton et al., 1989; Persons, 1989; Scott, Williams, & Beck, 1989).

Audio or Videotape Education

Reading, without accompanying clinical experience, will not usually provide an adequate background for learning CT. Staff are more likely to learn the methods and processes of CT when there is the opportunity to observe skilled clinicians *in vivo* or on videotape. Hospitals can enhance their employees' training in cognitive therapy by obtaining audio and videotapes that discuss or illustrate the principles and methods of effective CT. Catalogs of available audio and videotape training materials are available from the Centers for Cognitive Therapy mentioned earlier in this chapter.

Workshops

Workshops can provide didactic material on cognitive theory, case conceptualization, treatment methods, and management of complex patient issues. Also, CT workshops frequently offer the opportunity for hospital staff to role play various clinical situations with supervision by a workshop leader. Through these experiences, a workshop leader can shape staff members' skills, clarify misunderstandings about how the therapy is practiced, and help answer questions or suggest strategies to aid in the management of challenging cases.

Hospitals can sponsor workshops on-site specifically for their staff, or send treatment team members to programs presented elsewhere. The benefits of on-site workshops are that staff will often get more individualized attention than in a larger conference setting, and more staff members will be able to attend. On-site workshops can address directly the types of clinical issues and problems encountered at that hospital. Ongoing, inservice workshops are usually necessary to keep staff skills at a high level (Bowers, 1989).

Learning through Supervision

If a staff member is responsible for the hospital's CT program, individual supervision may be needed to help foster continued growth of his or her skills and to have assistance in solving complex patient problems. Individual supervision can be arranged either with a local CT expert or by phone with a specialist from outside of the community. In turn, this staff member can provide individual supervision and consultation with other therapists at the hospital. Clinicians who work intensively in the program (e.g., conduct individual, group, or family therapy with patients) may need supervision weekly or bimonthly, depending on their skill and experience as cognitive therapists.

Often, group supervision is an excellent and economical way to provide ongoing skill development and case management consultation for hospital staff. The advantages of group supervision include: (1) opportunities for staff to learn from many different people; (2) team-building; (3) identifying and solving program problems (e.g., communication between shifts); and (4) lower cost (i.e., when compared with the cost of individual supervision for each staff member). Of course, individual and group supervision can be used together in order to benefit from the advantages of each.

In both individual and group supervision, it is helpful for the supervisor to model the principle of collaborative empiricism (see Chapter 1). The supervisor typically collaborates with the supervisee in order to identify and solve problems. Instead of providing all the answers, a skilled supervisor uses guided discovery or Socratic questioning to help staff begin to apply the knowledge that they have about CT principles.

Modeling collaborative empiricism in the supervision process provides a good example of how staff can interact with patients. It helps create an atmosphere in which staff are likely to be actively involved in learning to solve problems (Childress & Burns, 1983). Collaboration also fosters an atmosphere of trust, so that staff can feel free to bring up difficulties openly. The empirical stance encourages staff to experiment with new interventions until desired treatment outcomes are attained. In addition, staff can be encouraged to examine their own beliefs that may limit their therapeutic effectiveness (Persons, 1989).

As an adjunct to supervision from more skilled therapists, and in situations where there is no external supervisor available, peer supervision can help staff develop better skills. One form of peer supervision that may be particularly helpful has been termed, by this author, "piggyback" supervision. Using this method, the most experienced staff members conduct group or individual sessions *in vivo*, via a one-way mirror or on videotape. After observing the CT session, all staff members discuss what happened, and the less experienced staff are encouraged to give feedback to the therapist based on what was observed. For example, a less experienced member may be asked to point out the aspects of the intervention that appeared to be good therapy, and why. Also, case formulations or interventions that didn't go well can be discussed and alternative strategies proposed. The staff members are more likely to be active observers when they know they will be participants in the discussion that follows.

To complete the piggyback method, less experienced staff subsequently move into the active intervention role when they are ready. Of course, for a peer supervision model to work well, at least one staff member needs to be well trained. Otherwise, staff may provide more misdirection than accurate feedback, and none of the therapists may know enough to tell the difference.

Intensive Education Programs

Some hospitals have begun their CTUs by first sending one or more staff members to intensive CT educational programs, such as postgraduate fellowships, extramural training, or visiting scholar programs sponsored by Centers for Cognitive Therapy. Several teaching centers in the United States and other countries (see Mooney, 1988) offer programs in which a limited number of therapists learn by participating in intensive postgraduate training. Therapists in such programs are enrolled full-time, usually at the training site, under the supervision of skilled cognitive therapists.

Most hospitals are not willing to delay opening a CT program until a staff member receives a year of postgraduate education (although hospitals have hired cognitive therapists after they have completed this training). As an alternative, intensive education can be acquired through extramural training and supervision. In these programs (usually at least one year in length) the staff member continues working at the hospital, while receiving periodic didactic education (via small workshops) along with weekly supervision. The Center for Cognitive Therapy at the University of Pennsylvania in Philadelphia has trained many therapists by using this approach. Supervision is usually done by phone, with the supervisor listening to or observing one session every week via audiotape or videotape.

Sometimes it is possible to secure a position as a visiting scholar at a training center for a period of time shorter than one year. Therapists from other countries wishing to learn CT in the United States often arrange several weeks or months of education by writing to a training center and requesting an individualized training program. In this way, mental health professionals have learned the basics of CT and returned to their home countries to set up inpatient programs. The availability of such arrangements is obviously limited, and it can be difficult to learn enough in a short amount of time to be able to begin an inpatient CT program. However, this model of learning can be employed when none of the others is feasible.

Continuing Education as the Program Develops

As stated earlier, at least one year of supervised experience is usually necessary for a therapist to become proficient in conducting CT at even an intermediate skill level. Therefore, regardless of the educational method employed, at a minimum, program staff will need ongoing guidance throughout the first year of the program. The intensive education models described above can be used to develop a staff member trainer, on whom the other staff will "piggyback" supervision. However, all staff may need outside, expert supervision on occasion, especially if the staff member has recently learned CT and can not confidently teach it to others.

Ongoing education can combine all of the above models for learning—reading, audiotapes, videotapes, workshops, and supervision. Whatever the mix of continuing education provided, some weekly discussion or observation of the therapy should be included. This can be provided by peers in a weekly staff consultation, or through supervision with an experienced cognitive therapist. If most of the supervision is done by peers, and there is no skilled cognitive therapist on staff, it is recommended that a consultant supervise the peer supervision at least once a month.

Education for Adjunctive Hospital Program Staff

Although there are no research data comparing inpatient CT programs operated by the "add-on" method (i.e., only a few staff are trained as group or individual therapists; see Chapter 3) with those involving all clinical services, several programs have been run successfully with active participation by all disciplines (Dubner, 1985; Perris et al., 1987). The primary advantage of involving all clinical services is that patients are exposed to a consistent point of view throughout their hospital stay. In addition, staff who work at hospitals with an integrated CT milieu report greater work satisfaction because team members speak the same "language," work together on the same set of identified treatment goals, and often experience an increase in professional competency (Dubner, 1985).

In some CT milieus, adjunctive therapists such as occupational therapists, pastoral counselors, recreational therapists, or expressive therapists are enrolled in the same training programs as the primary therapists. Adjunctive therapists can provide CT in their own area of expertise (see Chapter 3) and can also function as individual or group therapists.

Recreational and occupational therapists can easily integrate CT principles into their work. These adjunctive therapies provide ideal settings for patients to conduct behavioral experiments for testing beliefs that are central to their problems. For example, a depressed patient might believe, "If I try something new, I'll fail." An occupational therapist (OT) could encourage this patient to test this belief with an art project. Subsequently, the OT can help the patient identify negative thoughts that interfere with progress or diminish the positive aspects of completing the project.

Recreational therapists can ask a group of patients to predict the amount of enjoyment they will experience on an outing and then observe how much they actually enjoy themselves and what types of thoughts or behaviors interfere with enjoyment. These types of guided *in vivo* learning experiences are at the core of cognitive therapy and can easily be facilitated by occupational and recreational therapists educated in cognitive therapy.

In many inpatient programs, the adjunctive therapists have a more circumscribed role. In this case, the CT training program may include only a didactic series to present basic information on cognitive therapy and a brief series of experiential sessions to practice CT techniques with role-play exercises. When adjunctive therapists (or other staff members who are not primary therapists) are trained with this latter method, the educational sessions should be repeated at regular intervals (usually at least once every 12 to 24 months) to reinforce acquisition of CT principles.

EDUCATION FOR ADMITTING THERAPISTS

Many CTUs (e.g., "add-on" or staff models—see Chapter 3) treat patients who are admitted by psychiatrists or other therapists who are not cognitive therapists. These therapists do not need to know how to conduct CT in order for their patients to benefit from the program. However, some information about cognitive therapy is usually necessary before they will be willing to admit their patients to a CTU. Also, a basic orientation to CT may help prevent rivalries between disciplines or theoretical orientations from having a negative impact on patient care. At the very least, the admitting therapist who hasn't been trained as a cognitive therapist, should respect CT and be able to explain it's basic principles to his or her patients. An educational program on cognitive therapy may increase the likelihood that admitting therapists will encourage patients to apply themselves to the inpatient program and to practice acquired CT skills following discharge.

Education about CT is particularly important for therapists who have misunderstandings about what the CTU will, or will not, provide for their patients. In the following sections, some common misconceptions about CT are discussed, and information for admitting therapists is described. The orientation to CT for admitting therapists and other community referral sources (e.g., family practitioners, pastors, or community agencies) is probably best accomplished by brief workshops. Brochures and audio or videotapes may also be helpful.

Countering Myths About Cognitive Therapy

Cognitive Therapy Is Compatible with Other Treatments

First, the program staff will want to convey to admitting and referring therapists that CT is compatible with a broad range of other biological and psychotherapeutic approaches. Because CT helps patients understand the connections between cognition, emotion, behavior, biology, and environment (both current and past), the cognitive model can be used to support and explain other modes of treatment. For example, patients who are depressed can learn that the medication that has been prescribed works at a biological level and that these actions can occur in tandem with the behavioral and cognitive changes that are being stimulated by CT (see Chapter 7).

Cognitive Therapy Is Useful for a Wide Range of Patients

Some therapists may believe that only uncomplicated, major depressions can be helped by an inpatient cognitive therapy program. Earlier chapters in this book have detailed applications of CT for patients with many types of conditions, including personality disorders, substance abuse, eating disorders, and psychosis. Inpatient CTUs typically have diverse patient populations. Many inpatients in these programs have both Axis I problems (for example, depression, chemical dependency, or anxiety disorders) as well as Axis II personality disorders. Inpatients also frequently have histories of sexual and physical abuse, self-injurious behavior, and/or extreme interpersonal difficulties. These patients, contrary to the expectations of some therapists, can do quite well in cognitive therapy (see Chapters 4, 6, 12, and 14). The idea that CT is only appropriate for the mildly disturbed patient is an unfortunate misunderstanding.

Cognitive Therapy Does Not Minimize Affective Expression

Therapists with only a vague understanding of CT may believe that this therapy is an overly intellectualized approach in which emotion plays little or no role. In fact, cognitive therapists frequently help patients understand and recognize their emotions as a first step in the therapy. Patients who are avoidant of emotion are helped to develop greater tolerance for their feelings, whereas patients who are flooded with emotion are taught methods for controlling affective arousal. Beck has called emotions the "royal road to cognition" (1990a) and cognitions the "royal road to emotion" (1990b). These mirror quotes illustrate the interactional pairing of emotion and cognition in both cognitive theory and therapy. For some patients (e.g., those with compulsive or avoidant personality disorder or chemically dependent patients) a goal of therapy is to be able to tolerate more emotion, rather than to reduce emotional intensity. Indeed, CT can be used to help such patients test beliefs that "emotions are dangerous" or "intolerable," and lead to an increase in emotional expression (Beck et al., 1990).

Information on Cognitive Therapy Procedures

Referring therapists whose patients participate in CT programs usually appreciate receiving a brief description of CT principles and methods of self-help, especially if the referring therapist knows little about CT. Some therapists may want to learn how to help their patients continue to fill out thought records after they are discharged from the hospital. Basic education can be provided to admitting therapists in the form of periodic clinical demonstrations or introductory lectures. Although an hour or two of education will not prepare these therapists to conduct CT, such education will help therapists to become more conversant with their patients about the new skills the patients are acquiring and help therapists coordinate their aftercare treatment with the hospital's program (see Chapter 16).

PATIENT EDUCATION

One of the reasons hospital administrators may wish to open a CTU is the promise of improved patient outcome compared to a traditional milieu treatment program (Miller, Norman, & Keitner, 1989; Bowers, 1990). Moreover, as discussed in Chapters 1 and 16, CT also may have enduring, prophylactic benefits. Cognitive therapy's long-term effectiveness is linked theoretically to how well patients learn the therapy skills and continue to use these once treatment is concluded. Although skill acquisition has not been studied directly in an inpatient population, Neimeyer and Feixas (1990) found, at 6-month follow-up, that lower relapse among outpatients treated with group CT was associated with the level of therapy skills acquired by the end of the group. This chapter's final section discusses methods used to teach CT procedures to patients.

Patient Orientation to Cognitive Therapy

Ideally the orientation to CT will begin within the first hours after hospitalization. Some of the orientation may be done verbally by the admitting psychiatrist or by nursing or social work staff who are collecting initial information from the patient. Orientation can also occur through readings, video programs, or workbooks. The use of written or video materials is recommended because the patient may be quite emotionally upset and unable to concentrate when admitted to the hospital and thus may not remember information that is given verbally (Thase & Wright, 1991).

Reading

The basic reading assignment for all patients should include, at a minimum, a brief summary description of CT and an orientation pamphlet for the specific program. These materials should be written in simple, clear language because some patients will have poor reading skills, and most will have difficulty processing complex information because of their high levels of dysphoria and distress. Patients also benefit from the opportunity to discuss these readings with staff who can answer questions or clarify misunderstandings. Examples of brief pamphlets describing CT include *Coping with Depression* (Beck & Greenberg, 1974) and *Coping with Anxiety and Panic* (Beck & Emery, 1979). Program staff also may choose to write their own introduction to CT.

Many patients are interested in reading more about specific disorders or about cognitive therapy. A number of self-help books are available, and staff are urged to keep a well-stocked library of psychoeducational books for patients to read. However, it is important to screen these materials carefully to insure that they are compatible with the CT approach and are pitched at a level that can be understood by the patient. Examples of books that may enhance patients' understanding of CT include those written by Beck (for couples in distress, 1989), Burns (for depression and anxiety, 1989), Davis, Eshelman, and McKay (for stress reduction, 1988), and McKay and Fanning (for enhancing self-esteem, 1987).

Video Orientation

Some hospitals may wish to create a videotape orientation to their CT program. This format can provide a more personable and engaging orientation for new patients than can be accomplished with readings alone. It also can save staff time consumed by repeating programmatic information over and over to each new patient. In addition, patients can view the video more than once, thus enhancing retention and understanding of new material. If a video is used, it is important to have staff available to answer questions or discuss reactions to it after viewing. Although CT can be presented in standard ways to most patients, it is important that information be presented in a manner that is sensitive to each individual's issues and needs.

Learning and Practicing Cognitive Therapy

Cognitive therapy is most effective when patients ultimately learn to practice and apply skills in situations in which they are not directly supervised by a therapist or hospital staff. In order to maximize such learning, a variety of methods can be used that will help patients learn to apply therapy skills *invivo*. Moreover, it is important to provide ample opportunities to practice these skills repetitively (i.e., until the patient can apply them with confidence after discharge from the CTU).

Group Therapy as Education

In many hospitals, the primary opportunity for teaching CT skills is in group therapy. Group CT is economical, and has been found to be effective in treating outpatient depression (see, for example, the review by Hollon & Najavitis, 1988). Cognitive therapy groups are more structured and overtly educational than the traditional, process groups often conducted in hospital settings (Bowers, 1989). As described in Chapter 5, CT groups begin with an agenda, constructed in a collaborative fashion by the group members and leader. Sometimes the group has a goal of learning to use cognitive therapy techniques (e.g., to identify automatic thoughts or generate alternative explanations); other groups may focus on application of skills in coping with problems (e.g., hopelessness or victimization experiences).

It is important for the group leader to involve all of the patients in the learning experience. The leader might begin by constructing a thought record with one patient (or several patients with similar experiences) and ask everyone to join in by "personalizing" the thought record. The process of completing such thought records in group is very helpful for learning therapy skills. Whereas patients may have a difficult time discerning the distortions in their own thinking, they may be more adept at identifying distortions and providing alternative explanations for other group members.

One-on-One Education by Staff

In addition to group therapy, patients can benefit from additional, one-on-one assistance in learning CT skills. These meetings frequently are informal and impromptu, such as when a nurse notices that a patient is acutely upset or troubled (Thase & Wright, 1991). Other programs may schedule regular meetings for review of the patients' therapy workbooks and homework assignments. These meetings provide an opportunity to see how well the patient understands CT and to identify areas in which additional help may be needed. For example, in the first few days of hospitalization, a patient may need to: (1) define problems that will be worked on during the hospitalization; (2) review the cognitive model; and (3) begin to learn how to identify feelings and thoughts. A patient in the second or third week of hospitalization may be able to identify important automatic thoughts but may need help testing out beliefs, thinking of alternative explanations for distorted beliefs, and devising plans to solve real-life problems.

Written Practice

Most patients learn CT more readily if they practice the skills daily. For most patients, writing down thoughts and feelings makes it easier to examine these and to consider alternative explanations for events. Although patients can do this on single sheets of paper, it is generally more helpful if these experiences are recorded in a notebook so that an enduring body of knowledge is accumulated by the patient. A therapy notebook also provides a single source, from which written observations, thought records, logs of behavioral experiments, and other records of therapy material can be shown to an outpatient therapist. Often, the notebook can be used to integrate learning that occurs in the hospital with outpatient therapy. Notebooks completed in the hospital also facilitate the patient's ability to "take the program home." Many patients use and continue to add to their notebook long after discharge.

Workbooks

Instead of an individualized notebook, some hospital programs provide patients with a structured workbook to guide their learning in the hospital. These workbooks describe CT and give examples of different techniques. Workbooks often suggest skill-building exercises for the patient to complete.

There are many advantages to using a patient workbook as part of a CT program. Workbooks provide an organized format for patients to learn and allow patients to review principles and skills presented in therapy groups or individual sessions until these are mastered. At the beginning of the hospitalization, workbooks can help to provide an overview of CT and the cognitive model. During hospitalization, the workbook helps organize, structure, and direct patients' learning. In addition, workbooks can assist hospital staff in monitoring patient progress. Staff can help patients begin assignments in their workbook that can be followed up on the next shift. In groups, the therapist can assess each patient's skill level by asking how many assignments have been completed in the workbook. Several representative workbooks are described below.

The Feeling Good Handbook

Burns (1989) has updated his popular *Feeling Good* book, and has expanded it to include the application of CT to anxiety disorders and relationship problems. It also includes an easy-to-read chapter on common psychotropic medications. The book is written for both outpatient and nonclinical populations, so it does not address some of the more serious concerns of hospitalized patients. Whereas *The Feeling Good Handbook*'s strength for the general population is that it provides a good overview of the theory and techniques of CT, its weakness for inpatients is that it sometimes seems to suggest that most problems can be solved quickly, a tone that may be alienating or discouraging for those who have been admitted to a hospital.

The Benessere Center Workbooks

Billingsley and Billingsley have created patient workbooks and companion texts for their inpatients at the Benessere Center in Kansas. Their workbooks, *Depression: The Way Out* (1987) and *Eating Disorders: The Way Out* (1988), include extensive information on: (1) the theories of these disorders; (2) CT principles and methods; (3) worksheets for patients to use to identify feelings, automatic thoughts, and cognitive distortions; and (4) worksheets for developing behavioral plans for change. These workbooks are very elaborate in their explanations of the disorders. However, their academic and technical orientation may be overwhelming to some. For the highly educated, detailed discussions of physiological and biochemical aspects of clinical disorders might be welcome, but the biological explanations are unnecessarily complex for most patients. Conversely, the workbooks are less detailed in providing guidance to patients who may be struggling to learn CT skills.

Cognitive Treatment Workbook

A useful (but unpublished) workbook has been written by Eaves, Jarrett, and Basco (1989). This workbook emphasizes the cognitive tasks that patients need to learn, including identification of negative automatic thoughts, recognition of distortions, logical analysis of automatic negative thoughts, and various methods for testing the accuracy of automatic thoughts. In addition, the workbook includes sections on identifying and changing underlying assumptions and on increasing activity (emphasizing mastery and pleasure activities). Although it was written for outpatient applications, it appears to be readily adaptable to the inpatient setting. An appealing feature of this workbook is that patients are directed to make a problem list at the beginning of treatment and to record their progress on each problem at the beginning of each subsequent week. Although the workbook provides many useful worksheets for patients to complete, it would be even more useful if it included illustrations and sample responses so that patients could visualize methods of completing the exercises.

Cognitive Therapy: An Individualized Workbook

Another unpublished workbook has been written by Greenberger and Padesky (1990). This workbook uses a skill-building approach that breaks CT down into a series of small steps. It has been easily integrated into several inpatient programs, since it is divided into modules that can be read independently by patients, taught in individual sessions, or explained in group therapy. Furthermore, the workbook includes a skills checklist that can be used by both staff and patients to monitor progress on increasingly complex tasks and assignments. Each section of the workbook is two to five pages in length and emphasizes one or two cognitive therapy skills for the patient to practice. In addition to provision of sample responses for each exercise, the text is written in simple language to meet the needs of patients with poor reading skills. In progressively more comprehensive sections, patients learn a number of cognitive therapy skills: how to recognize feelings, techniques to examine the connection between behavior and emotion, identification of thoughts, ways to connect thoughts and feelings, identification of underlying assumptions, and methods of changing long-held, maladaptive schemas.

SUMMARY

An intensive training program for therapists is usually necessary to develop a cognitively oriented inpatient unit. If desired, CT skills can be learned by an entire multidisciplinary treatment team in order to create a comprehensive program that presents a consistent model for patients throughout the hospital stay. A variety of methods for educating staff are described in this chapter, including the use of readings, audio and videotapes, lectures, workshops, and ongoing individual or group supervision. The special challenge of orienting admitting therapists and other referral agents who are not cognitive therapists to CT is also discussed.

Patient education is a central goal of an inpatient cognitive therapy program. Learning CT principles may increase the likelihood that patients will have enhanced long-term functioning and lower relapse rates. Development of a high quality CTU requires an ongoing investment in both staff and patient education. The rewards of this effort can be a well-trained, effective staff and patients who are prepared to use cognitive therapy procedures as important tools for recovery.

REFERENCES

Baucom, D., & Epstein, N. (1990). *Cognitive–behavioral marital therapy*. New York: Brunner/Mazel.

Beck, A. T. (1989). *Love is never enough*. New York: Harper & Row.

Beck, A. T. (1990a, February). *Cognitive theory of personality disorders*. Paper presented at the Cognitive Therapy of Personality Disorders, Inpatients, and Complex Marital Problems Conference, Newport Beach, CA.

Beck, A. T. (1990b, February). *Cognitive therapy with depressed inpatients*. Paper presented at the Spend an Evening with the Experts program, Irvine, CA.

Beck, A. T. (1991). Cognitive therapy: A 30-year retrospective. *American Psychologist, 46*(4), 368–375.

Beck, A. T., & Emery, G. (1977). *Cognitive therapy of substance abuse*. Unpublished manuscript. University of Pennsylvania, Center for Cognitive Therapy, Philadelphia.

Beck, A. T., & Emery, G. (1979). *Coping with anxiety and panic*. Unpublished pamphlet. University of Pennsylvania, Center for Cognitive Therapy, Philadelphia.

Beck, A. T., Freeman, A., & Associates. (1990). *Cognitive therapy of personality disorders*. New York: Guilford Press.

Beck, A. T., & Greenberg, R. L. (1974). *Coping with depression*. New York: Institute for Rational Living.

Beck, A. T., Rush, J., Shaw, B. & Emery, G. (1979). *Cognitive therapy of depression.* New York: Guilford Press.

Beckham, E., & Watkins, J. (1989). Process and outcome in cognitive therapy. In A. Freeman, K. Simon, L. Beutler, & H. Arkowitz (Eds.), *Comprehensive handbook of cognitive therapy* (pp. 61–81). New York: Plenum Press.

Billingsley, M. L., & Billingsley, T. H. (1987). *Depression: The way out.* Unpublished workbook. Benessere Center, Shawnee Mission, KS.

Billingsley, M. L., & Billingsley, T. H. (1988). *Eating disorders: The way out.* Unpublished workbook. The Benessere Center, Shawnee Mission, KS.

Bowers, W. (1989). Cognitive therapy with inpatients. In A. Freeman, K. Simon, L. Beutler, & H. Arkowitz (Eds.), *Comprehensive handbook of cognitive therapy* (pp. 583–596). New York: Plenum Press.

Bowers, W. A. (1990). Treatment of depressed inpatients. Cognitive therapy plus medication, relaxation plus medication, and medication alone. *British Journal of Psychiatry, 156,* 73–78.

Burns, D. D. (1989). *The feeling good handbook: Using the new mood therapy in everyday life.* New York: William Morrow.

Childress, A. R., & Burns, D. (1983). The group supervision model in cognitive therapy training. In A. Freeman (Ed.), *Cognitive therapy with couples and groups* (pp. 323–335). New York: Plenum Press.

Dattilio, F., & Padesky, C. (1990). *Cognitive therapy with couples.* Sarasota, FL: Professional Resource Exchange.

Davis, M., Eshelman, E. R., & McKay, M. (1988). *The relaxation and stress workbook* (3rd ed.). Oakland, CA: New Harbinger Press.

Dobson, K., Shaw, B., & Vallis, T. (1985). Reliability of a measure of the quality of cognitive therapy. *British Journal of Clinical Psychology, 24,* 295–300.

Dubner, N. (1985). Cognitive therapy in a hospital setting. *International Cognitive Therapy Newsletter, 1*(2), 2–3.

Eaves, G. G., Jarrett, R. B., & Basco, M. R. (1989). *Cognitive treatment workbook.* Unpublished workbook, Department of Psychiatry, University of Texas Southwestern Medical Center, Dallas.

Fairburn, C. G. (1985). Cognitive–behavioral treatment for bulimia. In D. M. Garner & P. E. Garfinkel (Eds.), *Handbook of psychotherapy for anorexia nervosa and bulimia* (pp. 160–192). New York: Guilford Press.

Freeman, A. (Ed.). (1983). *Cognitive therapy with couples and groups.* New York: Plenum Press.

Freeman, A., Pretzer, J., Fleming, B., & Simon, K. (1990). *Clinical applications of cognitive therapy.* New York: Plenum Press.

Freeman, A., Simon, K., Beutler, L., & Arkowitz, H. (Eds.). (1989). *Comprehensive handbook of cognitive therapy.* New York: Plenum Press.

Garner, D. (1986). Cognitive therapy for anorexia nervosa. In K. D. Brownell & J. P. Foreyt (Eds.), *Handbook of eating disorders* (pp. 301–327). New York: Basic Books.

Garner, D. M., & Bemis, K. M. (1985). Cognitive therapy for anorexia nervosa. In D. M. Garner & P. E. Garfinkel (Eds.), *Handbook of psychotherapy for anorexia nervosa and bulimia* (pp. 107–146). New York: Guilford Press.

Glantz, M. D. (1987). Day hospital treatment of alcoholics. In A. Freeman & V.

Greenwood (Eds.), *Cognitive therapy: Applications in psychiatric and medical settings* (pp. 51–68). New York: Human Sciences Press.

Glantz, M. D., & McCourt, W. (1983). Cognitive therapy in groups with alcoholics. In A. Freeman (Ed.), *Cognitive therapy with couples and groups* (pp. 157–182). New York: Plenum Press.

Greenberger, D., & Padesky, C. (1990). *Cognitive therapy: An individualized workbook.* Unpublished workbook, Center for Cognitive Therapy, Newport Beach, CA.

Hawton, K., Salkovskis, P., Kirk, J., & Clark, D. (Eds.). (1989). *Cognitive behaviour therapy for psychiatric problems: A practical guide.* New York: Oxford University Press.

Hollon, S., Mandell, M., Bemis, K., DeRubeis, R., Emerson, M., Evans, M., & Kress, M. (1981). *Reliability and validity of the Young Cognitive Therapy Scale.* Unpublished manuscript, University of Minnesota, Minneapolis.

Hollon, S., & Najavits, L. (1988). Review of empirical studies of cognitive therapy. In A. J. Frances & R. E. Hales (Eds.), *American Psychiatric Press review of psychiatry,* Vol. 7 (pp. 643–666). Washington, DC: American Psychiatric Press.

Jarrett, R., & Nelson, R. (1987). Mechanisms of change in cognitive therapy of depression. *Behavior Therapy, 18,* 227–241.

Kendall, P. C. (Ed.). (1991). *Child and adolescent therapy: Cognitive–behavioral procedures.* New York: Guilford Press.

Kendall, P. C., & Braswell, L. (1985). *Cognitive behavioral therapy for impulsive children.* New York: Guilford Press.

McKay, M., & Fanning, P. (1987). *Self-esteem.* Oakland, CA: New Harbinger Press.

Meyers, A., & Craighead, W. E. (Eds.). (1984). *Cognitive therapy with children.* New York: Plenum Press.

Miller, I. W., Norman, W. H., & Keitner, G. I. (1989). Cognitive–behavioral treatment of depressed inpatients: Six- and twelve-month follow-up. *American Journal of Psychiatry, 146,* 1274–1279.

Mooney, K. A. (Ed.). (1988). *Cognitive therapy centers: Resource and referral directory.* Unpublished manuscript, Center for Cognitive Therapy, Newport Beach, CA.

Neimeyer, R., & Feixas, G. (1990). The role of homework and skill acquisition in the outcome of group cognitive therapy for depression. *Behavior Therapy, 21,* 281–292.

Perris, C., Rodhe, K., Palm, A., Abelson, M., Hellgran, S., Livja, C., & Soderman, H. (1987). Fully integrated in- and outpatient services in a psychiatric sector: Implementation of a new model for the care of psychiatric patients favoring continuity of care. In A. Freeman & V. Greenwood (Eds.), *Cognitive therapy: Applications in psychiatric and medical settings* (pp. 117–131). New York: Human Sciences Press.

Persons, J. (1989). *Cognitive therapy in practice: A case formulation approach.* New York: W. W. Norton.

Persons, J., & Burns, D. (1985). Mechanisms of action of cognitive therapy: The relative contributions of technical and interpersonal interventions. *Cognitive Therapy and Research, 9,* 539–551.

Sank, L., & Shaffer, C. (1984). *A therapist's manual for cognitive behavior therapy in groups.* New York: Plenum Press.

Schrodt, G., & Wright, J. (1987). Inpatient treatment of adolescents. In A. Freeman & V. Greenwood (Eds.), *Cognitive therapy: Applications in psychiatric and medical settings* (pp. 69–82). New York: Human Sciences Press.

Scott, J., Williams, J. M. G., & Beck, A. T. (Eds.). (1989). *Cognitive therapy in clinical practice: An illustrative casebook.* New York: Routledge.

Shaw, B. F. (1988). *Cognitive theory of depression: Where are we and where are we going?* Paper presented at the meeting of Contemporary Psychological Approaches to Depression: Treatment, Research, and Theory, San Diego, CA.

Teasdale, J. D., & Fennel, M. J. V. (1982). Immediate effects on depression of cognitive therapy interventions. *Cognitive Therapy and Research, 3,* 343–352.

Thase, M. E., & Wright, J. H. (1991). Cognitive behavior therapy manual for depressed inpatients: A treatment protocol outline. *Behavior Therapy, 22,* 579–595.

Truax, C. B., & Carkhuff, R. (1967). *Towards effective counseling and psychotherapy.* Chicago: Aldine.

Vallis, T. M., Shaw, B. F., & Dobson, K. S. (1986). The Cognitive Therapy Scale: Psychometric properties. *Journal of Consulting and Clinical Psychology, 54,* 381–385.

Wexler, D. (1991). *The adolescent self: Strategies for self-management, self-soothing, and self-esteem in adolescents.* New York: W. W. Norton.

Young, J., & Beck, A. T. (1980). *Cognitive therapy scale: Rating manual.* Unpublished manuscript, University of Pennsylvania, Philadelphia.

Young, J., Shaw, B. F., Beck, A. T., & Budenz, D. (1981). *Assessment of competence in cognitive therapy.* Unpublished manuscript, University of Pennsylvania, Philadelphia.

Chapter 16

Transition and Aftercare

Michael E. Thase, M.D.

This chapter discusses the transition from the inpatient to the outpatient treatment setting and aftercare procedures designed to reduce the chances of symptom recurrence. First, a brief overview of the goals of an inpatient admission is provided. In subsequent sections, methods are described for assessing the risk of relapse, coping with stigma, using the transition phase to enhance learning, and determining the level of appropriate aftercare. Throughout the chapter, cognitive models of psychopathology and treatment serve as the conceptual basis for understanding the problems patient's face as they prepare for discharge from a psychiatric inpatient unit.

BACKGROUND

Overview

The primary goals of an admission to a psychiatric inpatient unit are: (1) accurate diagnosis; (2) stabilization of acute psychosocial crises and symptomatic exacerbations; (3) initiation of appropriate treatment and, at the least, partial remission of the presenting disorder(s); (4) resolution of suicidal ideation or other forms of dangerous behavior; (5) psychoeducation about the disorder(s) and treatment(s); and (6) identification of issues, target symptoms, and vulnerabilities that warrant subsequent outpatient treatment. In addition to these universal goals, an inpatient treatment program that offers group or individual cognitive therapy provides education about the cognitive model of psychopathology and helps the patient learn to apply basic therapy techniques. When these tasks are accomplished in a collaborative fashion, the patient leaves the hospital with some degree of symptom relief, renewed optimism, and improved strategies to cope with both situational and symptomatic distress. Moreover, the patient will have acquired a coherent understanding of how his or her problems developed and what can be done in the future to prevent relapse.

It is clichéd but nevertheless true to assert that the process described above is complicated; it is easier said than done. Further, the high cost of inpatient treatment (and society's limited willingness and means to finance psychiatric hospitalization) mandates that the use of scarce funds allocated to pay for hospital care be carefully monitored. At times, aggressive methods are used by third party payers or their agents to lessen the length of hospitalization. Each day of inpatient treatment at a typical short-stay unit in the United States may cost between $500 and $1,500 (Craig, 1988). Thus, it should come as no surprise that the average length of stay for treatment of depression in the United States has decreased by 50% over the past 20 years (Black & Winokur, 1988). Although one may wish for a more generous Congress or an economic "peace dividend" resulting from the lessening international tensions, all available evidence points to the likelihood that the process of cost-containment and more efficient utilization of hospital care will continue into the next century.

General Issues

The major psychiatric disorders tend to be either episodic or chronic, and their treatments are more often successful at symptom control than cure. The natural history of nonbipolar major depression, a so-called good prognosis disorder, is a useful case in point. Although most individuals will recover from an episode of depression within 2 years of its onset, the probability of subsequent relapse or recurrence is quite high. At least 50% of persons suffering a first bout of major depression will subsequently have a second episode, and individuals with two or more prior episodes of depression have an 80% to 90% risk of further depressive episodes (Thase, 1990). Similarly, individuals with dysthymia (a milder but more chronically persistent mood disorder) may have as high as a 90% risk of suffering from a major depressive relapse during the 2 years after they first receive inpatient treatment (Keller & Shapiro, 1982). Relapse rates are high after termination of treatments for panic disorder and agoraphobia as well (Ballenger, 1991).

Patients who are hospitalized for treatment of mood and anxiety disorders are at particularly high risk for relapse for several reasons. First, disorders requiring hospitalization have a greater likelihood to be at the higher end of the severity continuum. Second, such patients often have failed to benefit from one or more standard treatments in an outpatient setting. Third, inpatients are more likely to have active suicidal ideation and/or recent self-destructive behavior. The accompanying marked level of hopelessness may have ominous long-term implications (Beck, Steer, Kovacs & Garrison, 1985; Beck, Brown, Berchick, Stewart, & Steer, 1990). Fourth, more severely depressed persons are likely to have significant comorbidity on Axes I, II, and III of the DSM-III-R (Thase, 1987). Although such complicating conditions do not render a patient untreatable, they do necessitate a broadening of the therapeutic focus, and, in the short run, reduce the chance for recovery from the principal disorder (Thase & Kupfer, 1987). Finally, the decision to hospitalize depressed or anxious patients may indicate that their social support systems have become dysfunctional or markedly stressed (Mezzich, Evanczuk, Mathias, & Coffman, 1984). Thus, individuals with mood disorders have a high risk of relapse in general, and such vulnerability is particularly pronounced for the recently hospitalized patient.

Two issues commonly interfere with the patient's preparation to face such risks. First, the potency of the inpatient experience *per se* tends to be underappreciated. A number of factors [e.g., respite from distressing problems and relationships, the license to temporarily assume the sick role, the benefits of following a structured routine (including stable meal and bed times), the remoralizing effects of receiving acceptance and understanding, and the opportunity to ventilate] all work in concert to create a milieu with powerful therapeutic effects. Furthermore, a collapsing social system may transiently reintegrate around the stress of a loved one's hospitalization, and, as a result, the patient's hope for the future may be buoyed by a significant other's well-intentioned promise to change his or her ways. Such factors tend to have transient benefits and may be likened to a psychological placebo effect. Second, there may be inadequate psychoeducation about the disorder(s) and the expectations for ongoing treatment. Thus, the individual may have unrealistically high expectations for maintaining improvement. Moreover, the patient may not fully appreciate the importance of maintaining aftercare treatment. Specific risk factors for relapse and recurrence are discussed in the following section.

ESTIMATING RISK OF RELAPSE OR RECURRENCE

The major risk factors for relapse and recurrence of depressive illness are summarized in Table 16.1. Relapse by convention is defined as (1) a worsening of depressive symptoms sufficient to again meet criteria for the disorder, and (2) the worsening has occurred temporally close to the time in which a depressed individual first remitted from the affective

TABLE 16.1. Risk Factors for Relapse and Recurrence of Depression

Relapse	Recurrence
Definite risk factors	
Chronicity	Multiple prior episodes
Residual symptoms	Withdrawal of pharmacotherapy
Inadequate treatment	Early age of onset
Personality pathology	Family history of bipolar disorder
Possible risk factors	
Aging	Seasonal pattern
Ongoing life stress	Aging
Poor social support	Life stress

Data from Thase (1990) and Belsher and Costello (1987).

episode (Prien, 1987; Thase, 1990). In practice, the term relapse typically is applied when the patient becomes symptomatic again during the first 6 months after having achieved symptomatic remission. Empirical studies have documented that the first 6 months following inpatient treatment represent a particularly "high-risk" time for symptomatic exacerbation or treatment failure (Keller, 1988). Specifically, the risk for relapse is highest when an individual has residual symptomatology, ongoing distressing life difficulties, inadequate social support, and/or a suboptimal level of follow-up treatment (see, for example, Keller, 1988 or Thase, 1990). With respect to depression, such residual symptoms may fall well within the range used to define treatment response on standard rating scales—a Hamilton Rating Scale for Depression (HRSD; Hamilton, 1960) score of 6 or a Beck Depression Inventory (BDI; Beck, Ward, Mendelson, Mock, & Erbaugh, 1961) score of 8 (Thase & Kupfer, 1987). Thus, with such low levels of residual symptomatology, all may appear "well" to both patient and clinician, perhaps leading to a lessening of the intensity of aftercare or premature reduction in the dose of antidepressant medication (Thase, 1990). Residual symptomatology and increased risk for relapse also may be reflected in persistently elevated scores on measures of cognitive vulnerability, such as the Dysfunctional Attitudes Scale (Eaves & Rush, 1984; Simons, Murphy, Levine, & Wetzel, 1986; Thase, Simons, McGeary, Hughes, & Harden, 1992).

Recurrence refers to development of a new episode of illness after a period of sustained recovery. For depressive and anxiety disorders, a period of 4 to 6 months of sustained, symptom-free status has been accepted by convention to define a recovery (Frank et al., 1991; Thase,

1990). In contrast to relapse, the principal risks of recurrence relate more closely to the natural history of the disorder being studied. For example, both an early age of onset of the illness (e.g., a first episode before age 25) and a large number of prior episodes (e.g., > 3 episodes) are robust indicators of risk for recurrence following recovery from a depressive episode (Thase, 1990). The distinction between relapse and recurrence can be summarized as follows: relapse represents the reemergence of the index episode (that has been suppressed or controlled by treatment), whereas recurrence describes a new episode of recurrent affective illness (Thase, 1990).

It is unclear to what extent life stress is associated with recurrence (as opposed to relapse). As reviewed in Chapter 1, a recent body of research indicates that schematic vulnerability (as inferred by extracted scores from the Dysfunctional Attitudes Scale or the Sociotrophy–Autonomy Scale, a new, unpublished measure developed by Beck's group) may predispose an individual to an increased risk of depression when he or she encounters a personally relevant life event. Thus, from a cognitive perspective, the depressogenic "toxicity" of life stress is presumed to be mediated by its personal relevance. Individuals with ongoing schematic vulnerability in areas such as interpersonal dependence or need for achievement may be at specifically elevated risk if they are exposed to "matching" adverse life experiences, such as romantic rejection or a failing business. If this line of research is confirmed in samples of fully recovered individuals, it will point to the possible prophylactic value of more extended courses of cognitive therapy aimed at identification and resolution of areas of schematic vulnerability.

PREPARING TO LEAVE THE MILIEU

For many patients, the experience of participating in the hospital's milieu has been quite positive. In some cases, the milieu may have provided the most explicit and consistent support the person has received in his or her adult life. For example, significant others may have been more attentive during hospital visits. Peers on the unit have been more understanding and less critical than friends or family members typically are, and professional staff have been available on almost a continuous basis. Problems that seemed overwhelming have been defined, explained, and addressed with a series of treatment interventions. In sum, the patient feels better, and optimism and morale have been restored.

It is not uncommon for patients to respond to these events with an unrealistically positive shift in cognitions and emotions. Indeed, our group has documented a somewhat distorted positive bias in affects and cognitions in a large proportion of remitted outpatients immediately prior to termination of cognitive therapy (Garamoni, Reynolds, Thase, Franks, & Fasiczka, 1992). In a well-functioning cognitive milieu, this response is recognized but does *not* require the use of pathological labels such as denial or "flight into health." However, therapists may help patients to relabel or normalize overgeneralized responses. For example, treatment team members may draw on widely relevant, personal experiences, such as one's recollections of attending church camp, a weekend retreat, or some other intense, yet uplifting experience. The lesson to be taught is that a "natural high" is likely to pass and that it will be helpful to prepare for future problems.

Conversely, it is important to address cognitions and behaviors that may reflect the patient's minimization of his or her own role in getting better. Although expressions of gratitude to the therapeutic team are normal human responses, attributions that affix the locus of change solely on the program or the primary therapist do not help future problem-solving, nor do they increase self-efficacy.

Some patients will suffer an exacerbation of symptoms in the days immediately prior to discharge. For these individuals, cognitive distortions such as selective abstraction, minimizing the positive, and catastrophization may be operative and may shape globally negative conclusions such as: "My improvement is just temporary. . . . I won't be able to make it after I leave. . . . I have too many overwhelming problems. . . . This improvement is just another false hope." Although dysphoric reactions in patients preparing for discharge are common to all inpatient settings, they can be managed systematically within the cognitive milieu with interventions that are more enduring than reassurance. The patient is encouraged to recognize that a downward shift in mood prior to discharge means that "hot" cognitions are operative. In both planned and impromptu sessions, the patient is helped to record these thoughts, test their veracity, recognize distortions, and develop more accurate alternatives and plans. This process is illustrated in a patient's Daily Record of Dysfunctional Thoughts provided in Table 16.2. Successful intervention around predischarge dysphoria often has a powerful, generalizable effect on the patient's confidence and may increase enthusiasm for ongoing participation in cognitive therapy. Nevertheless, the very existence of such a brief tailspin is suggestive that much work remains to be done in outpatient therapy following discharge.

The methods of CT during the discharge planning phase of treatment begin with identification of remaining areas of difficulty. These

TABLE 16.2. Predischarge Concerns: Sample Daily Record of Dysfunctional Thoughts

Situation	Emotion(s)	Automatic thought(s)	Rational response	Outcome
Describe: 1. Actual event leading to unpleasant emotion. 2. Stream of thoughts, daydreams, or recollection, leading to unpleasant emotion.	1. Specify sad/anxious/angry, etc. 2. Rate degree of emotion, 1–100%.	Write automatic thought(s) that preceded emotion(s)	1. Write rational response to automatic thought(s)	1. Rerate belief in automatic thought(s), 0–100% 2. Specify and rate subsequent emotions, 0–100%
Date:				
12/23 Packing my bags, thinking about going home.	Sad, 50 Anxious, 60	1. There's so much to be done at home.	1. There *is* a lot to be done. I'll need to ask for help and use an activity schedule to manage my time. Bob [husband] and my Mom both say that they don't mind helping.	Sad, 20% Anxious, 30%
		2. I won't be able to pull my share of the load.	2. I don't really know what I will or won't be able to do. If I can't work at 100% capacity at first, this will not be a tragedy. I am still recuperating, and it's okay to have help. It's normal to have some apprehension!	

3. I might get depressed again.	3. Yes, there is a chance of relapse. I know what the warning signs are, and I now can cope and manage symptoms a lot better. My therapist is available to help me if things get rough. Also, my antidepressant will help reduce the chance of relapse.
4. I'll let everyone down.	4. It's normal for people who care about me to be concerned about how I'm doing. However, my recovery is *not* something I owe *them.* If I'm not doing well, changes can be made in my treatment plan. Everything I know about my treatment indicates that the odds for doing well are very good.
5. I'll miss this place.	5. Missing my doctors, therapists, nurses, and other patients is okay. This is bittersweet. I've grown close to several people. Perhaps I can send a card or stop by later to say thank you. I can stay in touch with the new friends I've made.

problems often include both residual symptoms and areas of ongoing life distress. It is also helpful to begin to anticipate problems that may interfere with achievement of long-term goals. Examples of the latter include recognition of problematic patterns in relationships or skill deficits that may have interfered with happiness or inhibited vocational success in the past. Next, patients are encouraged to develop an inventory of their "assets" (i.e., resources available both to cope with current problems and build on in future undertakings). Such assets include new skills, techniques, and pragmatic solutions to life problems (e.g., shifts in child care responsibility, developing a budget, or temporarily dropping out of a class that was too taxing) learned during hospitalization as well as identification of resources available for ventilation, support, and practical help. The asset "ledger" also will include personal strengths (e.g., intellect, education, capacity for friendship, hobbies, income, or other talents). Patients are encouraged to answer the question "How has my inventory been strengthened over the past weeks?" They also may be asked to review their therapy notebook as a way of concretizing the gains made in therapy. As a final step in this process, patients are asked to match their assets against the list of ongoing or anticipated problems (see Table 16.3). This may be done as a homework assignment or explicated on a chalkboard during a group or individual therapy session. The advantage of completing such an assignment within a group therapy setting, of course, is the opportunity for other patients to benefit from social learning and to provide feedback.

Predischarge Passes

Therapeutic outings with staff and/or family provide particularly useful opportunities to test an individual's readiness for discharge. Initially, it is important to document if patients are comfortable outside of the hospital or if they show mood reactivity or enjoyment while participating in a potentially reinforcing activity. As such, an initial pass with family may have very simple goals (e.g., spend time with children or talk with spouse about material that is not emotionally charged). Subsequently, the goals of passes become more complex or demanding and, in the cognitive model of therapy, they may be construed as formal homework assignments. Such assignments typically may involve exposure (e.g., cope with anxiety while grocery shopping), assertiveness (e.g., speak with boss about delaying return to work), conflict resolution (e.g., conducting a family meeting), or depression "inoculation" (e.g., evoking a depressed mood outside of the hospital to test whether it can be alleviated using self-help methods).

TABLE 16.3. Sample Predischarge Homework Assignment: Problems Associated with Going Back to Work

Problems	Assets/solutions
1. Backlog of work	1. I can set more reasonable expectations. I can volunteer to work overtime. I can ask the supervisor for temporary help to get caught up. I have a better ability to cope now with guilt and pressure.
2. Facing co-workers; anticipating comments, questions, and criticisms	2. I know that my insecurities are my own responsibility; I can work on this in outpatient therapy. Some of my co-workers really care about me. I understand much more about mental illness and its treatment now than the average person, so I can't expect them to fully understand. I can tolerate a certain amount of ignorance or teasing, and I can get help from the union representative if their comments are too harsh. The assertiveness skills I learned in group will come in handy.
3. Resentment about being passed over for promotion last year.	3. I know how to prioritize, and this isn't the time to make waves. I can meet with my supervisor later for more feedback about why I didn't get that promotion. I can work on my irrational emotional responses to automatic thoughts about being rejected and overlooked. I can decide, once I'm reestablished, to look for another job. I can continue to explore my long-term goals in therapy to help decide the best course of action.

Interpersonal Aspects of Preparation for Discharge

During hospitalization, patients often develop relatively intense relationships with staff and other patients. One does not need to be too psychodynamically minded to observe that such *de novo* relationships may mirror more longstanding patterns or themes. Thus, the process of saying "good-bye" within the milieu can be quite informative and, when problems surface, germane for discussion and intervention. It is important to allow at least several days for recognition of such problems and implementation of treatment procedures. As is the case in coping with predischarge anxiety or dysphoria, the successful application of CT to address interpersonal problems generally enhances the salience of the treatment.

Empirical data are often lacking to justify common inpatient practices. However, most programs apply variants of at least three basic rules regarding the interpersonal aspects of termination: (1) patients are strongly discouraged (or even forbidden) from making social visits to the unit following discharge; (2) subsequent romantic involvement with peers met during a hospital stay is considered to be a hazardous endeavor; and (3) overreliance on friendships made during hospitalization (at the expense of the patient's broader social network) is discouraged. Some programs allow for patients' unspoken cognitions or fantasies *not* to terminate from the inpatient milieu by having periodic support group meetings for "alumni." Similarly, individuals may be invited to return as guest speakers for psychoeducational groups. The overall significance of the milieu experience for some patients should not be discounted. Indeed, for the markedly vulnerable patient, both the direct and symbolic value of the hospital as a coping resource must be recognized. From a cognitive perspective, this constellation of attitudes, thoughts, and feelings is akin to what has been referred to as institutional transference (e.g., Arieti, 1974).

Coping with Stigma

Although patients are often faced with the negative reactions of others early in their hospitalization, the prospects of impending discharge may elicit renewed concerns. More specifically, some patients anticipate the need to face family members, neighbors, and colleagues who may, or may not, know the details of the hospitalization. It is useful in all therapeutic encounters during the final week of hospitalization to inquire whether the patient has had thoughts, images, or even dreams pertaining to the reactions of others. This affords the opportunity to address automatic thoughts that typically convey themes of shame ("They all know I don't have my act together. I'm so embarrassed!"), failed responsibility ("I've really let my family down. I'm so weak."), unfairness ("Why can't people be more understanding?"), and rejection ("They're walking on egg-shells around me. No one wants to be with me now."). Such thoughts are often shaped by logical distortions and are thus amenable to standard cognitive interventions.

The rational basis for concerns about stigma also needs to be acknowledged. For example, some relatives' fears of psychiatric matters are such that they cannot differentiate a recovering depressed person from more severely ill psychiatric patients, whereas others may be unable to distinguish the concept of "depression" from notions of weakness or deserved punishment. Conversely, apparently well-meaning significant others may counsel dropping out of therapy or discontinuing antidepressant medication as means of proving one's strength. Of course, such advice also serves to help the family to deny that it has a problem. Mean-spirited and pejorative statements such as "nut-house," "loony bin," and the "men in white coats" also have not yet been extinguished from our culture's vernacular. Finally, institutional and actuarial practices may further reinforce the sense of stigma. For example, no matter how enlightened our society becomes in the foreseeable future, it is unlikely that we will elect a president who has previously received inpatient psychiatric treatment, nor would we invest heavily in an insurance concern that underwrites large, unrestricted policies for recently suicidal individuals. Because of these issues, it is wise to help patients grieve the loss of an idealized or invulnerable self-image and prepare to handle the occasions when they may encounter the ignorant, immature, callous, or unsupportive actions of others. Such preparation includes use of role-playing of assertive responses, mobilization of appropriately angry affects and responses (e.g., "If you refer to the hospital as a 'nut house' again I will report your harassment to our supervisor"), and the judicious use of humor (e.g., "You can come closer. I won't bite. And even if I did, my depression isn't contagious").

PLANNING FOR AFTERCARE

There are many more patients with mood disorders than there are cognitive therapists to treat them. Moreover, even at programs with strong outpatient components, not all patients can be followed by therapists who have been trained in cognitive therapy. There are several other reasons why cognitive therapy is not always continued after hospitalization: (1) many patients cannot afford a private therapist and must be seen at community mental health centers where there are no cognitive therapists; (2) not all patients embrace CT and some simply do not view it as a valuable endeavor; and (3) other patients with well-defined episodes of depression remit fully with antidepressant pharmacotherapy and receive a high degree of prophylactic success (i.e., 80%–90% efficacy rates) by maintenance pharmacotherapy (Prien, 1987; Thase, 1990).

The major experimental evidence for the prophylactic value of CT

TABLE 16.4. Indications for Continued Cognitive Therapy after Discharge from a CTU

- I. Definite indications
  - Inpatient treatment with CT alone
- II. Major indications[a]
  - A. Successful combined treatment with emphasis on CT
  - B. Partially successful combined treatment, with agreement between patient and treatment team that CT has been useful.
    - 1. Clinical indications
      - a. Recurrent depression
      - b. Chronic depression or dysthymia
      - c. Panic disorder
      - d. History of medication noncompliance
      - e. Past refusal of long-term medication strategies
    - 2. Psychosocial indications
      - a. Ongoing life stress
      - b. Schematic vulnerability
      - c. Patient desires continued CT
- III. Other indications[b]
  - A. Successful combined treatment with emphasis on pharmacotherapy
  - B. Rapid, full remission with excellent past response to maintenance medication.

[a]Cognitive therapy usually will be recommended.
[b]Cognitive therapy may be recommended in some cases, but patients in this category may do well with continuation pharmacotherapy and only limited CT follow-up.

has been derived from outpatient studies (see Chapter 1). However, two studies suggest that continued outpatient cognitive therapy (following initial inpatient treatment) may either enhance response or prevent relapse (Miller, Norman, & Keitner, 1989; Thase, Bowler, & Harden, 1991). The number of patients studied in these protocols is small (fewer than 40 patients), and, therefore, these findings should be considered preliminary. With these issues in mind, potential indications for patients likely to benefit from continued cognitive therapy are suggested in Table 16.4. At the University of Pittsburgh, we do not recommend offering intensive individual cognitive therapy as the only principal inpatient treatment (i.e., without pharmacotherapy) unless it seems likely that the patient will be able to participate in follow-up outpatient therapy (Thase, Bowler, & Harden, 1991).

Partial Hospitalization

Some patients may be suitable for continued CT after discharge, but their levels of residual depressive symptoms or functional impairment are too severe for conventional once- or twice-weekly therapy. Partial hospital treatment programs may be particularly useful in such cases

(Parker & Knoll, 1990). Although such programs have been traditionally underfunded, cost-containment efforts appear to be leading to a reemphasis on provision of partial hospital care (Parker & Knoll, 1990). A cognitive therapy program can be developed in a partial hospital setting using the various models described in Chapter 3. Among several such programs already in operation, Perris (1989) has established a comprehensive and continuous set of treatment services extending from inpatient, through partial hospitalization, to more traditional aftercare.

Targets for Outpatient Therapy

Continuation of cognitive therapy on an outpatient basis generally follows the treatment manual of Beck, Rush, Shaw, and Emery (1979), with appropriate accommodations for the material that already has been covered during inpatient treatment. Ideally, the primary inpatient therapist can continue to work with the patient following discharge. However, this arrangement often may not be practical. In the event that a transition in therapists is necessary, the first order of business is for the outpatient therapist to discuss the patient's history and case formulation with the referring inpatient therapist. Whenever possible, it is helpful if the "new" outpatient therapist is able to visit the patient on the unit before discharge. This is a particularly useful way to bridge the gap between the two different treatment settings. Ample time should be allowed during the initial session for establishment of rapport and development of a new working alliance, whether the session takes place on the unit or after discharge. No matter how excellent a discharge summary has been prepared by the inpatient treatment team, it is important for the new therapist to review the patient's background, past treatment experiences, and the events that led to hospitalization, as well as to ascertain the patient's appraisal of the active ingredients of the inpatient treatment program. This includes an open discussion of the patient's thoughts and feelings about changing therapists and elicitation of feedback about the patient's expectations of, and reaction to, the initial outpatient session. The outpatient therapist also may find it helpful to review the patient's therapy diary as an additional way of understanding the patient's knowledge and/or facility with cognitive therapy.

Primary agenda items for the first few outpatient sessions usually include: (1) tracking and managing target symptoms; and (2) recognizing thoughts and feelings that have emerged in relation to resumption of social and vocational roles. Such material typically is addressed by using basic behavioral and cognitive methods, such as graded-task assignments (for a progressively paced resumption of activities at home or at work) and Daily Record of Dysfunctional Thoughts (DRDT) worksheets (to facilitate recognition and modification of cognitive distortions and automatic negative thoughts engendered by the return to the home environment).

It has been our experience at the University of Pittsburgh program that at least one-half of the patients treated with inpatient cognitive therapy (without pharmacotherapy) experience an increase in symptomatology during the first month after discharge. Indeed, such symptomatic flurries are so common that we routinely inform patients about their likelihood in order to provide an adaptive attributional context for coping with feeling worse. We suggest that (1) the complexity and demands of everyday life will increase; (2) accumulated consequences of being away from home or work for several weeks will be encountered (e.g., a backlog of housework or a "mountain" of papers at the office); (3) the intensity of therapeutic support will diminish rather dramatically; (4) the interaction of such increased stress and diminished therapeutic support will, in all likelihood, lead to some greater level of distress and increased symptomatology; and (5) although uncomfortable and potentially discouraging, symptomatic flare-ups provide the opportunity to apply self-help skills in the natural environment.

An increase in symptoms can be likened metaphorically to the difficulties that might be encountered when an intermediate level skier first tries a more advanced slope or if a promising senior high school baseball star tries to bat against a tough college pitcher. In both examples, the difficulty is not a matter of personal incompetence or poor training; rather, in each case the problem is that an individual is *temporarily* overwhelmed by a situation that is too demanding for his or her level of training. Moreover, with additional practice, experience, and/or coaching, the individual will master the challenge. This contextual approach is of some benefit in preventing overgeneralized and catastrophic cognitions such as "I've wasted my time in therapy. It doesn't really work in the real world. I must not be using the therapy correctly. Why bother, I'm just going to relapse anyway." By contrast, the consequences of using cognitive therapy procedures for anticipating symptomatic exacerbations are patience, self-understanding, and continued work in therapy, instead of demoralization, "giving up" behaviors, or noncompliance with homework.

In concert with continuation of work on the issues and methods elaborated during inpatient treatment, the therapist and patient collaborate in order to identify long-term goals. They also need to work together to articulate more fundamental assumptions and schemas. As described in Chapters 1 and 4, useful strategies to address longstanding vulnerabilities include operationalizing the "unspoken" assumptions into written contracts, "rewriting" assumptive contracts based on the knowledge and experiences gained in adult life, acknowledgment of the advantages of assumptions and the associated costs of generating new rules of living (e.g., learning to live with loneliness or accepting a less than outstanding performance evaluation), and using homework assignments and experiments to challenge assumptions through actions that were previously prohibited or excessively inhibited (also, see Beck et al., 1979; Persons, 1989). One useful example of the latter strategy involves a cognitive–behavioral analogue of response prevention, in which the individual plans and carries out an assignment in a fashion contrary to that dictated by the assumption.

Usually, the time spent in therapy to address such inferred, "deep" cognitive structures is inversely proportional to the patient's level of acute symptomatic distress. Work on schematic issues requires an ability to develop perspective and as well as a capacity for abstraction. Nevertheless, the cognitive model of psychopathology suggests that therapy should continue until assumptive and schematic vulnerabilities are modified in order to derive maximum benefits. In working with patients who manifest longstanding patterns of difficulty, including dysthymia and Axis II personality disorders, therapeutic attention to multiple problematic schemas may constitute the bulk of therapy once the presenting symptoms of the acute major depressive or anxiety disorder have remitted (Beck, Freeman, & Associates, 1990).

Frequency of Aftercare Sessions

Outpatient group or individual cognitive therapy typically is provided in once- or twice-weekly visits over a time-limited course of 3 to 6 months postdischarge. Thus, patients may receive a predetermined aftercare program of 12 to 20 visits. Whereas this format is well-suited for use in research studies (i.e., a measured "dose" of therapy is provided during a time course that is roughly consistent with that employed in continuation pharmacotherapy), it may not be pertinent to the aftercare of former inpatients. For that matter, it may not be the best approach to treatment with all outpatients. For example, in an outpatient study of individual cognitive therapy of endogenous depression conducted by our group at the University of Pittsburgh (Thase, Simons, Cahalane, McGeary, & Harden, 1991; Simons & Thase, 1992; Thase & Simons, 1992a), we observed a 52% relapse rate during the first year of follow-up for those unmedicated patients who completed the 16-week therapy protocol in a partially recovered state (i.e., they had not achieved Hamilton Rating Scale for Depression scores < 6 for > 8 weeks by the time of termination of therapy) (Thase et al., 1992). By contrast, patients who maintained more durable remissions to the initial course of outpatient therapy had only a 9% relapse rate (Thase et al., 1992). Although this finding undoubtedly reflects the natural history of unipolar depressions (i.e., some cases are easier to treat than others), it also points to the importance of flexibility in assessing the length of continued outpatient treatment. As an example, our group has recommended that outpatient therapy should be continued on a regular and intensive basis until the patient has achieved a sustained remission of at least 2 months' duration (Thase & Simons, 1992b). During this time (in which Axis I symptomatology may be relatively quiescent), sufficient opportunity is available for modifying or weakening basic assumptions and schemas. Furthermore, it seems likely that the use of combined therapy (i.e., CT plus pharmacotherapy) may convey additional long-term prophylaxis for more vulnerable patients, such as recently hospitalized individuals. In a study by Miller and his colleagues (1989), maintenance of therapeutic gains was significantly greater when CT or social skills training were provided in combination with pharmacotherapy than observed in the pharmacotherapy alone condition.

Coordination of Cognitive Therapy and Pharmacotherapy

As discussed in Chapter 7, a majority of inpatients treated within a cognitive milieu will receive concomitant pharmacotherapy. An effective treatment team will have ensured that the patient understands that these two forms of therapy are compatible and potentially additive interventions. However, after discharge from the hospital, there may be the opportunity for friction between the providers of these key therapeutic modalities. This is particularly true when outpatient cognitive therapy and pharmacotherapy are provided by different mental health practitioners. In such cases, the two therapists need to constitute an outpatient treatment team so that their respective case formulations, along with plans and target symptoms for aftercare treatment, can be discussed. Examples of misalignments of the outpatient treatment team include a pharmacotherapist's advice for the patient not to complete a homework assignment ("Why don't you just take it easy for a while?") or a cognitive therapist's unilateral interventions when a patient confesses medication noncompliance. In the latter case, although it is true that cognitive therapy can be used to improve medication compliance (see Chapter 7), the alliance between the psychotherapist and pharmacotherapist would be strengthened if the patient's noncompliance and the use of such methods were discussed beforehand by both professionals.

It may be helpful to summarize briefly some of the current "basic assumptions" for long-term use of psychotropic drugs (see Prien, 1987, or Thase, 1990, for more detailed discussions). First, effective antidepressant and antipanic medications should be maintained for a minimum of 4 to 6 months in order to minimize the risk of relapse. Second, adjunctive medications (i.e., anxiolytics, neuroleptics, hypnotics, or lithium carbonate augmentation) usually should be tapered before primary antidepressant agents are withdrawn (Simons & Thase, 1990). Third, there is no good evidence that smaller dosages of antidepressants (i.e., so-called "maintenance" dosages) convey the same protection as the full dosage utilized in treatment of the acute episode. Fourth, persistent or residual symptoms mitigate against drug discontinuation even after a standard 4- to 6-month period of continuation pharmacotherapy has been completed. However, it is probably neither useful nor necessary to talk with patients about taking medication for their lifetime. Despite the appeal of comparing recurrent depression or anxiety disorders to other chronic medical illness (e.g., diabetes mellitus or hypertension), such comparisons may trigger worrisome associations for patients who are well-educated about long-term risks and complications of pharmacotherapy (e.g., retinopathy, renal disease, hypothyroidism). Furthermore, the best available evidence pertains to the benefits of antidepressants or lithium maintenance therapy over 1-, 3-, or even 5-year periods (Prien, 1987; Thase, 1990). Thus, we think that it is advisable to talk with patients about discrete time intervals for the continuation phase of pharmacotherapy.

Anticipating Flurries of Symptoms Following Termination of Outpatient Treatment

Patients may hold the implicit assumption that another episode of depressive illness or panic disorder would be a disaster. In such cases, the return of mild symptoms could trigger catastrophic cognitions that would reenvelop the patient in a downward spiral toward full recurrence. We thus attempt to "inoculate" patients against overreactions to symptomatic flurries by: (1) eliciting and modifying dysfunctional attitudes about recurrence; (2) reviewing relapse prevention procedures learned during the inpatient phase of treatment; and (3) using cognitive–behavioral rehearsal to prepare for the possibility of symptom outbreaks.

It also is useful prior to termination of therapy to consider whether the patient's past episodes of depression have had characteristic prodromal symptoms. In addition, the patient and therapist may examine whether or not there has been a coherent theme or pattern of life events or difficulties that preceded the onset of depression or panic attacks.

When taken together, these symptoms and circumstances may be organized into a set of warning signs or "yellow flags" for impending recurrence. The identification of such signals may then be used as the basis for intensified use of self-help exercises, resumption of antidepressant medication, or renewed psychotherapy. If a return to cognitive therapy is required, some patients may need only a few additional sessions, whereas others may benefit from resumption of an extensive course of outpatient therapy (Thase, 1990).

Alternatives to Terminating Cognitive Therapy

As suggested earlier, our group at the University of Pittsburgh does not advocate termination of outpatient therapy until an individual has achieved a stable and sustained remission (Thase & Simons, 1992b). Nevertheless, there are several options that may be considered when patients have not been able to reach a state of sustained recovery despite an extended course of outpatient individual therapy. One possibility is to begin to "thin down" the intensity of outpatient therapy—for example, by shifting from weekly to twice monthly sessions. Potential emotional reactions (e.g., apprehension or anxiety) or automatic thoughts associated with such a change may be elicited and modified, and the reduction in therapeutic intensity can be handled as an experiment. If the tapering doesn't work, weekly sessions can be resumed. Alternatively, some patients may benefit from a shift from individual to group therapy formats. Others may achieve a more stable remission following reevaluation and/or modification of their medication regimens. Third, even when terminating treatment seems appropriate after a long course of outpatient cognitive therapy (i.e., > 1 year), it is helpful to agree to ground rules for the patient to contact the therapist by telephone or request an emergency or "booster" session. Although an effective cognitive therapist does not wish to reinforce dependent behavior, the collaborative and empirical nature of the therapeutic relationship clearly allows for some ongoing contact if learning has been incomplete, new circumstances arise, or a previously "silent" pathological schema has become activated.

SUMMARY

The patient preparing for discharge from a psychiatric inpatient unit faces a host of distressing and realistic problems, including a high natural risk for relapse or recurrence. The cognitive milieu prepares an individual for these risks with a unique combination of treatment procedures such as psychoeducation, group and individual therapies, and self-help assignments. Results from a number of outpatient trials and several recent inpatient studies indicate that CT reduces the chances for depressive relapse. Moreover, a period of ongoing cognitive therapy, typically in combination with continuation and/or maintenance pharmacotherapy holds promise for reducing the risk of recurrent depression even further.

One of the important goals of cognitive therapy is to teach the patient new, more adaptive ways of thinking and behaving. If this effort is successful, patients are better prepared to respond effectively to future adverse events and to maintain the positive effects of hospitalization after discharge. Thus, patients should be able to leave the hospital anticipating substantial long-term benefits from their work in the cognitive milieu.

REFERENCES

Arieti, S. (1974). *Interpretation of schizophrenia*. New York: Basic Books.

Ballenger, J. C. (1991). Long-term pharmacologic treatment of panic disorder. *Journal of Clinical Psychiatry, 52*(S), 18–23.

Beck, A. T., Brown, G., Berchick, R. J., Stewart, B. L., & Steer, R. A. (1990). Relationship between hopelessness and ultimate suicide: A replication with psychiatric outpatients. *American Journal of Psychiatry, 147,* 190–195.

Beck, A. T., Freeman, A., & Associates (1990). *Cognitive therapy of personality disorders*. New York: Guilford Press.

Beck, A. T., Rush, A. J., Shaw, B. F., & Emery, B. (1979). *Cognitive therapy of depression*. New York: Guilford Press.

Beck, A. T., Steer, R. A., Kovacs, M., & Garrison, B. (1985). Hopelessness and eventual suicide: A 10-year prospective study of patients hospitalized with suicidal ideation. *American Journal of Psychiatry, 142,* 559–563.

Beck, A. T., Ward, C. H., Mendelson, M., Mock, J., & Erbaugh, J. (1961). An inventory for measuring depression. *Archives of General Psychiatry, 4,* 561–571.

Belsher, G., & Costello, C. G. (1988). Relapse after recovery from unipolar depression: A critical review. *Psychological Bulletin, 104,* 84–96.

Black, D. W., & Winokur, G. (1988). The changing inpatient unit: The Iowa experience. *Psychiatric Annals, 18,* 85–89.

Craig, T. J. (1988). Economic and inpatient care. *Psychiatric Annals, 18,* 75–79.

Eaves, G., & Rush, A. J. (1984). Cognitive patterns in symptomatic and remitted unipolar major depression. *Journal of Abnormal Psychology, 93,* 31–40.

Frank, E., Kupfer, D. J., Perel, J. M., Cornes, C., Jarrett, D. B., Mallinger, A. G., Thase, M. E., McEachran, A. B., & Grochocinski, V. J. (1990). Three year outcomes for maintenance therapies in recurrent depression. *Archives of General Psychiatry, 47,* 1093–1099.

Frank, E., Prien, R., Jarrett, R. B., Keller, M. B., Kupfer, D. J., Lavori, P., Rush, A. J., & Weissman, M. M. (1991). Conceptualization and rationale for consensus definitions of terms in major depressive disorder: Response, remission, recovery, relapse and recurrence. *Archives of General Psychiatry, 48,* 851–855.

Garamoni, G. L., Reynolds, C. F. III, Thase, M. E., Frank, E., & Fasiczka, A. L. (1992). Shifts in affective balance during cognitive therapy of major depression. *Journal of Consulting and Clinical Psychiatry, 60*, 260–266.

Hamilton, M. (1960). A rating scale for depression. *Journal of Neurology, Neurosurgery, and Psychiatry, 23*, 56–62.

Keller, M. B. (1988). Diagnostic issues and clinical course of unipolar illness. In A. J. Frances & R. E. Hales (Eds.), *American Psychiatric Press review of psychiatry,* Vol. 7 (pp. 188–212). Washington, DC: American Psychiatric Press.

Keller, M. B., & Shapiro, R. W. (1982). "Double depression": Superimposition of acute depressive episodes on chronic depressive disorders. *American Journal of Psychiatry, 139,* 438–442.

Mezzich, J. E., Evanczuk, K. J., Mathias, R. J., & Coffman, G. A. (1984). Admission decisions and multiaxial diagnosis. *Archives of General Psychiatry, 41,* 1001–1004.

Miller, I. W., Norman, W. H., & Keitner, G. I. (1989). Cognitive–behavioral treatment of depressed inpatients: Six- and twelve-month follow-ups. *American Journal of Psychiatry, 146*, 1274–1279.

Parker, S., & Knoll, J. L. (1990). Partial hospitalization: An update. *American Journal of Psychiatry, 147,* 156–160.

Perris, C. (1989). Cognitive therapy with the adult depressed patient. In A. Freeman, K. M. Simon, L. E. Beutler, & H. Arkowitz (Eds.), *Comprehensive handbook of cognitive therapy* (pp. 299–319). New York: Plenum Press.

Persons, J. B. (1989). *Cognitive therapy in practice: A case formulation approach*. New York: W. W. Norton.

Prien, R. F. (1987). Long-term treatment of affective disorder. In H. Y. Meltzer (Ed.), *Psychopharmacology: The third generation of progress* (pp. 1051–1058). Raven Press: New York.

Simons, A. D., Murphy, G. E., Levine, J. L., & Wetzel, R. D. (1986). Cognitive therapy and pharmacotherapy of depression: Sustained improvement over one year. *Archives of General Psychiatry, 43,* 43–48.

Simons, A. D., & Thase, M. E. (1990). Mood disorders. In M. E. Thase, M. Hersen, & B. A. Edelstein (Eds.), *Handbook of outpatient treatment of adults* (pp. 91–138). New York: Plenum Press.

Simons, A. D., & Thase, M. E. (1992). Biological markers, treatment outcome, and 1 year follow-up in endogenous depression: Electroencephalographic sleep studies and response to cognitive therapy. *Journal of Consulting and Clinical Psychiatry, 60*, 392–401.

Thase, M. E. (1987). Affective disorders. In R. L. Morrison & A. S. Bellack (Eds.), *Medical factors and psychologic disorders: A handbook for psychologists* (pp. 61–91). New York: Plenum Press.

Thase, M. E. (1990). Relapse and recurrence in unipolar major depression: Short term and long term approaches. *Journal of Clinical Psychiatry, 51*(6S), 51–57.

Thase, M. E., Bowler, K., & Harden, T. (1991). Cognitive behavior therapy of endogenous depression: Part 2: Preliminary findings in 16 unmedicated inpatients. *Behavior Therapy, 22*, 469–477.

Thase, M. E., & Kupfer, D. J. (1987). Characteristics of treatment resistant depression. In J. Zohar & R. H. Belmaker (Eds.), *Treating resistant depression* (pp. 23–45). New York: PMA Publishing.

Thase, M. E., & Simons A. D. (1992a). The applied use of psychotherapy to study the psychobiology of depression. *The Journal of Psychotherapy Practice and Research, 1,* 72–80.

Thase, M. E., & Simons, A. D. (1992b). Cognitive behavior therapy and relapse of nonbipolar depression: Parallels with pharmacotherapy. *Psychopharmacology Bulletin, 28*, 117–122.

Thase, M. E., Simons, A. D., Cahalane, J., McGeary, J., & Harden T. (1991). Severity of depression and response to cognitive behavior therapy. *The American Journal of Psychiatry, 148*, 784–789.

Thase, M. E., Simons, A. D., McGeary, J., Hughes, C., & Harden, T. (1992). Relapse after cognitive behavior therapy of depression: Potential implications for longer courses of treatment. *American Journal of Psychiatry, 149*, 1046–1052.

Appendix: Inpatient Cognitive Therapy Programs

Atlanta Center for Cognitive Therapy
Mark Gilson, Ph.D.
1772 Century Boulevard
Atlanta, Georgia 30345

The Benessere Center
Mary Billingsley, M.A.
4501 College Boulevard
Suite 150
Leawood, Kansas 66211

Bristol Regional Medical Center
Ridgeview Pavilion
John W. Ludgate, Ph.D.
209 Memorial Drive
Bristol, Tennessee–Virginia 37620

Butler Hospital
Ivan Miller, Ph.D.
345 Blackstone Boulevard
Providence, Rhode Island 02906

Center for Cognitive Therapy
Aaron T. Beck, M. D.
Room 754 Science Center
3600 Market Street
Philadelphia, Pennsylvania 19104-2648

University of Cincinnati
Marshall Ginsburg, M.D.
ML-59
Cincinnati, Ohio 45267

Clinique LaMétairie
Alexandra Konen, Lic. Psych.
Av. de Bois-Bougy
1260 Nyon, Switzerland

Grovelands Priory Hospital
David Veale, B.S.c., M.B.-B.S., M.R.C.Psych., M.Phil., Dip., C.A.C.P.
The Bourne
Southgate, London
N14 6RA England

The Hauser Clinic and Associates
Cal K. Cohn, M.D.
Mood and Stress Unit
7777 Southwest Freeway, Suite 1036
Houston, Texas 77074

Holliswood Hospital
Behavioral Disorders Unit
Andrew Levin, M.D.
87-37 Palermo Street
Holliswood, New York 11423

University of Iowa
Wayne A. Bowers, Ph.D.
1030 Fifth Ave., S.E.
Suite 3200
Cedar Rapids, Iowa 52403

University of Louisville—Geropsychiatry Unit
David A. Casey, M.D.
Norton Psychiatric Clinic
P.O. Box 35070
Louisville, Kentucky 40232

University of Louisville—Adolescent Unit
G. Randolph Schrodt, Jr., M.D.
Norton Psychiatric Clinic
P.O. Box 35070
Louisville, Kentucky 40232

University of Louisville—Adult Unit
Jesse H. Wright, M.D., Ph.D.
Norton Psychiatric Clinic
P.O. Box 35070
Louisville, Kentucky 40232

Mesa Vista Hospital
Ray Fidaleo, M.D.
7850 Vista Hill Avenue
San Diego, California 92123

Hospital of the University of Pennsylvania
William Ball, M.D., Ph.D.
11 Founders 14283, 3400 Spruce Street
Philadelphia, Pennsylvania 19104

University of Pittsburgh
Michael E. Thase, M.D.
Director of Mood Disorders Module
Western Psychiatric Institute and Clinic
3811 O'Hara Street
Pittsburgh, Pennsylvania 15213

The Royal Victoria Infirmary
Jan Scott, M.B., B.S., M.R.C.Psych.
Queen Victoria Road
New Castle Upon Tyne
NE 142 P England

Saint Louis University Medical Center
C. Alec Pollard, M.D.
1221 S. Grand Boulevard
St. Louis, Missouri 63104

CPC San Luis Rey Hospital
William Sparrow, M.S.W.
335 Saxony Road
Encinitas, California 92024

CPC Santa Ana Hospital
Susan Byers, Ph.D.
1801-G East Parkcourt Place
Santa Ana, California 92701

Skyline Psychiatric Associates, Inc.
Andrew B. Molchon, M.D.
5113 Leesburg Pike
Suite 209
Falls Church, Virginia 22041

Timberlawn Hospital
Roger Kobes, M.D.
4600 Samuel Boulevard
P.O. Box 11288
Dallas, Texas 75223

University of Umeå
Carlo Perris, M.D.
S-901 85 Umeå
Sweden

Westwood Lodge Hospital
Steven McDermott, Ph.D
45 Clapboardtree Street
Westwood, Massachusetts 02090

Yale University
Julio Lucinio, M.D.
Department of Psychiatry
School of Medicine
VA Medical Center 116A
West Haven, Connecticut 06516

Index

D

E